Physical Therapy for Intervertebral Disk Disease

A Practical Guide to Diagnosis and Treatment

Doris Broetz, PT
Physical Therapist
Private Practice;
University Hospital
Tübingen, Germany

Michael Weller, MD
Professor of Neurology and Director
Department of Neurology
University Hospital Zürich
Zürich, Switzerland

160 illustrations

Thieme
Stuttgart · New York · Delhi · Rio de Janeiro

Library of Congress Cataloging-in-Publication Data is available from the publisher.

This book is an authorized translation of the 3rd German edition published and copyrighted 2008 by Georg Thieme Verlag, Stuttgart. Title of the German edition: Diagnostik und Therapie bei Bandscheibenschäden

Translator: Gertrud G. Champe, Surry, Maine, USA
Illustrators: Doris Brötz, Tübingen, Germany; Angelika Kramer, Stuttgart, Germany

© 2016 Georg Thieme Verlag KG

Thieme Publishers Stuttgart
Rüdigerstrasse 14, 70469 Stuttgart, Germany
+49 [0]711 8931 421, customerservice@thieme.de

Thieme Publishers New York
333 Seventh Avenue, New York, NY 10001, USA
+1-800-782-3488, customerservice@thieme.com

Thieme Publishers Delhi
A-12, Second Floor, Sector-2, Noida-201301
Uttar Pradesh, India
+91 120 45 566 00, customerservice@thieme.in

Thieme Publishers Rio, Thieme Publicações Ltda.
Edifício Rodolpho de Paoli, 25° andar
Av. Nilo Peçanha, 50 – Sala 2508
Rio de Janeiro 20020-906 Brasil
+55 21 3172 2297 / +55 21 3172 1896

Cover design: Thieme Publishing Group
Typesetting by Thomson Digital, India

Printed in Germany by AZ Druck und Datentechnik, Kempten

5 4 3 2 1

ISBN 978-3-13-199761-6

Also available as an e-book:
eISBN 978-3-13-199771-5

Important note: Medicine is an ever-changing science undergoing continual development. Research and clinical experience are continually expanding our knowledge, in particular our knowledge of proper treatment and drug therapy. Insofar as this book mentions any dosage or application, readers may rest assured that the authors, editors, and publishers have made every effort to ensure that such references are in accordance with **the state of knowledge at the time of production of the book.**

Nevertheless, this does not involve, imply, or express any guarantee or responsibility on the part of the publishers in respect to any dosage instructions and forms of applications stated in the book. **Every user is requested to examine carefully** the manufacturers' leaflets accompanying each drug and to check, if necessary in consultation with a physician or specialist, whether the dosage schedules mentioned therein or the contraindications stated by the manufacturers differ from the statements made in the present book. Such examination is particularly important with drugs that are either rarely used or have been newly released on the market. Every dosage schedule or every form of application used is entirely at the user's own risk and responsibility. The authors and publishers request every user to report to the publishers any discrepancies or inaccuracies noticed. If errors in this work are found after publication, errata will be posted at www.thieme.com on the product description page.

Some of the product names, patents, and registered designs referred to in this book are in fact registered trademarks or proprietary names even though specific reference to this fact is not always made in the text. Therefore, the appearance of a name without designation as proprietary is not to be construed as a representation by the publisher that it is in the public domain.

Contents

Foreword

Back in the day, well, I was almost an athlete who'd won quite a few awards. But then there was my profession, and not so much sport. Things went along pretty well that way—for decades—and all the time I was sure that I was still in good condition. I have to confess though that I didn't think about my body very much, and it didn't give me much reason to.

But after a successful disc operation and four weeks of rehab, I suddenly noticed that some of my movements were rather rusty. My physical therapist handed down this decisive judgment: "*What we don't call on constantly—joint, muscle, and even brain—will fade and waste away. Use it or lose it!*", at which point I began to remember long-forgotten movements that I had obviously not performed, correctly anyway, for some time. And I'm not thinking of anything as brutal as knee bends or push-ups—no, just normal things: stooping, getting up out of a chair, and climbing stairs. My movements had clearly become more deliberate but much more limited.

Here was my question: Wouldn't a course of physical training be enough? Now I'm convinced that the answer is no. Even when I try hard to do my exercises correctly, I slack off, get sloppy, simplify them or leave them out altogether. At least for me, even after a few months of self-control, it's important to seek the advice and critical eye of my therapist and accept the new exercises she assigns me. She scolds me for neglecting my exercises and rewards me too, with the laconic comment: "*That was perfect.*" Sometimes I even score a real success, when I notice my progress and see my self-image improving.

But that doesn't mean that written instructions are useless. They help us find out, from someone who knows, how the spinal column is built and how it performs certain movements. Informative illustrations show how to maintain correct posture, avoid poor posture, and protect and train muscles, nerves, and joints. And what makes this book so useful is the presentation of step-by-step procedures and pointers for self-control.

Prof. Erich Koerber (Patient)

Author Biographies

Doris Broetz was born in Ulm, Germany in 1958; she is married and has two children. After completion of her secondary education (1978), she was trained as a physical therapist in Berlin and Tübingen (1978–82). From 1982 to 1986, she worked as a physical therapist at the trauma clinic of the Employers' Liability Insurance Association in Tübingen. Following an extended maternity leave, she worked first at the University Surgical Hospital in Tübingen and in 1993 moved to the Department of General Neurology at the University Hospital in Tübingen where she was chief physical therapist from April 2001 to September 2007 (Chairman: Prof. Dr. Johannes Dichgans; since October 2005 Prof. Dr. Michael Weller). Since October 2007 she has been active in studies on learning at the Institute for Medical Psychology and Behavioral Neurobiology (Chairman: Prof. Dr. Niels Birbaumer) at the Center for Functional and Restorative Neurosurgery (Director: Prof. Dr. Alireza Gharabaghi) and in her own practice. Since 1996, Doris Broetz has planned and conducted several studies of physical therapy diagnosis and therapy in patients with lumbar disk prolapse, working with Prof. Dr. Michael Weller to investigate the efficacy and quality optimization of therapy. On the basis of these studies, a new treatment was developed for patients with disk damage. In addition, the role of muscle relaxants during physical therapy treatment of patients with lumbar disk prolapse and changes in the MRI image of lumbar disk prolapse during physical therapy were investigated.

Doris Broetz is also interested in the analysis and physical therapy of patients with neurological diseases and research in motor learning background and motivation. She has developed diagnostic tests and physical therapy treatments for patients with ataxia, Pusher symptoms, and for the improvement of sensorimotor self-control of patients with hemiparesis.

Prof. Dr. Michael Weller was born in in Rheinbach, Germany in 1962. He is married and has

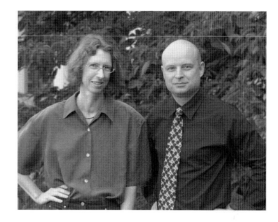

four children. He studied medicine in Cologne (1982–89) and received his training in neurology at the Department of General Neurology in Tübingen (1989–90) and the Department of Psychiatry in Würzburg (1991). He conducted research at the National Institute of Mental Health in Bethesda, Maryland, USA (1992) and the University Hospital, Zürich, Switzerland (1993–94) in the Department of Clinical Immunology. There he studied cerebral cell death processes and, in particular, experimental treatment of malignant brain tumors. In 1995, he returned to the Department of Neurology in Tübingen and completed his postdoctoral thesis (habilitation) in 1997 in the field of neuro-oncology. He became Deputy Chairman in 2001 and was appointed Chairman at the Department of General Neurology in October 2005. In addition to his research and clinical specialty of neuro-oncology, he has been the attending physician for the Pain Clinic of the Neurological Hospital. In collaboration with the Physical Therapy Department (D. Broetz), he established the specialty of conservative physical therapy treatment of disk problems in Tübingen, where he led clinical studies in this field. Since January 2008, he has been Chairman at the Department of Neurology at the University Hospital and University of Zürich.

1 Introduction

At least once in a lifetime, 80–90% of the population have back pain (Loeser and Volinn 1991; Waddell 1998) and about 66% have neck pain (Rao 2002). The causes of such problems originating in the spine are as numerous as the treatment options.

The many possible causes of back pain—tumors, spinal instability, foraminal or spinal stenosis, a prolapsed disk, inflammation, or trauma—can be diagnosed through the medical history, clinical examination, imaging, and laboratory tests. Symptoms that cannot be related to a specific illness by these means are usually interpreted as resulting from tension, sprain, facet pain, blockage of the sacroiliac joint, or as somatic expression of a psychosocial problem.

The usual medical treatment strategies include bed rest, chiropractic treatment, and oral or injectable analgesics and muscle relaxants. Physical therapists use fango treatments, massage, the sling table, and strengthening, usually in combination. Although the efficacy of most therapeutic strategies has not been assured, these treatments generate high healthcare costs (Hildebrandt et al 1996; Cherkin 1998; Chrubasik et al 1998; Williams et al 1998). In addition to the treatments themselves, disability and pension payments are a significant burden on public funds. In spite of increased investment in back pain research, little has changed in recent decades because the data are not reliable (Deyo and Phillips 1996; Van Tulder et al 1997; Cherkin 1998; Krismer and Van Tulder 2007; Vos et al 2012). Currently available guidelines make broad treatment recommendations for patients with back pain and radiating pain. Patient information, encouragement of normal activity, and the prescription of analgesics are cornerstones of these guidelines (Van Tulder et al 2006).

What can be done? First, the concept of "nonspecific back pain or neck pain" must be examined more closely and presented in more specific detail. It is no wonder that even precisely defined treatment methods, applied to a heterogeneous group of patients with the symptoms of back or neck pain in common but not their cause, lead to unsatisfactory results (Faas et al 1995; Malmivaara et al 1995; Cherkin 1998).

But how can disorders be studied and diagnosed if they cannot be unambiguously ascribed to an illness by imaging or laboratory tests? A special approach to this question was described by the New Zealand physical therapist McKenzie (2003, 2006), who used repeated spinal motion as a diagnostic strategy. A hypothesis about the causes of several back pain syndromes was developed on the basis of theoretical considerations regarding anatomy, tissue damage and healing, and knowledge of typical symptoms in certain diseases. McKenzie interpreted the clinical symptoms of *centralization* and *peripheralization* as an indication of disk damage. In this context, centralization means that while the spine is moving, the zone of radiating or radicular pain withdraws rapidly, in a central or proximal direction, toward or as far as the midline of the back. Peripheralization, on the other hand, develops in the opposite direction. That is, the pain radiation is shifted from the back to the periphery or distally.

Donelson et al (1997) described a significant correlation between the clinical sign of centralization in end-range movements and diskographically diagnosed tears in the anulus fibrosus. The clinical sign of peripheralization correlated with tears in the outer annulus (see Chapter 12 Selected Studies on the Topic of Spinal Disorders).

In diskography, after percutaneous injection of contrast medium into the nucleus pulposus, leakage of contrast medium into the anulus fibrosus is taken as evidence of structural damage. A diskogram is evaluated as positive if the pain familiar to the patient can be reproduced and if imaging shows tears in the outer third of the anulus with the outer edge still intact or completely torn.

Thus, disk damage might be diagnosed by means of repeated end-range movements of the spine, even if noninvasive imaging procedures such as computed tomography (CT) or magnetic resonance imaging (MRI) did not identify any damage. In this way, the patients with diagnosable disk damage could be filtered out from the large group of those with nonspecific back and neck pain.

Schwarzer et al (1995) used diskography to identify lumbar disk damage as a probable cause of problems in 39% of patients in whom the CT scan did not demonstrate lumbar disk prolapse. In a study by Laslett et al (2005) on patients with chronic back pain, some with radiating pain, a diskogram showed disk damage in 75% of patients. Consequently, in performing and interpreting diagnostic tests, experienced physical therapists may be able to filter out about half the patients in the group with nonspecific back pain and give them a specific diagnosis so that they can receive targeted physical therapy. This could also apply to patients with nonspecific neck pain, because of the anatomical and mechanical similarity of the different spinal segments. Up to now, the appropriate studies have not been conducted.

In patients with neuroradiologically confirmed disk prolapse, it can also be determined, by means of repeated end-range spinal movements, whether they can be expected to benefit from conservative treatment (Brötz et al 2001, 2003; Brötz, Burkard, Weller 2010).

The treatment described here is governed by changes in symptoms during the acute phase, and its success is evaluated on the basis of defined milestone targets. The measures used are spinal movements performed by the patients themselves. After the acute phase, movements of the extremities are added, with the objective of preserving or improving the mobility of the nerve roots and nerves. Spinal stability is restored by means of exercises that activate the tonic, stabilizing muscles. All therapeutic movements are very simple and can be easily performed by every patient. Only in very rare cases does the therapist supplement the effect of the exercises with passive movements.

Once the symptoms have largely subsided and no worsening occurs on loading, treatment aims at free mobility of the spine and extremities. Strengthening, coordination exercises, and fitness training finally bring the patient to normal movement, normal capacity, and ability to work.

Because patients experience rapid changes in their symptoms during the exercises they per-form themselves, they are motivated to share the work and the responsibility for their own recovery. The job of the therapist is as much to inform the patient explicitly about the pathogenesis of a disk prolapse as to instruct them precisely how to exercise and observe their symptoms. The patient learns how to modify their movement patterns and how to stress their body evenly, purposefully, and appropriately, so that the structures of the spine are not damaged but acquire stability as needed for a given load. In this way, the therapy described here can prevent development of a fear of pain that could result from movement or stress. This prevents chronification and relapses.

With time, the authors have changed and supplemented the strategies presented by McKenzie (1981, 1986, 1990) and for this reason the therapeutic program described here is called the BASE PT (behavioral, active, self-determined, evidence-based physio therapy). The possibilities and results of physical therapy according to the BASE PT have been systematically studied at the Neurology Clinic of the University of Tübingen in Germany from 1997 to 2010, in patients with lumbar disk prolapses. Patients with neurological deficits resulting from prolapsed disks were also included in the physical therapy studies.

The order of test movements was changed and now depends on which movement relieves the symptoms of the disorder assumed in the preliminary suspected diagnosis. Spinal rotation, both as a diagnostic test movement and as an exercise performed by the patient, is very important. In addition to the spinal movements, the concept includes movements of the extremities to prevent and treat limitation of nerve-gliding capacity and exercises to stabilize the spine. Observation and documentation of neurological disorders, signs of nerve stretching, and development of pain are given major attention.

The treatment design includes strengthening, coordination exercises, and fitness training, and brings the patient back to normal movement, load-bearing capacity, and ability to work.

2   General Principles

For the understanding and interpretation of disk prolapse symptoms, this summary presents the fundamentals of the *functional anatomy* of the spine and the nervous system, the *pathophysiology of disk damage* and its effect on nerve roots, and the *healing* process.

Pain and limited function in activities of daily living are the chief problems caused by disk damage. Assessment of pain and disability are necessary for evaluation of the effect of treatment and the course of the disease. Various measurement scales for this purpose are introduced.

The predisposing factors are of interest for prevention. Section 2.5 Epidemiology and Risk Factors sheds light on the controversial questions of whether certain activities lead to disk damage with particular frequency and which physical conditions or social circumstances promote these problems.

2.1   Anatomy of the Spine and Nervous System

The spine fulfills two different functions: it *carries the head and thorax* and *protects the spinal cord*. At the same time, a high degree of mobility is needed. The requirements of stability and mobility are in constant conflict. In order to perform both functions, the spine must display good interaction between its bearing and moving structures.

The *passive holding apparatus* consists of the vertebrae, disks, vertebral joints, ligaments, and articular capsules, while the *active holding apparatus* is made up of muscles and tendons. The *nervous system* registers the position, load, and stresses on the spine and controls the active system in order to fulfill the stability and mobility requirements (Waddell 1998). Malfunction in one of the three systems leads to a reaction in the other two systems. Adaptation, incorrect loading, pain, or loss of function can result.

2.1.1   Musculature

The active holding apparatus consists of numerous muscles and tendons. The muscles that move and actively stabilize the spine can be roughly grouped into back, abdominal, posterior and anterior neck muscles. Here we will discuss only the largest and most important muscles (**Table 2.1**).

2.1.2   Bony Spine and Ligaments

The spine is made up of seven cervical, 12 thoracic, and five lumbar vertebrae and the sacrum. The highest cervical vertebra is called the atlas and, in

Table 2.1 The chief muscle groups for stabilization and movement of the spine

Muscle	Origin	Attachment	Function	Innervation
Neck musculature				
Short, dorsal neck muscles	Atlas Axis	Linea nuchae Transverse process of atlas Jugular process of the occipital bone	Extension, rotation, and lateral flexion of the head	N. suboccipitalis (C1)
Scalene muscles	Ventrally at the transverse processes of the cervical vertebrae	1st–2nd ribs	Lateral flexion of the cervical spine with fixed head: elevation of the 1st and 2nd ribs	Cervical plexus Brachial plexus (C3–C8)

▶ (continued)

Table 2.1 The chief muscle groups for stabilization and movement of the spine (*continued*)

Muscle	Origin	Attachment	Function	Innervation
Prevertebral muscle group M. longus colli M. longus capitis M. rectus capitis anterior	Ventrally at all cervical vertebral bodies and the upper thoracic vertebral bodies Transverse processes of the cervical vertebrae	Atlas ventrally on all cervical vertebral bodies Transverse processes of the caudal cervical vertebrae Occipital bone	Flexion, rotation, and lateral flexion on the ipsilateral side of the cervical spine	Cervical plexus (C1–C6)
M. sternocleidomas-toideus	Sternum Clavicle	Mastoid process of the temporal bone Linea nuchae	Flexion of the caudal and extension of the cranial cervical vertebrae and the head joints (protraction) Rotation of the head to the contralateral side with fixed head: help in inspiration	N. accessorius Cervical plexus (C1–C3)
Back muscles				
Autochthonous back muscles: M. erector spinae (consists of many small muscle groups that connect transverse processes, spinous processes, and ribs)	Sacrum Iliac crest	Occipital bone	Extension, rotation, lateral flexion in individual sections and the entire spine Assurance of erect posture	Dorsal branches of spinal nerves (C2–L4)
M. trapezius	Linea nuchae Spinous processes of the cervical and thoracic vertebrae	Clavicle Acromion Spine of scapula	Cranial fibers: – Elevation of the shoulder blade – Rotation of the head to the contralateral side Medial fibers: – Retraction of the shoulder blade Caudal fibers: – Depression of the shoulder blade	N. accessorius Cervical plexus (C2–C4)
M. latissimus dorsi	Spinous processes from T7 to the sacrum 8th–12th ribs Iliac crest	Crista tuberculi minoris (humerus)	Inward rotation, "adduction," extension in shoulder joint with fixed arm (support): elevation of the pelvis	N. thoracodorsalis (C6–C8)
M. quadratus lumborum	Iliac crest Iliolumbal ligament	12th rib Lumbar vertebrae L1–L4	Pulls the 12th rib caudally Lateral flexion of the lumbar spine with fixed thorax: elevation of the pelvis	Muscular branches of the lumbar plexus N. intercostalis 12 (T12–L3)
Abdominal muscles				
M. rectus abdominis	5th–7th ribs Xiphoid process	Cranial edge of the pubic bone	Pulls the thorax toward the pelvis Bending the trunk or lifting the pelvis Antagonist of the long back extensor	Middle and caudal intercostal nerves (T5–T12)

▶ (*continued*)

Table 2.1 The chief muscle groups for stabilization and movement of the spine (*continued*)

Muscle	Origin	Attachment	Function	Innervation
M. obliquus externus	Exterior surfaces of 5th–12th ribs	Iliac crest Inguinal ligament Sheath of the rectus	Abdominal press Trunk bending Elevation of the pelvis Rotation of the trunk to the contralateral side	Caudal intercostal nerves (T5–T12)
M. obliquus internus	Iliac crest Thoracolumbar fascia Inguinal ligament	9th–12th ribs Linea alba	Abdominal press Trunk bending Elevation of the pelvis Rotation of the trunk to the ipsilateral side Lateral flexion of the trunk	Caudal intercostal nerves Branches of the lumbar plexus (T10–L2)
M. transversus abdominis	7th–12th ribs Transverse processes of the lumbar vertebrae Iliac crest Inguinal ligament	Sheath of the rectus abdominis	Retraction and tightening of abdominal wall Abdominal press	Intercostal nerves (T5–L2)

contrast to the other vertebrae, has no vertebral body. The second vertebra is called the axis and has an anterior projection (dens axis) that articulates with the atlas.

The vertebral bodies with the disks form the anterior portion of the spine. The vertebral arches with the transverse processes and the spinous processes enclose and protect the spinal cord laterally and posteriorly and form the posterior portion of the spine. The articulations between the vertebrae are formed anteriorly by the disks and posteriorly by the small vertebral joints (facet joints). The end plates of the vertebrae form the contact surfaces for the disks (**Fig. 2.1**).

The spaces between the vertebral bodies and the small vertebral articulations are the intervertebral foramina through which the nerve roots emerge from the spinal cord and run from the cervical spine to the arms, from the thoracic spine to the trunk, and from the lumbar spine to the legs. The sacrum forms the connection between the spine and the pelvis.

The spine is stabilized by three longitudinal ligaments:
- Anterior longitudinal ligament: runs anteriorly over vertebrae and disks.
- Posterior longitudinal ligament: runs posteriorly over vertebrae and disks.
- Ligamentum flavum: connects the vertebral arches of two adjacent vertebrae.

2.1.3 Intervertebral Disks

There are intervertebral disks between all vertebral bodies from cervical vertebral bodies C2–C3 to the transition between the lowest lumbar vertebral body (L5) and the first sacral vertebra (S1). They are attached to the end plates of the vertebral bodies (Bogduk 2000).

Each vertebral body is covered by an end plate consisting of hyaline and fibrous cartilage. Insertions of collagenous fibers from the intervertebral disk form the connection between the end plate and the disk. This connection is more stable than that between the end plate and the vertebral body.

Moreover, the disks are the connection between the end plates of two adjacent vertebral bodies. They consist of two parts (**Fig. 2.1**): the outer fibrous ring (anulus fibrosus) and the inner mucoprotein gel (nucleus pulposus). The two components are not sharply distinct from each other since the outer regions of the nucleus pulposus blend smoothly into the inner region of the anulus fibrosus (Bogduk 2000).

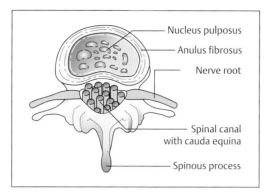

- Nucleus pulposus
- Anulus fibrosus
- Nerve root
- Spinal canal with cauda equina
- Spinous process

Fig. 2.1 Lumbar vertebra with disk. In the thoracic and cervical spines, the spinal canal contains the spinal cord instead of the cauda equina.

With increasing age, the structural and functional differentiation of the disk areas decreases. Both portions contain water, collagen, and proteoglycans in different concentrations.

The anulus fibrosus is 60% connective tissue (Type 1 collagen) arranged in an oblique ring. It creates the firm connection between the vertebral bodies, retains the gel mass between the vertebral bodies, and can cushion tensile stresses like axial spinal rotation (Hadjipavlou et al 1999).

The gel core consists largely of proteoglycans and glycosaminoglycans, which take up water and can carry loads and absorb shocks.

Physiological Compressive Stress

When the spine moves, the nucleus pulposus changes its shape and distributes pressure to the end plates and the anulus fibrosus. The nucleus pulposus is squeezed like a sponge by loading, and when pressure is released it absorbs water again (McMillan et al 1996; Wilke et al 1999; Race et al 2000).

Examples

- Wilke et al (1999) measured pressure for almost 24 hours in the middle of the disk between vertebral bodies L4 and L5, in a healthy 45-year-old subject. The patient performed various activities during this time and assumed a variety of positions. During a 7-hour sleep period, a pressure increase from 1 to 24 bar was measured. This was explained by regenerating water absorption by the disks.

- The increase of spinal pain and limitation of motion during the night in patients with disk damage could be related to this pressure increase and the greater volume occupied by the hydrated disk. At zero gravity, because of decompression, astronauts were up to 5 cm taller than under normal pressure conditions (Urban and McMullin 1988).
- Nachemson and Elfström (1970) investigated the pressure on intervertebral disks in nine subjects who assumed various body positions. Of these, six had had no back pain in the past, two had pains in the past, and one suffered from scoliosis. In each case, a probe was positioned in the middle of the L3–L4 disk.

Wilke et al's (1999) results were in many respects identical with Nachemson and Elfström's (1970): the lowest reclining disk pressure and the highest disk pressure while lifting loads with straight knees and bent spine, measured in both studies, were in agreement. Activity of the back muscles in all positions was associated with an increase in pressure (Nachemson and Elfström 1970; Wilke et al 1999). The intradiskal pressure also rises when traction is applied if the back muscles are activated in compensation at the same time (Andersson et al 1983).

In contrast to Nachemson and Elfström (1970), Wilke et al (1999) found no increase in pressure when the subject was sitting upright, as compared to when standing upright. When the subject was sitting in dorsal flexion, against a back rest, Wilke et al (1999) even observed a significantly lower pressure than when standing upright or sitting without a back rest.

This knowledge led to a wide-ranging discussion of the erect seated posture favored by physical therapists and in back schools (Reinhardt 1992; Brügger 1997; Nentwig et al 1997). Clinically, it has proven advantageous for patients with disk damage to avoid sitting as much as possible (see Chapter 9 Rehabilitation and Prevention).

Metabolism

Disks are the largest avascular structures in the body; they are characterized by low metabolism. Exchange of nutrients and metabolic products in the disk takes place passively by diffusion and osmosis through the blood vessels of the end plates and the anterior and posterior longitudinal ligaments (Holm et al 1981; Van den Berg 1999).

Repeated movement of the spine is thought to improve the exchange of nutrients and metabolic products in the disk (Holm and Nachemson 1983). This hypothesis is based on an animal experiment in which a group of dogs that performed repeated active movements of the spine during a controlled training program was compared with a control group (ibid.). In the group that performed repetitive spinal movements, there was increased oxygen consumption in the external portion of the anulus fibrosus and the nucleus pulposus, with a lower lactate concentration than in the control group.

Innervation

The question of whether disks have sensory innervation was controversial for a long time. Free nerve endings that make the sensing of pain possible were at first found only in the skin, the facet joints, the sacroiliac joint, the anterior and posterior longitudinal ligaments, the ligamentum flavum, the periosteum of the vertebrae and the vertebral arches, the fasciae and tendons, the dura mater, and the dural sheaths of the nerve roots.

Bogduk et al (1981, 1983, 1988) described sensory innervation in the anulus fibrosus as well. The posterior portion is supplied by the sinuvertebral nerve, the lateral areas by the communicating gray branches of the ventral branches of the spinal nerves.

Palmgren et al (1996) found both sensory and autonomic nerve endings in surgically removed disk tissue. The fact that the anulus fibrosus contains pain receptors endorses the interpretation that back pain can be triggered by injury to the anulus fibrosus.

Indahl et al (1997) triggered action potentials in the longissimus and the multifidus muscles of 23 sedated pigs by applying electrical stimuli to the posterolateral anulus fibrosus. After local stimulation of the small vertebral joints by injection of physiological saline, the action potentials triggered by electrical stimulation of the anulus fibrosus were weakened. This indicates that there is a reflex mechanism between the anulus fibrosus, the back muscles, and the facet joints such that stimulation of the small vertebral joints decreases muscle tone

rather than increasing it. We will return later to the possible significance of this mechanism for the interpretation and treatment of back pain (see 2.2.3 Disk Damage and Muscle Tension).

The disks have the following functions:
- Firm connection of two vertebral bodies.
- Facilitation of movement.
- Bearing the weight that is transmitted by the vertebrae lying above.
- Shock absorption.

2.1.4   Nervous System

Depending on its location and function, the nervous system is divided into the *central* and the *peripheral nervous system*. The central nervous system (CNS) consists of the brain and the spinal cord. It serves to receive and process information and initiate appropriate reactions.

As soon as they emerge from the spinal cord, structures become part of the peripheral nervous system. This system serves to conduct sensory impulses from the periphery to the central nervous system and motor impulses from the central nervous system to the periphery.

In addition, depending on the function, a distinction is made between the *somatic* and the *autonomic nervous system*. This classification applies chiefly to the peripheral nervous system but also to the central nervous system.

The somatic nervous system serves to control voluntary motion and conscious perception of sensory stimuli. The autonomic (visceral, vegetative) nervous system consists of the sympathetic and the parasympathetic systems and controls (unconscious) events in the internal organs (e.g., breathing, digestion, blood pressure). It plays only a subordinate role in disk prolapse and will therefore not be discussed further.

Spinal Cord, Cauda Equina, and Nerve Roots

The spinal cord is part of the central nervous system and runs through the spinal canal. It is connected to the brain, specifically the medulla oblongata, at the level of the foramen magnum of the occipital bone and extends down as far as the first lumbar vertebra. Below this point, the nerve roots run inside the vertebral canal and only emerge through the intervertebral foramina in lower segments. They resemble a horse's tail, reflecting the anatomical Latin designation, *cauda equina*.

The anterior (motor) roots emerge between the anterior and lateral strands of the spinal cord and the posterior (sensory) roots emerge between the lateral and posterior strands. They join at the level of the intervertebral foramina to form the spinal nerves. The sensory spinal ganglion associated with each spinal nerve is located in the corresponding intervertebral foramen.

In the cervical region, the nerve roots are named for the vertebra that forms the lower boundary of the intervertebral foramen. Thus the root between the fifth and sixth cervical vertebrae is called C6; yet the root between the seventh cervical vertebra and the first thoracic vertebra is called C8. Consequently, the nerve roots from the first thoracic vertebra are numbered after the vertebra forming the upper boundary of the intervertebral foramen. The root between L5 and S1 is called L5.

Spinal Nerves and Peripheral Nervous System

Eight cervical, 12 thoracic, five lumbar, and five sacral spinal nerves on both sides emerge from the various spinal cord segments. The thoracic nerves run throughout the thorax and provide the sensory and motor supply for the back, chest, and abdomen. The spinal nerves from the cervical and lumbar spine, as well as those from the sacral segments, unite in the paravertebral plexuses that divide into individual peripheral nerves further along their course. The skin area supplied by the fibers of a given nerve root is called a *dermatome*.

As a result of the interconnection of nerve root fibers in the plexuses with the formation of peripheral nerves, in cases of sensory disorders it is possible to distinguish between areas corresponding to a root lesion (segmental innervation) or to the area of innervation of a peripheral nerve (peripheral innervation; **Fig. 2.2a, b**). Most muscles

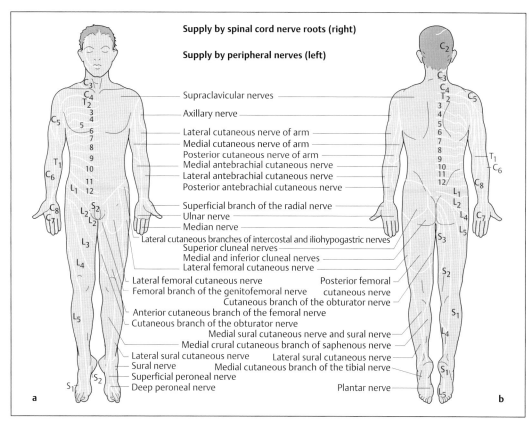

Fig. 2.2 Sensory innervation of the skin. The right half-body shows the sensory innervation by nerve roots (segmental innervation); the left half-body the sensory innervation by peripheral nerves (peripheral innervation). **(a)** Front. **(b)** Back.

are supplied by fibers from several nerve roots. Sometimes a single nerve root predominates to such an extent that a *segment-indicating* muscle can be ascribed to it (**Table 2.2**).

In a nerve root syndrome, the associated pain and sensory disorders occur in the dermatome that is supplied by the affected nerve root and paresis and reflex weakening occur in the corresponding segment-indicating muscles (**Table 2.3**). Pain and sensory disorders can extend laterally over the neck or back from the corresponding spinal segment.

Table 2.2 Segment-indicating muscles

Segment-indicating muscles	Segments
Deltoid muscle	C5
M. biceps brachii M. brachioradialis	(C5) C6
M. triceps brachii	C7
Muscles of the hypothenar eminence Mm. interossei	C8
M. quadriceps femoris M. tibialis anterior	(L3) L4
M. extensor hallucis longus	L5
M. triceps surae	S1

Table 2.3 Signs and symptoms of root syndromes (predominant pareses and impaired functions are printed in bold type)

Root	Pain and hypesthesia area	Paresis	Functional impairment	Reflex
C2–C4	Between shoulder blades Back of neck	**Trapezius**	**Elevation** and retraction of the shoulder blade	
C5	Outside of upper arm (upper third)	**Deltoid** **Biceps brachii**	**Abduction of shoulder joint more than 30°** Flexion in elbow joint	Deltoid reflex Biceps tendon reflex
C6	Shoulder Arm to radial side of lower arm Fingers I and II	**Biceps brachii** **Brachioradialis**	**Flexion in elbow joint**	Biceps tendon reflex Brachioradialis reflex
C7	Shoulder Arm to fingers II–IV volar and dorsal, especially finger III	Pectoralis major **Triceps brachii** Opponens pollicis	Adduction in shoulder joint **Extension in elbow joint** Opposition of thumb	Triceps tendon reflex
C8	Shoulder Arm Lower arm ulnar side Fingers IV–V	Flexor carpi ulnaris Abductor digiti minimi **Interossei dorsales**	Volar flexion with ulnar abduction in wrist Abduction of the little finger **Spreading fingers**	Finger flexor reflex
T1	Inner side of upper and lower arm	–	–	–
T2–12	At corresponding level in the trunk	–	–	–
L1	Groin	**Iliopsoas**	**Hip flexion**	
L2	Groin	**Iliopsoas** Hip adductors	**Hip flexion** Hip adduction	Adductor reflex
L3	Front of thigh to knee	Iliopsoas Adductor magnus and brevis **Quadriceps femoris**	Hip flexion Hip adduction **Knee extension**	Adductor reflex Patellar tendon reflex
L4	Front of thigh Knee Inner side of lower leg Inner ankle Medial edge of foot	Quadriceps femoris **Tibialis anterior**	Knee extension **Dorsal extension in ankle**	Patellar tendon reflex

▶ (continued)

Table 2.3 Signs and symptoms of root syndromes (predominant pareses and impaired functions are printed in bold type) (*continued*)

Root	Pain and hypesthesia area	Paresis	Functional impairment	Reflex
L5	Posterior exterior thigh Outer lower leg Medial dorsum of foot Toes I–II	**Extensor hallucis longus** **Gluteus maximus, gluteus medius, gluteus minimus**	**Dorsal extension of great toe** **Hip abduction and extension**	Tibialis posterior reflex
		Tibialis posterior	Plantar flexion/supination in ankle	
		Tibialis anterior	Dorsal extension in ankle	
S1	Posterior thigh Posterior lower leg Heel Sole of foot Outside edge of foot to toes III–V			Achilles tendon reflex
		Peroneal muscles	Pronation and plantar flexion in ankle	
		Triceps surae	**Plantar flexion/supination in ankle**	
		Gluteus maximus, gluteus medius, gluteus minimus	**Hip abduction and extension**	

All root syndromes of roots C5–T5 can cause pain between the shoulder blades, and syndromes of roots L1–S1 can cause pain in the lumbar spine, lateral back, and buttocks. **Table 2.3** shows only the distal pain and hypesthesia areas typical for individual nerve root syndromes.

Tissues of the Nervous System

Nervous tissue is made up of nerve cells (neurons) and glial cells. Neurons conduct and process excitation. For this purpose, they have special processes that are not found in other cell types. Each neuron has a neurite (axon) and several dendrites. Neurites conduct signals from the cell (efference) and dendrites receive signals from other cells (afference).

Glial cells have a supporting function that provides structure; they also participate in exchange of nutrients between neurons and blood as well as in conduction of stimuli. A specialized form of glial cell—oligodendrocytes of the central nervous system and the Schwann cells of the peripheral nervous system—surrounds the axons and forms myelin sheaths.

The inner subarachnoid spaces are lined with ependymal cells. The musculature is innervated by motor neurons of the spinal cord, whose neurites form the motor anterior roots (**Fig. 2.3**).

Peripheral nerves consist of nerve fibers and the connective tissue that surrounds them. Several axons and dendrites, enclosed in myelin sheaths, are called nerve fibers (fascicles) and are embedded in the endoneurium. The perineurium gathers the nerve fiber bundles. Several nerve fiber bundles are embedded in the epineurium and form the peripheral nerve (**Fig. 2.4**).

Elasticity and extendability of the nerves depend on the sheath tissues of the fascicle, while the epineurium protects against *compression* like a cushion. Every nerve contains several bundles of fascicles, each of which provides sensory or motor innervation to a specific area. Individual axons run wavelike within the fascicles, the fascicles run in waves in the epineurium, and the nerves run in waves in their sheaths (Sunderland 1990). This makes adaptation possible in case of extension during physiological movement sequences.

The thickness of the epineurium varies along the course of the different nerves. Nerves consisting of only a few fascicles and copious epineurium (e.g., the tibial nerve) are better protected against pressure and mechanical stress than those with many fascicles and less epineurium (e.g., the peroneal nerve). The epineural and perineural tissue structures of nerve roots are not distinct; the nerve fibers are parallel and the endoneurium is finer than along the course of the nerves. These structural conditions make nerve roots particularly sensitive to compression and extension.

In the spinal canal, the nervous system is surrounded by a hard covering referred to as the dura

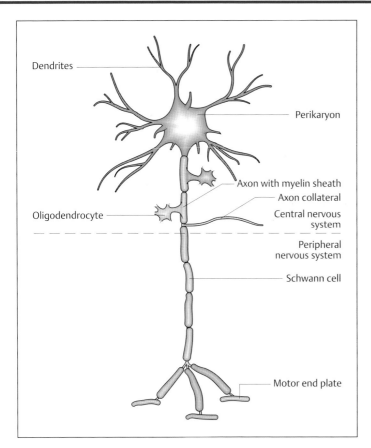

Dendrites

Perikaryon

Axon with myelin sheath

Axon collateral

Central nervous system

Peripheral nervous system

Oligodendrocyte

Schwann cell

Motor end plate

Fig. 2.3 Motor neuron from the anterior horn of the spinal cord. The dotted line marks the boundary between the central and peripheral nervous systems.

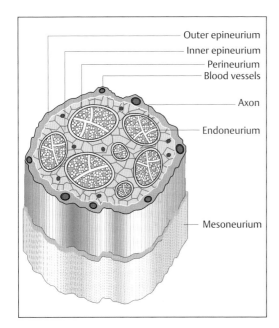

Outer epineurium

Inner epineurium

Perineurium

Blood vessels

Axon

Endoneurium

Mesoneurium

Fig. 2.4 Connective tissue of a nerve.

mater. Cranially, it is attached to the foramen magnum and caudally it is attached to the coccyx by the filum terminale. The dura mater is connected to the spinal cord internally by ligaments, via the arachnoid membrane and a soft cerebrospinal coverage referred to as the pia mater, and externally to the bony surroundings (**Fig. 2.5**). In this way, the spinal cord is safely suspended and protected from elastic stress by ligaments and the dura mater. The spinal fluid in the subarachnoid space is a flexible, protective cushion for the nervous system. Anteriorly, the dura mater is connected to the posterior longitudinal ligament and posteriorly, to the ligamentum flavum.

Stimulus Conduction

The chief function of the nerve cells is reception, processing, and communication of signals from the periphery (afference) as well as transmission back to the periphery of signals generated

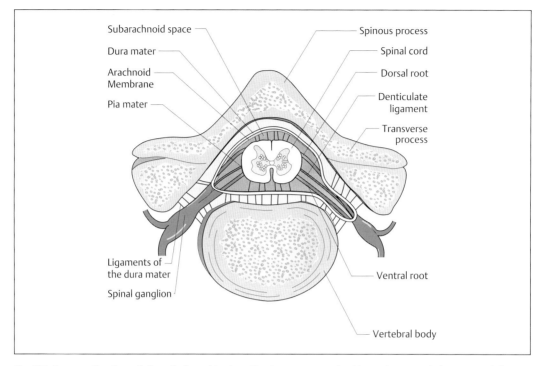

Fig. 2.5 Cross-section through the spinal canal to show the dura mater, arachnoid membrane, and pia mater, and the ligaments that suspend the spinal cord and nerve roots.

in the brain and spinal cord (efference). Peripheral nerve endings register touch, temperature, pressure, pain, and position of body parts. The signals are transmitted electrically in the form of potential changes in the membrane of the nerve cell processes (dendrites, axons). Communication between nerve cells takes place when these potential changes lead to the release of transmitter substances (messenger substances, neurotransmitters) that produce another potential change in a downstream nerve cell.

Nerve cells are differentiated from other cells of the body by their partially very long cell processes that, for the motor neurons of the sciatic nerve, for instance, extend along the length of the leg as far as the distal muscle innervated by this nerve. The metabolism of these cell processes is ensured by antero- and retrograde transport systems that enable the transport of various molecules through the cell processes. Growth factors such as nerve growth factor (NGF) are secreted in the periphery by the target structures of the nerves and transported back over long distances

as far as the nuclei of the nerve cells. It is suspected that mechanical damage to nerves and nerve roots, such as caused by a prolapsed disk, interferes with such transport processes through the effect of pressure.

Blood Supply

The nervous system consumes 20% of the oxygen made available to the body by the circulating blood, but the nervous system only represents 2% of the total body mass (Dommisse 1986). The blood supply of the nerve roots and the peripheral nerves is provided through a special vascular system (vasa nervorum). Spiral supply vessels branch from the main vessels that run parallel to the nerves and enter the nerve. Additional collateral safety systems ensure oxygen supply in case of disruptions in individual vessels (Lundborg 1975; Bell and Weddell 1984).

A grid-like collagen structure protects the blood vessels from extension and compression damage

(Breig 1978). By this structure, blood supply to the axons and dendrites that run through the nerves and to cellular components (e.g., Schwann cells) is ensured for every movement and sustained position.

In studies on rabbit sciatic nerves, slowing of blood flow was observed at 8% extension and interruption of blood flow was observed at 15% extension (Lundborg and Rydevik 1973). Such an extension is not likely to occur under physiological conditions, but if nerve mobility is impaired (e.g., in the form of a fibrosed nerve root after a disk prolapse), an extension with impairment of the blood flow is conceivable. This could explain the occurrence of sensory disorders in nerve tension tests.

Innervation

The connective tissue sheaths of the nervous system are innervated and can be the cause of pain (Hall and Elvey 1999). A fine nerve web (sinuvertebral nerves) supplies the dura mater, dural root sac, posterior longitudinal ligament, periosteum, blood vessels, and anulus fibrosus (Bogduk 2000).

Free nerve endings were also found in the connective tissue of peripheral nerves and called nervi nervorum (nerves of the nerves) by Horsley in 1884. Already in 1883, Marshall assumed the existence of such nerves and established the hypothesis that the substances secreted during an inflammation irritate these nerves and thus trigger neuralgia (Sugar et al 1990). This hypothesis is supported by indications of inflammatory processes and pain mediators in the nervi nervorum (Zochodne 1993; Sauer et al 1999).

The significance of the innervation of the nerves and their sheaths in the occurrence of neurological symptoms, especially radiating pain, has remained unclear.

2.1.5 Biomechanics of the Nervous System and the Spine

Movements of the Nervous System

In movement, the individual tissue layers of a nerve glide against each other (Elvey 1997), while at the same time, nerve roots and networks as well as the spinal cord are unfolded or folded

(Breig 1978; **Fig. 2.6a, b**; **Fig. 2.7a, b**). Longitudinal, transverse, and rotational movements can be distinguished. When the extremities are moved, first the waves in the nerves are smoothed out, but not in the fascicles, so that these are protected from overextension. Human nerve roots and peripheral nerves can compensate for 6 to 20% extension before they tear. The degree of elasticity depends, among other things, on the intensity, duration, and speed of the force applied (Sunderland 1990).

Movements of the extremities cause tension changes in the peripheral nerves that are transmitted to the central nervous system via the nerve roots. In the same way, movements of the spine cause tension changes in the central and peripheral nervous systems (**Fig. 2.8**). When nerves are extended, the nerve fibers unfold and thus become

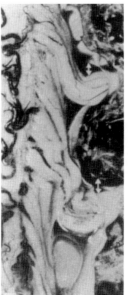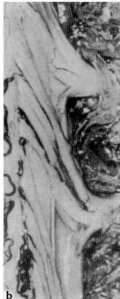

Fig. 2.6 Changes in the nervous system in movement of nerve roots, dura mater, and spinal cord. **(a)** In full extension of the spine, the dura mater, the nerve roots, and the spinal cord are relaxed. The nerve roots have no contact with the dural sacs (lower arrow); the dural sacs have no contact with the vertebral arches (upper arrow). **(b)** In full flexion of the spine, the dura mater, the nerve roots, and the spinal cord are tensed. The nerve roots are in contact with the dural sacs and the dural sacs are in contact with the vertebral arches. (Images reproduced courtesy of Breig 1978.)

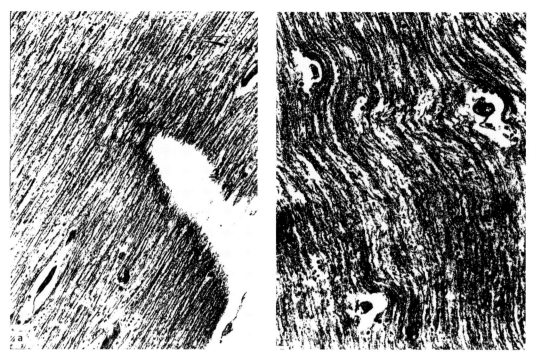

Fig. 2.7 Changes in the nervous system during movement in the spinal cord. **(a)** Elongation of the spinal cord in flexion of the spine. **(b)** Shortening of the spinal cord in extension of the spine. (Images reproduced courtesy of Breig 1978.)

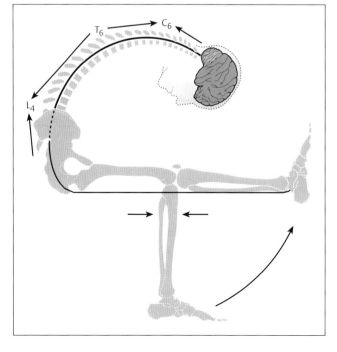

Fig. 2.8 Maximal tension on the nervous system. In spinal flexion and simultaneous hip flexion with knee extension, the entire nervous system is tensed. A particularly intense tension is generated at tension points C6, T6, L4, and in the hollow of the knee. (Image reproduced courtesy of Butler 1991.)

longer and thinner. The pressure inside the nerve fibers rises, and the blood circulation is decreased (Sunderland 1990). The collagenous connective tissue and the glial cells limit the mobility of the nervous system in contraction (Breig 1978). Because of the three-dimensional folding of the nerve fibers of the spinal cord that takes place in this movement, their diameter in extension of the spine is greater than in flexion.

The flexibility of the nervous system is externally influenced by various anatomical features. Bony structures bound the nervous system, for instance in the skull, spinal canal, intervertebral foramina, ulnar sulcus, and at the head of the fibula. The connective tissue surrounding the nervous system creates contact surfaces that permit the movement of nervous structures under physiological conditions.

The denticulate ligaments connect the nerve roots with the dura and thus transmit tension from the nerve roots to the spinal cord. In movement, increased tension is transmitted over these ligaments to their points of attachment and at the same time they protect the nerve roots from over-extension.

Butler (1998) observed that patients regularly reproduced symptoms at specific points during nerve tension tests, in spinal cord segments C6, T6, and L4, in the hollow of the knee and the crook of the elbow. He proposed the hypothesis that in these areas, very little movement is possible for the nervous system and this leads to a sensitive reaction to tension. He explained that from the anatomical point of view, this could be due to the fact that the spaces between spinal cord and vertebral canal are particularly narrow (ibid.). However, contemporary computed tomography (CT-) or magnetic resonance imaging (MRI-) based data to support this view are not available.

In the hollow of the knee and the crook of the elbow, particularly robust connections between neural structures and surrounding structures via nerve branches and penetrating blood vessels lead to elevated tension upon movement.

Spinal Movement

Spinal movements are complex combinations of individual components, of which the most important are flexion, extension, rotation, and lateral flexion. The movement patterns are different in different spinal segments and different from each other. They can proceed differently if performed with or without stress (Bogduk 2000).

Movement of the Lumbar Spine

In *flexion*, lumbar lordosis disappears. In this movement, the vertebrae change their relative positions such that the vertebral bodies lie parallel to each other. A further convergence of the anterior vertebral edges, beyond parallel, and thus additional flexion, is only possible in the upper lumbar spine (Bogduk 2000). At the same time, the vertebrae are shifted forward. In flexion, there is anterior compression of the disks and a release of compression in the facet joints.

Extension is the opposite of flexion. The posterior edges of the vertebrae converge and the vertebrae are shifted posteriorly. The disks are compressed dorsally and the facet joints are compressed. The spinous processes and the disks limit the range of motion. Extension trauma usually leads at first to injury of the spinous processes before the disks are injured, thus disk damage without damage to the spinous processes is unlikely (Adams et al 1988).

Upon *rotation*, the disks are subjected to torsional stress and the facet joints are pushed into each other. The maximal rotational capacity of a disk before injury is 3°. The facet joints only permit a small degree of movement (1–2° per segment), thus protecting the disks from overload by rotational movements. The rotation of the upper three lumbar vertebral segments is associated with lateral flexion to the contralateral side. In segment L4–L5 there is no stereotypical combination of movements. Rotation in the joint between L5 and S1 is associated with ipsilateral lateral flexion.

In *lateral flexion*, complex combinations of movements occur that have not yet been studied in detail. Lateral flexion of the upper lumbar segments is associated with rotation to the contralateral side. In segment L4–L5 there is no stereotypical combination of movements. Lateral flexion between L5 and S1 is accompanied by ipsilateral rotation (Bogduk 2000).

Movement of the Thoracic Spine

The thoracic spine is considerably less mobile than the lumbar or the cervical spine because of its connection to the ribs. Slight flexion (thoracic kyphosis) is the natural position of the thoracic spine.

Mobility in *extension* is limited by the spinous processes, which are longer in this region than in the lumbar or cervical spine and therefore present a greater mechanical impediment.

Lateral flexion is limited chiefly by the ribs. The greatest leeway in movement is in *rotation*.

Movement of the Cervical Spine

Because of different anatomical situations and different postural and movement patterns, division into upper (C1, C2) and lower (C3–C7) cervical spine is useful.

Flexion and *extension* take place in the atlantooccipital joint, while *rotation* is barely possible. At the level of C2–C3, mobility in *rotation* is greater than in the lower segments.

Lateral flexion takes place chiefly in the lower segments of the cervical spine, where rotation is less possible than in the upper cervical spine. As in the lumbar spine, rotation and lateral flexion are complex movement sequences that are always associated with each other.

Clinically relevant combination movements of the cervical spine are retraction and protraction. In *retraction* the occiput is moved dorsally and the chin is moved caudally. This movement is associated with flexion of the upper and extension of the lower cervical spine.

In *protraction* the face moves ventrally. This movement is associated with extension of the upper and flexion of the lower cervical spine. In flexion of the entire cervical spine, there is more flexion in the lower cervical spine than in protraction. In extension of the entire cervical spine there is more extension in the lower cervical spine than in retraction (Ordway et al 1999).

Relationship Between Movements of the Spine and Movements of the Nervous System

Spinal Flexion

- Spinal cord, meninges, and nerve roots are unfolded and are subject to tension (**Fig. 2.6**; **Fig. 2.7**).
- The nerve roots come into contact with the vertebral arches (**Fig. 2.6**).
- The spinal cord is moved ventrally in the spinal canal.

- The cross-section of the spinal canal is enlarged.
- The intervertebral foramina are enlarged by 30% (Butler 1998).

Spinal Extension

- Spinal cord, meninges, and nerve roots are approximated, folded, and released from tension (**Fig. 2.6**; **Fig. 2.7**).
- The nerve roots are not in contact with the vertebral arches (**Fig. 2.6**).
- The spinal cord is moved dorsally in the spinal canal.
- The cross-section of the spinal canal is reduced.
- The intervertebral foramina are reduced by 20%.
- The spinal canal is elongated by 5 to 9 cm from maximal spinal extension to flexion (Breig 1978).

Lateral Flexion of the Spine

- Spinal cord, meninges, and nerve roots are approximated on the concave (flexed) side and extended on the convex side.
- The intervertebral foramina become narrower on the concave side and wider on the convex side.

Spinal Rotation

The effects of rotational movements on the spinal canal have not yet been extensively studied. The flexion, extension, and lateral flexion movements associated with spinal rotation decisively modify the effects of rotation on the nervous system.

2.2 Pathophysiology of Disk Damage

As a general rule, degenerative processes in the disks develop over a period of many years (Weber 1994; Waddell 1998; Von Strempel 2001). Patients with prolapsed disks can usually remember numerous episodes of back or neck pain and sudden limitation of movement suffered in the past. Traumatic disk damage tends to be an exception rather than the rule.

Disk prolapses can occur from youth to old age, but almost never (unless they are traumatic) in childhood. They occur most frequently in middle age, between age 30 and 50 (McKenzie 1981, 1986,

1990, 2003; Weber 1994; Von Strempel 2001), because at a younger age (under 30) the degenerative process is not yet advanced, and with increasing age (over 50) the elasticity of the disks has decreased to such an extent that displacement of the nucleus pulposus occurs less frequently. In addition, there is typically less stress on the spine after the age of 50.

Fractures of the end plates can cause degenerative processes within the disks. The end plate is less able to withstand pressure than the anulus fibrosus. Fractures lead to a loss of height in the disk and an increase of tension in the posterior region of the anulus fibrosus. This significantly decreases the resistance of this region, which is always particularly stressed in activities of daily living (Adams, Freeman et al 2000; Bogduk 2000).

The buffering function of the intervertebral disk depends on its water content. Pressure stress, for instance in standing, causes a 13 to 36% decrease in the water content of the nucleus pulposus. This shifts the pressure stress from the nucleus pulposus to the anulus fibrosus. This can lead to acute and chronic pain and in the long term to degenerative processes in the disk (Adams et al 1996). For this reason, a low proteoglycan content, and the associated low water uptake capacity of the disk, promotes degenerative processes (Pearce et al 1987).

The areas that are the most mechanically stressed are the transitions from mobile to stable segments. For this reason, disk prolapses are most frequent at vertebral levels L5–S1 and C6–C7 (Mundt et al 1993; Elfering et al 2002; Witt and Stöhr 2003).

2.2.1 Mechanism of a Disk Prolapse

With every movement, the disks also move passively. Repeated one-sided movements or maintaining a position for a long time causes the gel nucleus to move away from the one-sided pressure and migrate in the opposite direction (Adams and Hutton 1985; Fennell et al 1996). In activities that require stooping (e.g., sitting, lifting, gardening) there is continual ventral pressure on the disks. The gel mass moves to the back and presses on the sensitive fibrous ring (**Fig. 2.9**; **Fig. 2.10**) that is simultaneously overextended posteriorly (Adams et al 1994). This effect on the fibrous ring is most likely responsible for back pain after a long period of stress.

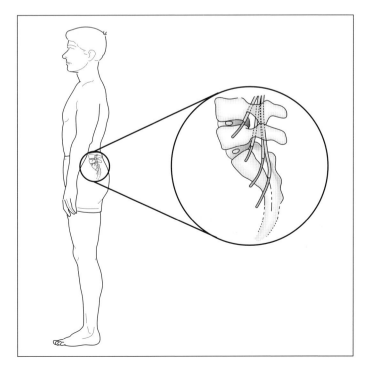

Fig. 2.9 Erect posture. The *sacral spine* has a slight forward curve and the posterior edges of the vertebral bodies are approximated. The gelatinous nuclei are located in the middle between the anterior and posterior edges of the vertebral body.

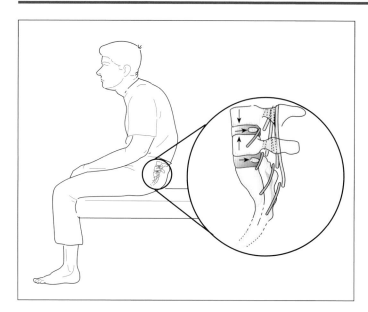

Fig. 2.10 Stooped posture. The vertebral bodies are parallel to each other. The gelatinous nuclei deviate posteriorly.

Repeated incorrect loading can produce tears in the fibrous rings. With further stooping, the gelatinous nucleus deviates so sharply to posterior that when the subject stands up again, it is caught between the posterior edges of the vertebral bodies. This limits extension and the subject feels forced into a stooped posture that is maintained because it is so painful to stand erect. Sustained stooping can shift the gelatinous nucleus so far to the back that the fibrous ring finally tears (Adams and Hutton 1985). The gelatinous mass protrudes partially through this tear and a disk prolapse results, with or without compression of a neighboring nerve root, depending on the location and size of the tear (**Fig. 2.11**).

Examples

Hamburger Effect
Everyone is familiar with the following situation. You want to take a bite of a hamburger. To make it fit into your mouth, you squeeze it on one side, and the meat slides out the other side (**Fig. 2.12**). This is a good way to imagine the mechanics of a disk prolapse.

Nerve root compression often causes radiating pain that emanates from the lumbar spine over the buttocks to the thigh, corresponding to the dermatome supplied by the affected nerve root. In the case of the L5 root the pain typically radiates as

Fig. 2.11 Disk prolapse. There is a tear in the anulus fibrosus. The nucleus pulposus is displaced to the rear and presses on the nerve root.

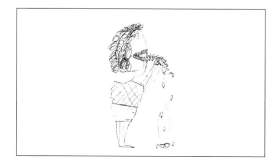

Fig. 2.12 Hamburger effect. Like the hamburger, the disk moves away from the one-sided pressure and is shifted to the opposite side.

far as the great toe. From the cervical spine, pain radiates over the shoulder blade into the upper arm and finally into the fingers. Strong pressure on the nerve roots causes sensory disorders in the area supplied by the nerve. In addition, the muscle it supplies can be weakened. Sometimes the back pain remits at this point.

A disk prolapse in the thoracic spine causes radiating pains along the ribs. Disk prolapses that compress the spinal cord or the cauda equina are rare (see 2.2.4 Nerve Damage Associated with a Prolapsed Disk). In this case, a cross-sectional spinal cord syndrome develops at the affected level. It is commonly incomplete.

A disk prolapses ventrally only at high pressure and concomitant hyperextension of the spine. This is very rare (Adams et al 1988).

In activities of daily living, the spine is chiefly loaded in a stooped position: in the morning, one gets up, sits at the breakfast table, brushes one's teeth, and sits in the car, to sit at work or work physically in a stooped position. In the evening, one sits in the car, drives home, sits at dinner, and finally, for relaxation, sits in front of the TV. Up to that point, one may probably not have extended the spine all day. The spine loses its mobility. The disks are constantly being pushed posteriorly. As a result of this typical everyday loading, extending the spine is probably the most important exercise, and pain-free mobility in extension is a central goal of treatment.

2.2.2 Classification of Intervertebral Disk Damage

Classification is based on the two criteria of *degree of severity* and *position of the displaced disk tissue*.

Degree of Severity

- Anular tear: tear in the anulus fibrosus that can only be visualized with diskography.
- Bulging disk and protrusion: slight forward bulging of disk tissue that can be visualized with CT or MRI. Judging by the severity of the disorder, it is assumed that the outer layer of the anulus fibrosus is usually intact.
- Extrusion, disk herniation: pronounced forward bulging of the disk tissue in which it is assumed,

judging by the severity of the disorder, that the anulus fibrosus is torn.
- Sequestration: the disk tissue is displaced upward or downward beyond the edge of the vertebral body and has lost continuity with the rest of the disk tissue. In this case, the anulus fibrosus must be torn.

This is the classification recommended by the North American Spine Society. In this classification, other parameters important for the evaluation of the degree of severity of the disease and the prognosis (e.g., decrease in height of the intervertebral space and signal intensity in MRI; see Chapter 3 Medical Diagnosis and Treatment) are not taken into account (Kotilainen et al 2001).

Position of the Displaced Disk Tissue

- Median: toward the middle of the spinal canal. Nerve roots can be compressed on both sides, as well as the spinal cord or cauda equina, depending on size.
- Mediolateral: to one side of the spinal canal (most frequent position). On one side, one or more nerve roots (in rare cases the spinal cord or cauda equina as well) can be compressed.
- Foraminal: extending into the intervertebral foramen. The nerve root at the affected level is compressed.
- Extraforaminal: displaced to the side, beyond the intervertebral foramen. The nerve root exiting at the affected level is compressed.

2.2.3 Disk Damage and Muscle Tension

In patients with prolapsed disks, increased tone is usually observed in the lumbar extensor spinae muscles. An abnormal posture of the spine with reduction of physiological lordosis is typical of diskogenic disorders. It is often associated with lateral shift of the spine (see Chapter 5 Therapy; McKenzie 1986; Maitland 1986, 1994; Waddell 1998).

Indahl et al (1997) observed action potentials in the paravertebral musculature and in the latissimus dorsi after local electrical stimulation of the posterolateral anulus fibrosus. This could be an indication that the tension in the paravertebral musculature is a physiological protective mechanism when the anulus fibrosus is injured. Muscle tension dorsal to the spine prevents movements that would increase the disk prolapse, usually stooping, partially combined with lateral displacement of the spine. The patient is thus not drawn into incorrect posture by the increased muscle tone but protected from moving even further in the damaging direction.

McKenzie (1986) considered the incorrect spinal posture in patients with a prolapsed disk to be a mechanical deformation. According to him, displacement of the gelatinous nucleus causes a limitation of movement in the direction of the displaced mass. This means that, for instance, repeated bending of the spine causes backward displacement of the gelatinous nucleus and thus mechanically prevents extension of the spine.

Waddell (1998) interpreted the loss of lordosis and lateral shift of the spine as the effect of a muscle spasm. However, it is questionable how increased tone of the erector spinae muscles can cause a loss of spinal lordosis, since in this situation lordosis should in fact be promoted.

Thus, the pathogenesis and significance of the increased paravertebral muscle tone in patients with diskal prolapse remains controversial. Since there are no convincing explanatory models for the muscles as the cause of back and neck pain (Bogduk 2000; Rao 2002), a critical reappraisal is necessary as to whether muscle-relaxing measures such as muscle relaxants, massage, or fango are helpful or harmful.

2.2.4 Nerve Damage Associated with a Prolapsed Disk

Symptoms

Cross-sectional Paralysis

Dorsally, the disks are protected by the posterior longitudinal ligament and for this reason, disk prolapses directly to posterior (median) with the resulting compression of the spinal cord or cauda equina rarely occur. Cross-sectional paralysis above L1 resulting from a median disk prolapse leads to central paralysis because, formally, the central nervous system ends at this level with the spinal cord and the peripheral nervous system begins with the cauda equina.

After the acute phase of spinal shock, central cross-sectional paralysis is characterized by elevated tone and increased reflexes of the affected muscles. In the acute phase, the bladder is disturbed, with urinary retention and high amounts of residual urine. Later, a spastic bladder develops that empties spontaneously in small volumes, with a clinical picture of stress incontinence.

With a lesion below L1, there is peripheral paralysis with decreased tone and reduced reflexes in the affected muscles. This is associated with a bladder disorder of residual urine collection and an overflow bladder with incontinence.

Nerve Root Compression

Mediolateral or foraminal diskal prolapses are much more frequent than clinically relevant median prolapses. The former lead to irritation or damage of specific nerve roots. In the lumbar spine, the nerve roots run past the disk far dorsolaterally before they leave the spinal canal through the intervertebral foramen one segment below (**Fig. 2.13**).

As a result of this anatomical configuration, in most cases the nerve root affected is the one that emerges one segment lower than the prolapsed disk. A disk prolapse at L4–L5 leads to compression of root L5 in approximately 80% of cases. Root L4 is only affected if the prolapse is located laterally or foraminal.

In the thoracic and cervical spine, in case of a disk prolapse, the nerve root usually affected is the one that lies in the same segment. A disk prolapse at C5–C6 leads to compression of root C6; at T1–T2, a prolapse leads to compression of root T1.

Bony Anatomy

The severity of the symptoms and the prognosis for successful conservative treatment are closely related to the additional narrowing applied to the affected nerve roots by bony structures. In the case of a disk prolapse, the nerve root, swollen as a result of compression, is also mechanically impaired by the bony limitation in the intervertebral foramen. If there is an unfavorable relationship between the severity of the swelling and the width of the intervertebral foramen, there is nerve compression here as well, and potential permanent damage. Especially if the disk prolapse is located toward the foramen, damage to the nerve root is likely (Aota et al 2001).

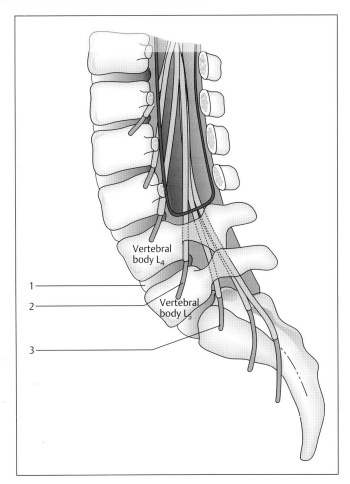

Fig. 2.13 The lateral view of the lumbar spine shows the relative positions of disk and nerve roots. (Images reproduced courtesy of Trepel 1995.)
1 = Disk between L4 and L5 (L4–L5)
2 = Nerve root L4, lateral to the disk (L4–L5)
3 = Nerve root L5, behind the disk (L4–L5)

Vertebral body L4

Vertebral body L5

A narrow spinal canal also contributes to a relatively unfavorable prognosis because there is little space for the nerve to move out of the way if space is also taken up by a disk prolapse (Saal and Saal 1989).

Pathophysiology of Nerve Damage

Course of the Nerve Damage

Sunderland (1976) described three stages of nerve damage resulting from constant pressure:
- First the venous return is impaired causing hypoxia of the axon and development of edema.
- The resulting increased impairment of venous return destroys the capillary endothelium.
- The intrafascicular pressure rises, activating fibroblasts and causing scar formation. Pain,

sensory disorders, paresis, and painful limitations of movement can result.

Effect of Compression and Extension

Breig (1978) considered damage to the spinal cord or a nerve root by compression as the result of extension. Pressure (e.g., in case of disk prolapse) causes tension in the immediate surroundings. Blood vessels and nerve fibers are not compressed but extended, and can tear. Thus extension is the decisive damaging force. It can arise as local stress and deformation, pinching, or occupation of space. The damage resulting from extension depends on its extent and duration. Where there is acute pressure, the nervous system should not be stressed with additional extension. In this case, flexion of the spine must be avoided and extension of the spine should be the goal.

Extension (elongation by 20%) of the sciatic nerve in rats led to reduction of retrograde transport by 43% and of the blood flow in the vasa nervorum by 50%. Extension of a peripheral nerve seems to inhibit retrograde axonal transport. The chief reason for this appears to be limitation of blood supply (Tanou et al 1996).

In experiments in pigs, 3-hour compression (50 mm Hg or 6.7 kPa) by means of an inflatable balloon placed on the exposed cauda equina resulted in damage to Schwann cells, hyperemia, and bleeding (Byröd et al 1998). An inflammatory reaction developed in the epineural tissue, with infiltration of mast cells and leukocytes. The function of motor fibers of the corresponding nerve roots was measured in the form of muscular action potentials and had not been disturbed after 3 hours of compression (ibid.).

After nerve damage, the destroyed portions of the axon and the myelin are biodegraded by macrophages and Schwann cells. This lowers the tension within the endoneural sheath. The nerve shrinks, becoming shorter and thinner. This process takes place over a period of 3 months (Sunderland 1990).

Breig (1960, 1978), Breig and Marions (1963), and Breig and Troup (1979) investigated the effect of motion on the dura mater and the sacral nerves of recently deceased individuals. When hips and knees were flexed, the sacral plexus remained relaxed. In contrast, when knees were extended the plexus and the nerve roots were tensed and the fascia surrounding the nerve roots was pulled caudally. When a disk prolapse was simulated, the nerve root and its surrounding fascia were pulled up through the intervertebral foramen. Thus in vivo fibrosis and shrinking of the root sac as well as local adhesions could be the result of disk prolapses (see Chapter 12 Selected Studies on the Topic of Spinal Disorders).

Clinically, these changes are marked by positive signs of nerve extension. The patient's familiar pains are triggered or increased by passive movement of the extremities and the spine. At the same time, sensory disturbances can be triggered or intensified.

Chemical Nerve Stimulation or Inflammation

Compression damage promotes formation of cytokines with pro- (interleukin 6) and anti-inflammatory (transforming growth factor-β) effects (Specchina et al 2002). Because wounds to the disk tissue have a poor healing capacity in animal models, it was postulated that soluble mediator substances from the injured tissue can promote chronic pain (Hampton et al 1989). There is still controversial discussion as to whether compression or irritation by inflammatory mediators is the dominant pain trigger (Hampton et al 1989; Saal et al 1990; Vucetic et al 1995; Kayama et al 1996; Olmarker et al 1996; Zwart et al 1998; Furusawa et al 2001; Specchina et al 2002).

In patients with prolapsed lumbar disks, morphological changes were observed in the multifidus muscle in the form of atrophied type 1 and type 2 fibers (Yoshihara et al 2001). The connection between muscle weakness, positive straight leg raise test, and inflammatory cells in patients with prolapsed disks has been studied repeatedly. The presence of macrophages, T and B lymphocytes, and activated T lymphocytes in the resected disk tissue of 96 patients did not correlate with nerve extension pain (straight leg raise test) or muscle weakness (Gronblad et al 2000; Brisby et al 2002).

Since the nucleus pulposus is not vascularized, it is usually not affected by immunological processes. Some authors suspect that a disk prolapse changes this situation because the disk tissue comes into contact with the immune system so that an autoimmune reaction against the disk tissue could develop (Gertzbein et al 1977; Satoh et al 1999). In autoimmune reactions, immune cells lose their tolerance for the body's own tissues, as in multiple sclerosis.

Ikeda et al (1996) doubt this theory, since signs of inflammation in the form of macrophage and lymphocyte infiltration were already found in the first episode of a disk injury (without previous immunization).

2.2.5 Regeneration Processes and Recovery of Disk and Nerve

Wound Healing Phase

The wound healing process that begins immediately after an injury is divided into three phases:
- Inflammation phase.
- Transitional phase.
- Stabilization phase.

Inflammation Phase

Tissue injuries are always associated with an inflammatory reaction. Mediator substances from the damaged tissue lead to local changes in vascular permeability and invasion of leukocytes and macrophages. These cells, like the damaged tissue itself, release substances such as prostaglandins, bradykinin, and proinflammatory cytokines like interleukins and tumor necrosis factor-α. The peripheral nociceptors secrete neuropeptides such as substance P, neurokinin A, and calcitonin gene-related peptides. These mediators modulate the subjective pain stimulus and also precapillary vasodilation and postcapillary plasma extravasation, which support inflammation and lead to tissue swelling.

The activated macrophages resorb injured disk tissue and mediate the recruitment and activation of fibroblasts, which complete the wound healing process and scar formation. Type 3 collagen is formed first, to close the wound quickly. However, it is not very strong. In the normal course of healing and without further damage, the inflammatory reaction is complete in 5 days.

Transitional Phase

The number of monocytes, leukocytes, and lymphocytes and macrophages decreases within 5 days after an acute injury, while the number of fibro- and myofibroblasts in the injured tissue increases. Then collagen is synthesized in large amounts. The organization and orientation of the newly formed tissue depends on stress stimuli (Van den Berg 1999; Schünke 2000). In the normal course of wound healing, the transitional phase is complete after 21 days.

Stabilization Phase

Collagen, glycosaminoglycans, and proteoglycans are synthesized to an increasing extent. Fibroblasts transform Type 3 collagen into Type 1 collagen. This leads to greater resistance to tensile and pressure stress. After 60 to 360 days, healing is normally complete and the strength of the tissue is largely restored.

Special Events in the Healing of Disk Tissue

The specific characteristics of disk tissue create some distinctive features in the process of regeneration after mechanical injury. Hampton et al (1989) studied regeneration of the anulus fibrosus in animal experiments. The disk was surgically injured and the healing process was observed after 3, 6, 9, and 12 weeks. Large wounds—through the entire thickness of the anulus fibrosus, reaching as far as the nucleus pulposus—showed a good tendency to heal. Defects were closed with fibrous tissue. Small puncture wounds through the anulus fibrosus, approximately comparable to naturally occurring tears, exhibited a significantly weaker tendency, if any, to heal. Fibrous tissue formed only in small amounts in the outer anulus fibrosus (ibid.). The authors suspect that chemical substances could escape outward from the nucleus pulposus and cause nerve root irritation. However, there are no experimental data to support this hypothesis.

Macrophages, neovascularization, and granulation tissue were found in surgically excised disk tissue as a sign of inflammation. The nucleus pulposus exhibited more macrophage infiltration than the anulus fibrosus. According to these results, disk prolapses are resorbed by phagocytic cells, especially macrophages (Ikeda et al 1996).

Special Events in the Healing of Nervous Tissue

In studying the healing of a peripheral nerve, regeneration of the axon and restoration of function must be considered separately. Even if the structure of the axon is reconstructed, reinnervation of the area it supplies can remain impaired. Nerve tissue is exposed to special difficulties in the healing process. The swelling associated with the inflammatory phase can increase nerve compression. The regrowth of axons is slow and depends on an intact connective tissue guide structure that is not deformed by scar formation. An axon does not grow more than 2 to 3 mm a day. Consequently, regeneration after nerve damage can last many months or even years.

Fibrosis

The connective tissue surrounding the nervous system provides contact surfaces that play a part in movement, and in pathological events (e.g., scar formation) may be the cause of symptoms (Butler 1998; Bogduk 2000). At the end point of the movement or if physiological nerve gliding is hampered by neighboring structures, the nervous system is subject to tension. The cross-section of the nerve becomes smaller and the intraneural pressure is elevated (Breig 1978; Sunderland 1990). The result is pain and possible neurological deficits.

Fibrosis of the nerve root is predominantly discussed in association with surgery (Saal and Saal 1990; Jonsson and Stromqvist 1996; Devulder 1998; BenDebba et al 1999; Brotchi et al 1999; Ross 1999; Spencer 1999; Vogelsang et al 1999; Krappel and Harland 2001). Introduction of modern surgical techniques, especially microsurgery, has led to a decrease of scarring-associated, chronic postoperative lumbago and sciatica. However, nerve scarring can also be caused by chronic mechanical injury (Butler 1998).

Friction and inflammation of the nerve root near a prolapsed disk can trigger the formation of fibrous tissue, just as after an operation the scar tissue can become a space-occupying mass that compresses the nerve. Most of all, the natural gliding movements of the individual tissue layers are prevented to such an extent that movement exerts a pull on the nervous system.

Regeneration of Nervous Tissue

The regeneration capacity of nervous tissue is rather limited in comparison to that of other tissues in the body. This is true not only for the central but also for the peripheral nervous system. How and under what conditions a regenerating axon can grow back into its original sleeve structures and can thus reach its original target organ again, remains unknown.

Some observations speak against a truly goal-directed growth, since regenerating axons also develop outside fascicular structures. Motor axons grow into the endoneurium of sensory fibers and vice versa. It can thus be a matter of chance whether a regenerating axon reaches the distal end of its endoneural sleeve. Irreversible endoneuronal shrinking as a result of scar formation can also be a reason why reinnervation often remains incomplete. As a result, the nerve fibers cannot grow to their original size and degree of myelination (Sunderland 1990).

On the biochemical level, the regulation of nerve regeneration is incompletely understood. Some findings indicate that the mechanisms that developmentally ensure the survival of axons and their arrival at their goals also play a role in healing of lesions in the mature nervous system. For instance, *nerve growth factor* (NGF) is a neurotrophic factor that has definite significance for the development of the nervous system and possible significance for regeneration.

Possibly, *vascular endothelial growth factor* (VEGF), which is also formed in the spinal dorsal ganglia, plays a role in the repair of nerve injuries. It stimulates axonal growth, Schwann cell proliferation, and the formation of blood vessels (Sondell et al 1999).

The muscles affected by *denervation* (decoupling from the nervous system) in a nerve injury remain vital for up to 1 year (Sunderland 1979) and if reinnervation is successful, their function may be restored. Pareses triggered by a disk prolapse usually resolve with both conservative and surgical treatment (Weber 1983; Weber et al 1993; Brötz et al 2001, 2003; Brötz, Burkard, Weller 2010).

In a nonrandomized study (Dubourg et al 2002), paresis improved (strength grade 3 and worse) within 6 months in 53% of a group of patients receiving surgical treatment. This included complete recovery (strength grade 5). In the group of patients receiving conservative treatment, the paresis improved (strength grade 3 and worse) in 56% of patients within 6 months. This included complete recovery (strength grade 5) in 40%.

2.3   Pain

Pain is an unpleasant sensory or emotional experience associated with actual or potential tissue damage. It is a common impairment of well-being associated with disk damage. Sensory disorders, muscle weakness, and limited range of motion, on the other hand, are often considered minor by patients. Pain can have a variety of qualities. It can be deep or superficial, burning, cutting, pulling, piercing, compressive, or dull, have different intensities and be constant or fluctuating. It is a subjective experience, perceived and mastered variably, depending on personality, education, and earlier illnesses.

The *physiological basis of pain* is the stimulation of nociceptors by mechanical or chemical stimuli in the course of tissue injuries (Loeser 1999, 2000). Pain is primarily the sensation perceived when nociceptors are stimulated. Yet, it can be felt without tissue injury, for example in the case of central pain after disturbed blood supply in the thalamus or in the exceptional case of phantom pain, which is projected into a lost (amputated) limb.

Suffering: this concept covers the unpleasant emotional response to a pain stimulus and other emotional stimuli. Suffering is not only associated with pain stimuli but can also be elicited by stress, grief, fear, or depression.

Pain behavior: this includes all actions demonstrating that a person is in pain. Pain behavior can be expressed by speaking, sighing, groaning, facial expression, limping, taking pain medications, frequent visits to a physician, and disability. In a broad sense, pain behavior is one aspect of the overall illness behavior.

> **Note:** In studying pain, Loeser distinguishes between its somatic, cognitive, and behavioral aspects.

2.3.1   Location of Pain

In diseases of the intervertebral disks, pain is experienced as central, near the spine, or radiating from the roots. According to clinical experience, the degree of severity of disk damage or associated nerve root compression correlates with the topographic extension of the projected pain. This means that distal extension of the projected pain is considered an exacerbation of the disease.

The pathophysiology of the radiating pain has hardly been investigated up to now. It is often assumed that the further the pain radiates, the stronger the suspected pressure on the nerve root. However, this assumption has not been confirmed experimentally. In addition, there is the observation that the topographic change of sensory disorder behaves precisely in reciprocal fashion. This means that while movement of the pain in a central direction within the affected dermatome indicates that the disease is improving, central extension of a sensory disorder indicates worsening.

A classification should be physiologically plausible, clinically useful, and simple. Moreover, the classification should be able to include, as much as possible, all patients with the same symptoms. Such a classification can be used for better evaluation of the necessity of expensive or invasive tests, the intensity of medical care, the prognosis, and the patient's ability to work.

The *Quebec Task Force* suggests a classification for spine and spinal cord diseases in 11 categories (McKenzie 1990), of which the first four are largely based on the location of the pain:
- *Pain in the lumbar, dorsal, or cervical region:*
  - No radiation below the gluteal fold or over the shoulder blade.
  - No neurological findings.
- *Pain in the lumbar, dorsal, or cervical region:*
  - With radiation below the gluteal fold or over the shoulder blade, but not below the knee or the elbow.
  - No neurological findings.

- *Pain in the lumbar, dorsal, or cervical region:*
  - With radiation to below the knee or the elbow.
  - No neurological findings.
- *Pain in the lumbar, dorsal, or cervical region:*
  - With radiation to below the knee or the elbow.
  - Additional neurological findings (paresis, asymmetry of reflexes, dermatome-related sensory or bowel or bladder disorders).

Selim et al (1998) selected a classification of lumbar pain syndromes into the following four degrees of severity:
- Only back pain (without radiation into one leg).
- Back pain radiating as far as the thigh.
- Back pain radiating to below the knee joint with negative straight leg raise test.
- Back pain radiating to below the knee joint with positive straight leg raise test.

The prognostic significance of radiating pain was studied on the basis of this classification. The intensity of the back pain, the degree of disability, and the number of sick days increased from group 1 to group 4. In addition, the validity of the classification was borne out by the fact that higher degrees of severity were associated with greater use of medication, CT and MRI, and surgery (ibid.).

McKenzie (1986, 1990) defined a classification with six degrees of severity (*Derangement 1–6*) for disk damage with injury of the posterior anulus fibrosus. He described anterior displacement of a disk as a rare exceptional case (*Derangement 7*).
- *Derangement 1:*
  - Central or symmetrical spinal pain.
  - Rarely radiating to the thigh or elbow.
  - Without spinal deformation.
- *Derangement 2:*
  - Central or symmetrical spinal pain.
  - Rarely radiating to the thigh or elbow.
  - Additional deformation by loss of lordosis.
- *Derangement 3:*
  - Unilateral spinal pain.
  - Radiating at most to above the knee or elbow.
  - Without spinal deformation.
- *Derangement 4:*
  - Unilateral radiating spinal pain.
  - Radiating at most to above the knee or elbow.
  - With additional lateral deformation (shift).
- *Derangement 5:*
  - Unilateral radiating spinal pain.
  - With or without pain in thigh or upper arm.

- Pain below the knee or elbow.
- Without spinal deformation.
- *Derangement 6:*
  - Unilateral radiating spinal pain.
  - With or without pain in thigh or upper arm.
  - Pain below the knee or elbow.
  - Additional lateral deformation (shift).

The three classifications described here take into account the location of the pain (centrally–radiating as far as the knee or elbow–radiating beyond the elbow or knee). In each case, a different additional finding is evaluated: neurological deficit, sign of nerve extension, deformation by loss of lordosis or shift.

All three additional findings are of equal significance and should be taken into account. Since they are not stereotypically associated with specific pain patterns, they must be evaluated independently of the pain classification.

If possible, such classifications are meant to facilitate the mapping of all clinically relevant syndromes, that is, those that occur with assured certainty. However, none of the classifications describes a set of pain symptoms with purely radiating pain, without spinal pain. Since this situation is often observed in patients with prolapsed disks, it should be taken into account in a classification. For this reason, the authors find the following classification of pain locations, used in current studies, useful:

- Central, symmetrical spinal pain, or symmetrical spinal pain.
- Pain radiating from the spine (usually only in one extremity), at most to the knee or elbow.
- Pain radiating from the spine (usually only in one extremity), to beyond the knee or elbow.
- Distal pain only, usually only in one extremity, without spinal pain.

In root compression syndromes of the upper cervical spine (C3–C5) and the upper lumbar spine (L1–L3), category 3 is not applicable since on the basis of the peripheral supply area of these roots, the maximal pain radiation of these roots can only reach as far as the knee or elbow joint. The additional significance of a change in pain location for mechanical diagnosis and therapy will be discussed in detail in Chapter 4 Diagnosis in Physical Therapy.

2.3.2   Pain Measurement

In the following, we will introduce various methods for the measurement of pain perception, but experimental stimulation methods based on the use of defined electrical, mechanical, thermal, or chemical stimuli will not be discussed.

Numerical Analog Scale (NAS)

A range of 0–10 has proven useful for this purpose. The patient ranks the intensity of their pain (0 = no pain, 10 = the greatest imaginable pain). This scale can be easily used without a special form. Usually patients are well able to express their pain numerically.

Visual Analog Scale (VAS)

In this visual scale, the patients themselves can record the intensity of pain they experience. Usually the scale is exactly 10 cm long and can be used with or without subdivisions.

Both scales are frequently used for clinical studies (Melzack 1987; Selim et al 1998; Brötz et al 2001, 2003; Brisby et al 2002; Brötz, Burkard, Weller 2010; Brötz, Maschke, Burkard et al 2010).

Other Measurement Methods

Changes in pain intensity can also be expressed in percentages. For this purpose, the patient reports their pain in comparison to the pain experienced at the beginning or the most intense period of the disease.

Sensory and emotional adjectives are also used to document pain. Roland and Morris (1983) provided a kind of diagrammatic thermometer, divided into six pain units: no pain, slight pain, moderate pain, fairly intense pain, very intense pain, and unbearable pain. The patient checks the pain level they experience at the moment.

McGill Pain Questionnaire

This questionnaire (Melzack 1987) consists of a table (**Table 2.4**) that gives the degree of severity corresponding to sensory and emotional adjectives that apply to the patient: not severe, slight, moderate, and intense.

2.3.3   Time Course of the Pain

The time period over which the pain has already existed, according to the patient's history, is of great significance for the selection of treatment strategies and the prognosis (Van Tulder et al 1997; Cherkin et al 1998; Waddell 1998). For this reason, in the evaluation of clinical studies, in which the development of painful diseases is investigated, the duration of the disease before the start of treatment must be taken into account.

There is no agreement in the literature about the period that should be considered *acute, subacute,* or *chronic.* Waddell (1998) described the following division as the traditional clinical pain classification, based on criteria for the patient's history:
- *Acute:* duration of the current episode of less than 3 months.
- *Recurrent:* duration of the current episode of less than 3 months but with similar previous episodes.
- *Chronic:* duration of the current episode of longer than 3 months.

The following division is common as well (Faas 1996; Van Tulder et al 1997; Selim et al 1998):
- *Acute:* duration of the current episode of less than 6 weeks.
- *Subacute:* duration of the current episode between 6 and 12 weeks.
- *Chronic:* duration of the current episode of longer than 12 weeks.

The Quebec Task Force recommends the following classification (McKenzie 1990):
- *Acute:* pain felt for less than 7 days.
- *Subacute:* pain felt for 7 days to 7 weeks.
- *Chronic:* pain felt for longer than 7 weeks.

Pain lasting for longer than 3 months without interruption is almost always considered to be chronic (Nachemson 1994; Faas 1996; Van Tulder et al 1997; Selim et al 1998; Waddell 1998).

In addition, documentation of pain over the course of 24 hours (how many hours, of what intensity) and the frequency of pain episodes in the course of the past weeks, months, and years is important in evaluating the course of disease (Maitland 1986, 1994; Selim et al 1998; Waddell 1998). In addition, the average and maximal pain intensity in a specified time period can be recorded.

2.3.4   Pain Physiology

Pain is a warning signal essential for life. If there is a danger of tissue damage or it has already occurred, or if there is inflammation, it immediately triggers a protective reaction. Once the protective mechanisms have set in, the pain normally decreases.

The nociceptors are terminal branchings of peripheral nerve dendrites that signal pain in response to mechanical, thermal, or chemical stimuli. They are present in great numbers throughout the entire body. Their afferent fibers are myelinated only slightly or not at all, and have a conduction speed of 1 to 15 m/sec. This means that they are significantly slower than sensory mechanoreceptors (60 m/sec).

The first afferent pain perception neuron is located in the dorsal ganglion of the dorsal nerve roots. Pain stimuli are transmitted in the dorsal horn of the spinal cord from the first to the second neuron. The majority of pain conductors cross to the contralateral side as they enter the spinal cord and run via cord and brainstem to the thalamus and finally, via a third neuron to the cerebral cortex. Presumably, after the information is processed in somatosensory cortical areas such as the postcentral gyrus and the parietal operculum, the pain and its location are consciously perceived.

Table 2.4 Sensory and emotional adjectives that grade the pain perception (selection from the McGill Pain Questionnaire).

Sensory adjectives	Emotional adjectives
Spreading, radiating, penetrating, piercing	Tiring, exhausting
Tight, numb, squeezing, drawing, tearing	Sickening, suffocation
Cool, cold, freezing	Fearful, frightful, terrifiying
	Punishing, grueling, cruel, vicious, killing

The emotional processing probably takes place in the limbic system. Information from the nociceptive tracts is forwarded in the spinal cord to neurons connected to somatomotor and autonomic reflex arcs. For instance, flight reflexes and sweat secretion are regulated here. Descending inhibitory tracts that control nociceptive stimuli in the dorsal horn and influence spinal autonomic and somatomotor reflex arcs run along the brainstem.

Pain episodes are often associated with inflammation that can have traumatic, infectious, or immunological causes. In their course, the stimulation threshold of the nociceptors is decreased by the release of hyperalgesic endogenous chemical mediators. These include, among other substances, peptides (e.g., substance P, neurokinin A, and calcitonin gene-related peptides) that originate in the nociceptors themselves, as well as prostaglandin, bradykinin, and proinflammatory cytokines (e.g., interleukin 1a and 1b).

In addition, there are pain-inhibiting systems in the peripheral tissue that exert a negative control over the sensitivity of this warning system. Interleukin 1, *corticotropin-releasing factor* (CRF) and stress induce the release of endorphins, for example from the pituitary gland and the hypothalamus. Endocannabinoids and γ-aminobutyric acid (GABA) ergic and catecholaminergic neuronal projection systems also inhibit the activity in pain processing systems.

In an inflammation, immune cells play not only the activating pacemaker role but also participate with a counter-regulatory effect in pain and inflammation relief. Not only inhibitory cytokines like interleukin 4, 10, and 13 are formed, but opioid peptides are also formed by the immune cells themselves (endorphins, enkephalins) that function as pain-inhibiting agonists on opioid receptors. In this way, opioids decrease the excitability of peripheral nociceptive nerve endings and thus the conduction of action potentials to the spinal cord (Rittner et al 2002).

2.3.5 Pathophysiology of Pain— Chronification

Damaging stimuli such as tissue injury and inflammation can change the function and structure of the peripheral and central nervous system. This can be seen from the fact that pain or oversensitivity to pain can remain, even when the damaging

mechanisms have been eliminated. Pain perception from the past flows into the pain felt at the moment.

A chronified pain syndrome, with changes on the neuronal level, must be distinguished from chronic pain that is simply defined on the basis of its duration for more than 3 months (Loeser 1999). The tendency to such chronification mechanisms differs among individuals (Loeser and Volinn 1991; Loeser 1999).

The nervous system is plastic. Even after a few minutes of nociceptive stimulation, the activity of the spinal nerve cells changes. With constant stimulation, structural changes in individual nerve cells can be triggered in a few days. New dendrites sprout, contributing to the creation of new connections between projection tracts.

These structural changes are found chiefly in the dorsal horn of the spinal cord and in the thalamus. They can cause hyperactivity in the tracts that process nociceptive stimuli or disturb descending inhibitory mechanisms. This gives rise to a pain experience independent of mechanical or chemical stimulation (Loeser 1985, 1991; Loeser and Volinn 1991; Diener and Leonhardt 1998; Tölle and Berthele 2001).

Hyperactivity of pain processing areas in the brain can be visualized with the use of imaging techniques such as functional MRI or positron emission tomography (PET). This hyperactivity presumably represents the result of multilayered sensory, cognitive, and emotional processing mechanisms.

These physiological mechanisms can be used to explain numerous clinical findings. In peripheral nerve or root lesions, the original circumscribed pain can expand over a larger area that can no longer be ascribed to the peripheral supply area of a single nerve or dermatome (Tölle and Berthele 2001). After repeated surgeries or injections, the pain can be intensified by summation of the stimuli and inflammatory reactions. Even after surgical elimination of the afferent neuron, the chronified pain persists if plastic changes in the dorsal horn or thalamus have resulted in so-called pain memory (Diener and Leonhardt 1998; Tölle and Berthele 2001).

Psychosocial aspects of the pain that are often associated with chronic pain conditions are discussed in Chapter 11 Psychosocial Risk Factors.

In order to avoid structural changes in the nervous system and thus the chronification of the pain, early efficient pain relief (ideally freedom from pain) should be aimed for, through adequate doses of pain medication, using peripherally and centrally acting analgesics. The information described here is also valuable for physical therapy. Rapid and lasting reduction of acute pain should be the primary goal (see Chapter 4 Diagnosis in Physical Therapy).

Varied activities, in which pain is blocked as much as possible, and behavioral therapy are promising treatments for chronified pain syndrome (Basler et al 1997; Pfingsten et al 1997; Diener and Leonhardt 1998; Loeser 1999). Such therapeutic approaches attempt to eliminate pain memory by means of afferent stimuli and positive experiences.

2.4 Functional Limitation: Objective and Subjective Aspects and Questionnaires

Functional limitations and associated disabilities should be considered apart from pain. In the first place, additional impairments such as pareses and sensory disorders can lead to functional limitations. Second, the patient's challenges in activities of daily living and their personality play a decisive role. A person who works at a desk and likes to read in their leisure time will not experience a disability from a sensory disorder in the sole of their foot. On the other hand, a roofer, who needs good balance, can become disabled by the same deficit.

Recovering the ability to work in the shortest time possible is the most important goal of therapy, not only from an economic point of view. Assessment of the ability to work can be facilitated by objectifiable and subjective factors as well as by questionnaires and made independent of the investigator's clinical impression.

The World Health Organization (WHO 1976) defines a disability as follows: "A disability is any impairment or lack (resulting from injury) of the ability to perform an activity in the form or to the extent that is considered normal."

This definition is problematic since it connects every case of disability with a health deficit. Yet, in the case of pain, this is not necessarily the case and with the methods presently available, is not objectifiable. Moreover, "normal" covers a broad range and is thus not appropriate for this kind of definition.

It is useful in determining the degree of functional limitation to take both objectifiable factors and the patient's subjective evaluation into account.

2.4.1 Objectifiable Factors

In studying the patient's disability, pain is only *one* factor among many. Although even the objectifiable factors always depend on the patient's cooperation, they still offer good information about the severity of the functional limitation. Since many closely related parameters are available, the actual disability can be easily evaluated.

Behavior that can be ascribed to psychosocial factors that can obscure the patient's actual functional capacity will be discussed in Chapter 11 Psychosocial Risk Factors. Some objective findings that only depend on the patient's cooperation slightly or not at all, such as neuroradiological findings and examination of the rate of nerve conduction and muscle activity, will be explained in Chapter 3 Medical Diagnosis and Treatment.

The following can be considered as potentially objectifiable parameters:
- Muscle function.
- Signs of nerve extension.
- Mobility.
- Spontaneous posture and movement patterns.

2.4.2 Subjective Factors and Questionnaires

Questioning patients about their disability concentrates more on limitation in activities of daily living than on pain. In this context, it is of the greatest interest which activities the patient can pursue and only of secondary interest whether they cause pain while pursuing them.

The most frequently used questionnaires (Deyo and Phillips 1996; Waddell 1998) are the *Roland-Morris Questionnaire* (Roland and Morris 1983; **Fig. 2.14**) and the *Oswestry Questionnaire* (Fairbank et al 1980; Fairbank and Pynsent 2000; **Fig. 2.15** showing modified questions). Both of these questionnaires were validated by studying whether their results agree with objectifiable clinical results. Moreover, their reliability was investigated in a test–retest procedure. According to these studies, both questionnaires, developed especially for patients with back pain, are valid and reliable (Fairbank et al 1980; Roland and Morris 1983). This also applies to the German translation of the Roland-Morris Questionnaire (Wiesinger et al 1999).

Roland-Morris Questionnaire

The questionnaire uses 24 statements of patients with back pain about their functional limitations. The respondents check the statements that apply to them. Each check mark receives 1 point and statements that are not checked receive a 0.

Questionnaire regarding functional limitation in cases of low back pain

Patient Name: _____

Date: _____

Disabled: ☐ Yes ☐ No (please check one)

Please read instructions: When your back hurts, you may find it difficult to do some of the things you normally do. The list of questions below contains statements by people who have suffered back pain. If you suffer from pain radiating into the buttocks or legs, please apply the questions about low back pain to your radiating pain. Mark only the sentences that describe you today.

☐ I stay at home most of the time because of my back.

☐ I change position frequently to try to get my back comfortable.

☐ I walk more slowly than usual because of my back.

☐ Because of my back, I am not doing any jobs that I usually do around the house.

☐ Because of my back, I use a handrail to get upstairs.

☐ Because of my back, I lie down to rest more often.

☐ Because of my back, I have to hold on to something to get out of an easy chair.

☐ Because of my back, I try to get other people to do things for me.

☐ I get dressed more slowly than usual because of my back.

☐ I only stand up for short periods of time because of my back.

☐ Because of my back, I try not to bend or kneel down.

☐ I find it difficult to get out of a chair because of my back.

☐ My back is painful almost all of the time.

☐ I find it difficult to turn over in bed because of my back.

☐ My appetite is not very good because of my back.

☐ I have trouble putting on my sock (or stockings) because of the pain in my back.

☐ I can only walk short distances because of my back pain.

☐ I sleep less well because of my back.

☐ Because of my back pain, I get dressed with the help of someone else.

☐ I sit down for most of the day because of my back.

☐ I avoid heavy jobs around the house because of my back.

☐ Because of back pain, I am more irritable and bad tempered with people than usual.

☐ Because of my back, I go upstairs more slowly than usual.

☐ I stay in bed most of the time because of my back.

Many thanks for your participation!

Instructions:

1. The patient is instructed to put a mark next to each appropriate statement.

2. The total number of marked statements are added by the clinician.

3. Clinical improvement over time can be graded based on the analysis of serial questionnaire scores. If, for example, at the beginning of treatment, a patient's score was 12 and, at the conclusion of treatment, their score was 2 (10 points of improvement), we would calculate an 83% ($10/12 \times 100$) improvement.

Fig. 2.14 Roland-Morris Questionnaire.

Questionnaire based on the Oswestry Questionnaire

Name: _____ Address: _____

Date: _____

Date of Birth: _____ Age: _____

Occupation: _____ Hospital No. _____

How long have you had back pain?   Years   Months Weeks

How long have you had leg pain?   Years   Months Weeks

Please read the following paragraph before answering:

This questionnaire was designed to give the physician information about how much your back pain affects your ability to perform the activities of your daily living. Please answer each section and in every section check only the *one* option that applies to you. You may find that in one section, two statements apply to you; nevertheless please check *only the one option that describes your problem most precisely.*

Section 1: Pain intensity

☐ I can tolerate my pain without needing pain medication.

☐ The pain is bad, but I can manage without pain medication.

☐ Pain medication takes away my pain completely.

☐ Pain medication relieves the pain to a certain extent.

☐ Pain medication does not relieve the pain very much.

☐ Pain medication has absolutely no effect and I don't take any.

Section 2: Independence (washing, dressing, etc.)

☐ Normally I can take care of myself without additional pain.

☐ Normally I can take care of myself but it causes me additional pain.

☐ The activities of daily living cause me pain, and I perform them slowly and carefully.

☐ I need a little help in daily activities, but I can do most of them alone.

☐ I need help every day for most activities of daily living.

☐ I don't dress myself, wash myself only with effort, and stay in bed.

Section 3: Lifting

☐ I can lift heavy objects without additional pain.

☐ I can lift heavy objects but it causes me additional pain.

☐ I cannot lift anything heavy from the floor because it is so painful, but if a heavy object is in a good place, like on a table, I can lift it.

☐ I can't lift anything heavy because it's so painful, but I can lift something light or moderately heavy that is well placed.

☐ I can only lift very light things.

☐ I cannot lift or carry anything at all.

Section 4: Walking

☐ Pain does not prevent me from walking as far as I like.

☐ Pain prevents me from walking more than 2 km.

☐ Pain prevents me from walking more than 1 km.

☐ Pain prevents me from walking more than 500 m.

☐ I can only walk with a cane or crutches.

☐ I am in bed most of the time and have to crawl to the toilet.

Section 5: Sitting

☐ I can sit on any chair as long as I want.

Fig. 2.15 Questionnaire based on the Oswestry Questionnaire.

▶ (continued)

☐ I can only sit on my favorite chair as long as I want.

☐ Pain prevents me from sitting for more than 1 hour.

☐ Pain prevents me from sitting for more than 30 minutes.

☐ Pain prevents me from sitting for more than 10 minutes.

☐ Pain prevents me from sitting at all.

Section 6: Standing

☐ I can stand as long as I want without additional pain.

☐ I can stand as long as I want but it causes me additional pain.

☐ Pain prevents me from standing for more than 1 hour.

☐ Pain prevents me from standing for more than 30 minutes.

☐ Pain prevents me from standing for more than 10 minutes.

☐ I have so much pain that I cannot stand at all.

Section 7: Sleeping

☐ Pain does not prevent me from sleeping well.

☐ I can sleep if I take some pills.

☐ Even when I take pills, I sleep less than 6 hours.

☐ Even when I take pills, I sleep less than 4 hours.

☐ Even when I take pills, I sleep less than 2 hours.

☐ I have so much pain that I cannot sleep at all.

Section 8: Sex life

☐ My sex life is normal and causes me no additional pain.

☐ My sex life is normal but causes me a little additional pain.

☐ My sex life is almost normal but very painful.

☐ My sex life is greatly limited by pain.

☐ Because of pain, I have almost no sex life.

☐ Because of pain, I have no sex life at all.

Section 9: Social life

☐ My social life is normal and causes me no additional pain.

☐ My social life is normal but increases my pain.

☐ Pain does not affect my social life decisively, except that it limits my physically more active interests, such as dancing.

☐ Pain limits my social life and I don't go out very often.

☐ Pain limits my social life to home.

☐ Because of pain, I have no social life.

Section 10: Travel

☐ I can travel all over without additional pain.

☐ I can lift travel all over but it causes me additional pain.

☐ The pain is bad, but nevertheless, I can manage to be on the road for 2 hours.

☐ Because of pain, I travel less than 1 hour at the most.

☐ Because of pain, I travel only for necessary errands and less than 30 minutes.

☐ Because of pain, I do not travel, except to the doctor and the hospital.

Comments:

_____

_____

Evaluation (not seen by patient)

Fig. 2.15 Questionnaire based on the Oswestry Questionnaire (*continued*)

▶ (continued)

The highest possible score for each section is 5. If the first statement is checked, the score is 0; the last statement is scored at 5 points. If all 10 sections are answered the total score is calculated as follows:

Example: $\dfrac{16\ \text{point target}}{50\ \text{(total possible point score)}} \times 100 = 32\%$

If a section is not filled out or cannot be evaluated, the overall score is calculated as follows:

Example: $\dfrac{16\ \text{point target}}{45\ \text{(total possible point score)}} \times 100 = 35.5\%$

Fig. 2.15 Questionnaire based on the Oswestry Questionnaire (*continued*)

Thus 0 points correspond to no disability and 24 points to the most severe disability.

For patients with a disk prolapse that causes no back pain but only leg pain, it can be difficult to interpret the statements in a way that gives equal importance to back pain and leg pain. Moreover, for patients who cannot walk because of their pain, it is not unambiguously clear whether or not they should check activities that are absolutely impossible at the moment.

Examples

- The fifth statement reads: "Because of my back, I use a handrail to get upstairs." A patient who is unable to climb stairs can only imagine that if they tried, they would certainly hold on. But if they do not check the statement, because it does not apply to them, the questionnaire gives a false, overly positive result.

For patients in this condition, an additional explanation is needed. Moreover, the questionnaire is inappropriate for patients whose problems originate in the thoracic and cervical spine.

Oswestry Questionnaire

This questionnaire contains statements about 10 activities of daily living that the patient evaluates in six categories. The first statement is always scored as 0 and indicates that there is no disability. The sixth statement is always scored as 5 and indicates that the disability is severe.

Using this questionnaire, it is possible to determine the severity of the disability also for patients whose problems originate in the thoracic and cervical spine.

2.5 Epidemiology and Risk Factors

Epidemiology deals with the distribution throughout the population of transmissible and nontransmissible diseases. The physical, chemical, psychological, and social interrelationships of disease causes and consequences for the population are studied.

Frequency of Disk Damage in the Population

Definition of Prevalence: The concept applies to the relative number of individuals within a population who suffer from a disease or symptom; it is expressed in percentages. Prevalence is the measure of frequency of a disease at any given point in time.

Definition of Incidence: This parameter gives the number of new cases of a certain disease within a specified period (usually 1 year) in a specified population.

Approximately 80 to 90% of the population of Western industrialized nations suffer acute back pain once in their lives. This results in significant healthcare costs and loss of work time (Loeser and Volinn 1991; Waddell 1998). The most frequent causes of these problems are structural, degenerative, or inflammatory spinal disease. In the Global Burden of Disease Study 2010, Vos et al (2012) showed that, worldwide, the most frequent cause of years lived with disability is back pain. This was the case in 2010 as it was in 1990.

Social Factors

There is a high correlation between the frequency of back and neck pain on the one hand and the nationalization and development of the healthcare system on the other (Loeser and Volinn 1991; Carragee et al 1996; Volinn 1997; Waddell 1998; Rasmussen et al 2001; Hee et al 2002). Both retrospective and modern epidemiological studies arrive at the conclusion that back pain has not become more frequent or more intense and that the pathophysiological basis has not changed (Leino 1994; Leboeuf-Yde and Lauritsen 1995).

By contrast, in a comparison of disability on grounds of back pain in Finland between 1978–79 and 1991–92, there was an increase of 340% (Leino 1994). This suggests that psychosocial factors have contributed to this epidemic rise. Dissatisfaction with one's job, low income, low social status, job loss, and dissatisfaction within the family seem to promote the occurrence of back and neck pain (Boos et al 1995; Pope et al 1998; Waddell 1998; Borenstein 1999; Thomas et al 1999; Lutza et al 2000; Hasenbring et al 2001).

On the other hand, the development of the healthcare system promotes the frequency of reported disability as a result of such problems. The decision to stay away from work depends on the social consequences of the decision (Waddell 1998).

Gender

Earlier, disability due to back pain was chiefly a problem for men, but in recent years this has changed (Waddell 1998). A Norwegian study of disability because of back pain showed a significantly higher 1-year incidence for women (2.7%) than for men (1.9%; Hagen and Thune 1998).

A study of pain showed that women suffer from pain more often, more intensely, and longer than men (Plass et al 2014 from the Years Lived with Disability Study 2010). The most frequent complaints were about head, neck, and shoulder pain (Chrubasik et al 1998). However, it seems that men suffer more frequently from radiologically confirmed disk prolapse than women (Weber 1983; Zitting et al 1998).

Age

Disk prolapses occur most frequently in middle age, between age 30 and 50 (Weber 1994; Von Strempel 2001). This is believed to be because before this middle period of life, at a younger age (under 30), the degenerative process is usually not so pronounced and that later, with increasing age (over 50), the elasticity of the disks decreases to such an extent that a shift of the nucleus pulposus occurs less frequently and the mechanical load on the spine is less in daily activities. In most studies of disk prolapse, the median age of affected patients was approximately 40 (Cherkin et al 1998; Ten Brinke et al 1999; Brötz et al 2001, 2003 ; Brötz, Maschke, Burkard et al 2010).

Occupation and Hobbies (Frequency of Bending, Sitting, Lifting)

In looking for predisposing factors for the development of disk damage in relation to activities of daily living, occupational and leisure activities must be given equal consideration. The mechanical loads that cause disk damage have already been listed (see 2.2 Pathophysiology of Disk Damage).

Many studies have identified frequent or constant flexion of the spine, flexion combined with turning, and heavy lifting as causative factors for disk damage (Adams and Hutton 1982, 1985; Adams et al 1996; Adams, Freeman et al 2000; Bogduk 2000). Sudden, unfamiliar physical stress can also lead to disk damage (Adams and Dolan 1997; Bogduk 2000). Various study results are available about the stress of pressure on the disk while sitting (Nachemson and Elfström 1970; Wilke et al 1999). It is possible that flexion of the spine associated with sitting, not pressure stress, is the cause of problems.

Clinically, it can be observed that patients with confirmed disk damage who suffer from back, neck, or radiating pain experience an increase of their symptoms when sitting or standing up. Conversely, these patients often experience a pronounced improvement in their problems as soon as they stop sitting.

Forward movement in all kinds of vehicles can be a cause of back and neck pain, as well as favoring lumbar and cervical disk prolapse. Responsibility for this is ascribed to vibrations of the whole body added to the already unfavorable sitting position. The vibrations tire the muscles so that they can only react slowly to a sudden exposure to a load. In this situation the spine is insufficiently protected against excessive pressure. Accordingly, truck drivers, for example, who carry heavy weights after driving are at greater risk of spinal damage than bus drivers. In addition, with vibration a greater decrease in the height of the disks was measured than in sitting without vibrations (Pope et al 1998).

There is controversy in the literature as to whether heavy physical labor leads to more back pain and disk damage; nevertheless, individuals doing heavy physical labor are more frequently on sick leave and disabled longer than individuals with a different kind of work (Waddell 1998).

Body Weight

Although the relationship between body weight and back pain has been investigated in many studies, it has not been proven that overweight causes back pain (Leboeuf-Yde 2000). The relationship between disk damage and body weight is also unclear. For instance, obese individuals tend to exhibit pronounced lumbar lordosis because of the weight of their abdomen. In addition, the volume of the abdomen limits the flexion capacity of the lumbar spine. On the basis of these facts, it is conceivable that corpulent individuals are less likely to suffer lumbar disk prolapse than slender individuals.

Difference in Leg Length

Differences in leg length are common. The average difference in leg length of a healthy population is 5.5 mm (Grundy and Roberts 1984). The exactitude of the measurements is controversial, but it is easy to see which leg is shorter and which is longer (Friberg et al 1988).

Ten Brinke et al (1999) found that in patients undergoing a lumbar disk operation the pain in almost 60% of affected patients radiated into the shorter leg. This relationship was only statistically significant in patients with a difference of 1 mm or more.

It is biomechanically conceivable that in standing and walking on the side of the longer leg, a side bias develops with an increase in pressure on the disk. This results in a shifting of the nucleus pulposus to the side of the shorter leg and possibly a disk prolapse to this side.

Smoking

Smoking is a risk factor for the development of back pain and disk prolapse (Waddell 1987; Scott et al 1999). It may even promote the degeneration of the disks by reduced metabolism, and smoker's cough leads to increased mechanical stress.

After a 2-hour exposure to cigarette smoke, diffusion of sulfates and oxygen in the disk was decreased by 50% in pigs (Holm and Nachemson 1988).

Physical Fitness

In a stress test of disks in young men who had died in accidents, tears in the anulus fibrosus occurred at greater stress in individuals who had been physically active in daily living than in less active individuals (Porter et al 1989).

In an epidemiological study of patients with lumbar and cervical disk prolapse, disk prolapse was less frequent in individuals who regularly worked out than in individuals who did not engage in any sport (Mundt et al 1993; Elfering et al 2002).

In an animal model, the metabolism of the disk (see 2.1.3 Intervertebral Disks) was activated by spinal movement (Holm and Nachemson 1983). These findings suggest that physical activity can guard against changes in the disk tissue.

Inheritance and Familial Clustering

In an investigation of close relatives of individuals operated on for disk prolapse, significantly more indications of degenerative disk changes were found than for individuals without cases of disk surgery in the family (Matsui et al 1998). MRI studies of the cervical and lumbar spine of 172 identical and 154 fraternal twins led to the hypothesis that hereditary factors are responsible for over 72% of radiologically confirmed degenerative changes in the spine (Sambrook et al 1999).

It is often impossible to associate neck and back pain with a single disease entity. This kind of pain is ascribed to muscles, tendons, ligaments, bones, joints, disks, and nerve roots. Approximately 85% of patients with back pain receive unspecific diagnoses. In 6% of patients, disk prolapse or spinal canal stenosis are diagnosed and in approximately 9% of patients, diagnoses such as aortic aneurysm, scoliosis, or tumor are established (Deyo and Phillips 1996).

For the rest, symptoms or syndrome names that do not lead to firm conclusions about the presumed cause are often used as diagnoses. Cervical and shoulder-neck syndrome or cervicalgia are diagnoses for disorders in the cervical spine; lumbago or sciatic pain in the lumbar spine; and polytopic pain syndrome or chronic pain syndrome can stand for pain throughout the whole body. Fibromyalgia and related disorders are another group of diagnostic classifiers related to polytopic pain that remain controversial entities.

In addition to structural changes in the spine, somatization of psychosocial problems is also often made responsible for pain, particularly back pain (see Chapter 11 Psychosocial Risk Factors; Waddell et al 1980; Waddell 1987, 1998; Boos et al 1995; Hildebrandt et al 1996; Hasenbring et al 1999). Thus many diagnoses remain hypothetical and thus disallow specific, disease-oriented treatment. Modern methods of imaging such as computed tomography (CT) and magnetic resonance imaging (MRI) have done little to change this situation.

CT is a computer-supported radiological procedure based on the fact that Roentgen radiation is attenuated to different degrees in different tissues. After summation of such attenuation effects, various tissues can be defined in a way that is far beyond the capacity of conventional radiological diagnosis.

MRI does not use Roentgen radiation; it is an electromagnetic process in which changes in the orientation of hydrogen nuclei in the body, produced by application of a strong external magnetic field, can be recorded by the emission of electromagnetic waves. In this process, various modes of imaging are used, designated, for instance, as T1- or T2-weighted sequences. T1-weighted sequences are used chiefly to detect the uptake of contrast medium. T2-weighted sequences are suited to determine changes in the water content of tissues or the internal structure of tissues.

In both CT and MRI, contrast medium can considerably improve the information content of the examination technique, for instance, by demonstrating inflammations or tumors.

Both procedures have created new dimensions for the diagnosis of most neurological diseases. However, the diagnostic validity is limited if no clear relationship between the clinical symptoms and the imaging findings can be established. CT and MRI of asymptomatic individuals may show forward-bulging disks and degenerative changes in the facet joints, especially in older patients.

In individuals older than 60 years with no history of symptoms in the lumbar spine, disk prolapses were found in 36% and spinal canal stenosis in 21% of patients (Boden et al 1990). A similar MRI study of 60 asymptomatic individuals aged from 20 to 50 years showed that disk protrusions and T2 signal changes in the intervertebral space were so common that they are not suitable as correlations of clinical problems. On the other hand, asymptomatic individuals of this age group only rarely had disk prolapse with sequestration and root compression or end plate changes (Weishaupt et al 1998).

In the cervical spine, young asymptomatic individuals often had changes, but only disk prolapses, not protrusions or degenerative changes, correlated with a history of neck pain (Siivola et al 2002). Thus in patients with neuroradiologically confirmed disk protrusion or degenerative changes of the facet joints it cannot always be assumed that these findings are also responsible for the symptoms. For this reason, careful elicitation of the medical history and conduct of the clinical neurological examination are of primary importance in investigating spinal syndromes. And finally, it seems likely that the potential of mechanical diagnosis by physical therapy methods is still underestimated and the methods underused.

3.1 Medical History and Clinical Examination

3.1.1 Medical History

Usually a carefully taken medical history makes it possible to establish the diagnosis of a disk prolapse and distinguish it from the most important differential diagnoses. If there is no prolapse, but just a protrusion or damage to the disk that causes fluctuating problems in the form of lumbago or sciatica, the diagnosis can be more difficult.

The onset of symptoms indicates whether the problem is a classic lifting trauma (e.g., carrying crates of bottles, moving house). Intensification of symptoms resembling sciatica, by coughing, sneezing, or straining, is a characteristic indication of a prolapsed disk. It is likely that this phenomenon is based on elevation of local intraspinal pressure caused by venous backflow. This can be explained by the elevated intra-abdominal pressure associated with these maneuvers. On the other hand, in many patients coughing, sneezing, or straining causes spinal flexion and thus intensification of the symptoms.

The different manifestations of the problems, depending on the body position and physical stress, provide valuable information about the cause. For example, patients with lumbar or cervical disk prolapse experience relief of symptoms when lying down or at rest, and patients with lumbar disk prolapse report an increase in pain when sitting or getting up from a seated position.

For patients with *spondylolisthesis* (formation of sliding vertebrae) in whom loosening and structural changes in the small vertebral joints cause one vertebra to slide over the other (usually the fourth over the fifth lumbar vertebral body or the fifth lumbar vertebral body over the first sacral vertebral body), sitting is usually the most uncomfortable position. In addition, they often describe an increase in symptoms when standing for a long while or walking downhill.

A clear dependence of sciatica on load, with almost complete absence of pain while reclining and increase of pain while sitting and particularly in standing and walking for a long time, is characteristic of lumbar *spinal canal stenosis*. The distance the patient is able to walk is limited by either pain or a feeling of weakness. Patients can experience pain relief while sitting or in standing and leaning forward on a railing but they prefer to lie down.

If pain is the leading complaint, notably distally in the legs, the differential diagnosis must consider peripheral *arterial occlusive disease*.

If the medical history neither provides information about the onset of symptoms nor reveals a significantly fluctuating course, the pain symptoms are more likely to be caused by *chronic degenerative disease* of the motor apparatus or a *tumor*. In case of undesired weight loss, generalized unwellness, fatigue, and a history of tumor, tumor recurrence must be excluded.

If the history includes a fall or another source of injury, a *fracture* must be ruled out radiographically. If, in addition to complaints in the cervical spine, head movement causes neurological symptoms like vertigo and, in individual cases, visual disorders, the cause can be a (rare) bony-mechanical *impairment of blood flow* in the vertebral or basilar artery caused by degenerative change in the cervical spine.

If the history is markedly inconsistent or not very precise, *psychosocial factors* that contribute to or support the pain symptoms should be considered. The longer pain symptoms exist, the more the patient's environment has adjusted to the situation, with potential primary and secondary gains, and therefore the consequences for the patient if their pain was successfully treated may be more challenging. For instance, if disability payments because of back pain are a possibility and this is exactly what the patient wants, no treatment of the symptoms that would justify such payments will be very successful.

3.1.2 Neurological Examination

All patients with back pain should undergo a complete neurological examination to rule out neurological deficits that the patients themselves have not become aware of.

The status of the cranial nerves is normal in patients with isolated disk problems. Analysis of standing and walking provides information about pain severity and about protective postures the patient may not know they have assumed. It can also provide differential diagnostic evidence of other diseases, for example hip problems.

In addition to examination of normal stance and walk, more complicated stance and walking tests are performed. Walking on tiptoes and on the heels, for instance, can reveal paresis of the muscles supplied by L5 and S1 (see Chapter 6 Lumbar Spine).

Tightrope walker's gait, in which the patient walks heel to toe in the straightest line possible, is a global test of coordination that may disclose polyneuropathy or cerebellar disease. In the *Romberg test*, the feet are placed side by side and parallel to each other and the eyes are closed. Insecurity in this test indicates a primary disorder of the sensory (afferent) information about the position in space of the lower extremities, caused, for example, by peripheral neuropathy in diabetes mellitus or chronic alcohol abuse.

In addition, cerebellar disease leads to a coordination disorder in standing and walking. In the *Unterberger step test* patients are asked to walk on the spot with their eyes closed. This test checks the function of cerebellum and inner ear. Both the Romberg and Unterberger tests should be normal in patients with disk disease, but movement can be so painfully limited that the patient refuses to carry out the test.

The *finger to floor distance test* is usually used in neurological examinations to determine spinal mobility. This distance, depending on age and other mechanical factors such as obesity, is usually zero or not more than 20 cm. The test is not supposed to trigger pain in the spine or the legs. Several other chapters (see Chapters 4–9) discuss the diagnostic significance of nerve extension signs.

The *straight leg raise (Lasègue)* and the *prone knee bend (reverse Lasègue) tests* are performed in recumbent position (see Chapter 6 Lumbar Spine). These maneuvers are also meant to test free mobility in the hip joint, in order to rule out a hip problem. A differential diagnostic indicator in cases of radiating hip and leg pain is a painful *sacroiliac joint*. Since none of the medical or physical therapy diagnostic examination methods can provide a reliable diagnosis of pain syndrome of the sacroiliac joint (Dreyfuss et al 1996), a diagnostic pain blockade of the joint may have to be performed for clarification.

Strength Test

The *gross strength test* in the segment-indicating muscles has special significance for the neurological examination of patients with suspected disk disease (see Chapters 2, 6, and 8). Strength is determined according to the classification in **Table 3.1**.

Table 3.1 Classification of the strength grades

Strength grade	Definition
5	(Five times) full range of motion against strong resistance over the trajectory and at the end
4	Full range of motion against moderate resistance over the trajectory and at the end
3	Full range of motion against gravity
2	Full range of motion without gravity
1	Visible or palpable muscle tension without motion
0	No visible or palpable muscle tension

In case of doubt, especially with lower-grade paresis, it is important to document what the patient could and could not do. Subdivisions such as pareses of strength 5–, 4–, or 4+ are not standardized and are less helpful than the precise documentation of the deficit; that is, recording the extent to which the patient exhibited a deficit when performing a given movement.

Compression of a nerve root leads to peripheral paresis marked by flaccid muscle tone, reduction or loss of proprioceptive reflexes, and, in the long term, by muscular atrophy. A thoracic or cervical disk prolapse can result not only in a peripheral paralysis at the level of the affected segment but also in spinal cord transection symptoms caused by median compression. The latter case is a central paresis, usually symmetrical, of both legs, which is marked by elevated muscle tone, increased reflexes below the level of the lesion, and development of pathological reflexes (pyramidal tract signs) after the acute phase has subsided.

Sensory Tests

These tests usually examine the following senses:
- Touch.
- Pain and temperature.
- Sense of position.
- Perception of vibration (pallesthesia).

Test of the Sense of Touch (Esthesia)

In this test, the skin is touched with a defined stimulus (usually the examiner's own fingertip) at the extremities, with direct side-by-side comparison. The sensitivity to touch can be reduced (*hypesthesia*) or absent (*anesthesia*). Sometimes spontaneous or unpleasant paresthesia is reported (*dysesthesia*). *Allodynia* is the experiencing of pain from stimuli that normally do not trigger pain.

Test of Pain and Temperature Perception

Pain perception is tested with a sharp object (e.g., a straightened paper clip), with comparison of sides.

There are specific testing devices for investigation of temperature perception, with the qualities hot and cold. They are not needed in the clinical routine because pain testing is usually sufficient.

Sensitivity to touch and pain or temperature is tested from distal to proximal and then on specific skin areas that the patient says have sensory abnormalities. Such an area is defined by finding the boundaries from inside toward the outside and from outside to inside in all directions. It should be documented on a body map on paper.

Test of Sense of Position and Vibration Perception

Sense of position (*kinesthesia*) and perception of vibration largely engage the same structures of the nervous system. The test of vibration perception is more sensitive; that is, patients with an intact sense of position can certainly exhibit deficits in the test of vibration perception (*pallesthesia*) but not vice versa, at least not in the case of peripheral lesions of the nervous system. The examination begins distally at the toe or fingertip joints.

The sense of position is tested by changing the position of the joint (upward or downward) and the patient must be able to recognize the change without being able to see it. If the sense of position is intact, even minimal changes in joint position are perceived.

Pallesthesia is tested using a tuning fork divided into eighths, with which it is possible to test at which intensity of oscillation the vibration is still perceived. A young, healthy subject achieves 8/8; in patients older than 60 years pallesthesia is often reduced without signs of disease. The loss of vibration perception is called *pallanesthesia*.

Interpretation of Findings

Symmetrical sensory disorders that are more pronounced distally and begin at the toes and feet are found chiefly in patients with polyneuropathies. In disk prolapses with root compression syndrome, on the other hand, there are typically circumscribed areas with reduced sensitivity (touch, pain, temperature) that are associated with a specific dermatome, whereas sense of position and vibration perception are intact.

A particular syndrome associated with disk pain is the often symmetrical sensory disorder of the sacral segments that is called *saddle anesthesia* because of its topography (loss of sensation restricted to the area of the buttocks, perineum, and inner surfaces of the thighs). Saddle anesthesia is an important symptom that points to compression of the cauda equina, chiefly as the result of a large lumbar disk prolapse and thus requires immediate further examination and intervention.

In cord compression due to cervical or thoracic disk prolapse, there can be symmetrical impairment of all sensory qualities below the level of the lesion. These usually begin distally and do not always rise to the level of the lesion. Since with large medial disk prolapses there is a danger of impairment to bladder and bowel function, such disorders should be specifically explored when taking the history. Since urinary retention appears earlier in such patients, as an acute symptom, and is much more frequent than urinary incontinence but is often unnoticed, it is important to determine—using a single-use catheterization or sonography—after a voluntary attempt at maximal bladder emptying, whether complete bladder emptying, with no residual urine, is possible. Healthy individuals do not exhibit residual urine; amounts greater than 100 ml cannot be tolerated long term.

Rectal function can be tested as part of the clinical-neurological examination by examining the anal sphincter tone and by triggering the anal reflex. Since the strength of the anal reflex is variable, testing it is less helpful than checking the sphincter tone. In case of doubt, the patient's report of bowel emptying is decisive.

3.2   Technical Diagnostic Procedures

3.2.1   Electromyography (EMG)

Additional electrophysiological diagnosis plays a subordinate role to medical history, clinical-neurological examination, and imaging procedures in diagnosing disk prolapses. In electromyography, a thin needle electrode introduced into the muscle is used to measure the electrical activity of the muscle at rest and during voluntary tension. Introducing the needle into the muscle may be painful. After the examination, pain may be felt in the tested muscle for 1 to 2 days. Resting healthy muscle shows no electrical activity. After a certain degree of damage of motor nerves or nerve roots, pathological spontaneous activity can be demonstrated as florid *denervation*. Since this pathological pattern only develops when there has been structural degeneration of axons spreading distally, the electromyogram will not show this result until approximately 10 days after appearance of paresis. For this reason, electromyography is not suitable for evaluation of acutely occurring paresis, yet it can be useful in evaluating the extent of previous chronic damage and for distinguishing between motor fiber loss and pure dysfunction (conduction block) or between nerve root lesions and damage to peripheral nerves. If neuropathy has existed for some time, the electromyogram shows changes that follow the distribution pattern of peripheral nerves and correspond to changes on electroneurography.

3.2.2   Electroneurography (ENG)

The differential diagnosis of root compression with disk prolapse versus polyneuropathy is obtained more easily with electroneurography than with electromyography.

Electroneurography examines the conduction velocity of the nerves and the amplitude of the sensory nerve action potentials or the compound muscle action potentials upon peripheral nerve stimulation. The peripheral nerve is electrically stimulated at suitable points on the skin and the response to the stimulus is measured at another point along the course of the same nerve or at the target muscle.

Reduction of nerve conduction velocity is found in demyelinating neuropathy because the myelin sheaths are responsible for the high conduction speed of peripheral myelinated axons. As long as the integrity of the axons is not impaired, the amplitude of the nerve action potential remains normal. On the other hand, if neuropathy primarily involves the axons, the sensory nerve or muscle compound action potential are reduced without a change in nerve conduction velocity.

In acute root compression, the conduction speed and amplitude of the nerves that this root supplies are unchanged because the stimulation and measurement in this method take place in the periphery, considerably distal to the nerve root. However, if axons are destroyed by chronic root compression, the motor amplitude can in fact be reduced. In this case, the sensory amplitudes are usually not affected because the first nerve cell bodies of the sensory (afferent) tract lie in the extraforaminal dorsal root ganglia. Because of this position, the afferent fibers that are measured in neurography are not affected by compression.

Neurography is particularly valuable if, in spite of careful clinical examination, it remains open whether (chiefly) paresis of the great toe is caused by a peripheral lesion of the peroneal nerve or compression of the L5 root.

3.2.3   Evoked Potentials (EPs)

There are *motor-evoked potentials* (MEPs) and *sensory evoked potentials* (SEPs). Peripheral conduction time is usually determined by means of an F-wave examination that, with peripheral stimulation, gives the retrograde conduction time to the spinal cord and back to the periphery. The central motor conduction time can be measured with magnetic stimulation (MEPs): a stimulus is applied with a magnetic coil over the motor cortex from the outside, and conduction time can be recorded distally at the hand or foot. Subtraction of the peripheral motor conduction time gives the time for the impulse to travel from the motor cortex to the anterior horn motor cells of the spinal cord. This time can be longer if a cervical or thoracic disk prolapse is causing a spinal cord compression.

In a similar way, the measurement of *sensory-evoked potentials* (SEPs) with peripheral stimulation over the tibial, ulnar, or median nerves can be used, with fractionated recording before the impulse enters the spinal cord, at various levels of the spinal cord, and at the cerebral cortex, to demonstrate a conduction delay in the sensory tracts when the spinal cord is compressed.

3.2.4 Examination of the Cerebrospinal Fluid (CSF)

The cerebrospinal fluid surrounds the brain and spinal cord and protects them from mechanical damage during movement or external force. The *blood–cerebrospinal fluid barrier* and the *blood–brain barrier* are special cellular or tissue layers that prevent uncontrolled movement of protein and also small molecules (e.g., medications) from the blood into the brain and the cerebrospinal fluid.

In patients with disk disorders, examination of the cerebrospinal fluid usually yields normal results or an elevation of the protein concentration, which can be ascribed to disturbance of the blood–cerebrospinal fluid barrier in the area of the root compression. The cell count is normal. This examination is routine when myelography (see 3.2.5 Radiological Diagnosis—Myelography) is to be performed for diagnostic workup or as part of preoperative preparation.

The examination of the cerebrospinal fluid is recommended if clinical and imaging findings are not in agreement or if clinical examination points to the involvement of several affected roots. Such patients may be suffering from polyradiculitis, for example if they suffer from borreliosis, and the analysis may reveal strongly elevated protein levels and increased inflammatory cell counts or both.

3.2.5 Radiological Diagnosis

Conventional Roentgen Diagnosis

Conventional radiographic images of the spine have lost importance since the introduction of CT and MRI, which serve to confirm injuries, instabilities, and degenerative arthritic changes in the spine. Functional images of the lumbar spine in flexion and extension are useful to confirm spondylolisthesis, whereas images of the cervical spine

(**Fig. 3.1a, b**) are used to confirm instability, for instance after whiplash trauma. A disk prolapse cannot be diagnosed with conventional radiographic imaging.

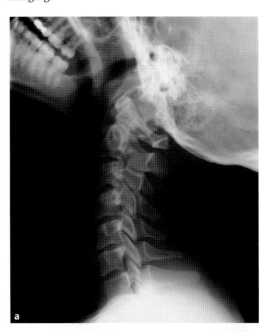

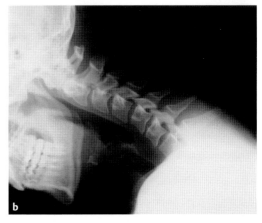

Fig. 3.1 Functional imaging of a 25-year-old patient with flexion trauma acquired while jumping on a trampoline. Conventional radiographs show a distinct limitation of motion but a gross disk prolapse was only diagnosed by magnetic resonance imaging (see also Fig. 3.4). **(a)** Extension, clear motion deficit in reclining. **(b)** Flexion, straightening of the lower cervical spine and angular kyphosis at intervertebral level C3–C4; no sign of instability. (Images provided courtesy of Dr. W. Küker, Department of Neuroradiology, University Hospital Tübingen, Germany.)

Computed Tomography

CT is a rapidly accessible cross-sectional imaging procedure that presents disk prolapses very clearly in axial sections (**Fig. 3.2a, b**; **Fig. 3.3**). A prerequisite for its useful application is the definition of the levels to be examined on the basis of the clinical examination, since compared to MRI (see below) it has the drawback that images in the sagittal plane are not easily acquired.

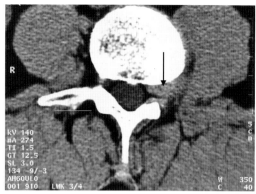

Fig. 3.3 Imaging of a 59-year-old patient with acute root compression L3 left, grade 3 adductor paresis and sensory loss in dermatome L3. CT shows a large disk prolapse into the intervertebral foramen and a disk prolapse extending beyond it at intervertebral level L3–L4 left. (Images provided courtesy of Dr. W. Küker, Dept. of Neuroradiology, Univ. Hospital Tübingen, Germany.)

When focused on bony structures, CT produces particularly good resolution of neuroforaminal narrowing.

Finally, the procedure is used in association with myelography (see below) (myelo-CT) to produce images of spinal cord or nerve root compression after contrast medium has been introduced into the subarachnoid space.

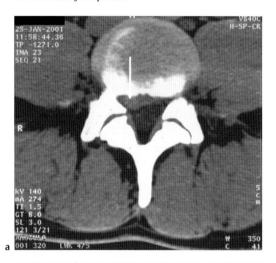

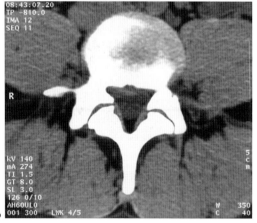

Fig. 3.2 Imaging findings in a 37-year-old patient with compression of the right L5 root, grade 2 weakness of the dorsal foot flexor, and grade 4 weakness of the toe flexor. **(a)** CT shows a right caudally sequestered disk prolapse at intervertebral level L4–L5 with compression of the L5 root in the lateral recessus. **(b)** Finding after 10 months with complete resolution of symptoms. (Images provided courtesy of Dr. W. Küker, Dept. of Neuroradiology, Univ. Hospital, Tübingen, Germany.)

MRI

This procedure has the advantage of clearer visualization of details and pathological changes in all planes (**Fig. 3.4a, b**; **Fig. 3.5a, b**). Disadvantages are the higher costs and a tendency for artifacts (errors in the perception or representation of visual information) to appear in the analysis of bony structures, for instance in the examination of foraminal narrowing. Further limitations include the inability to examine the majority of patients with cardiac pacemakers and metallic implants.

Myelography

Contrast medium is introduced into the subarachnoid space (cerebrospinal fluid space) by lumbar puncture. As soon as the contrast medium is distributed throughout the subarachnoid space, the compression of the dural sac or the

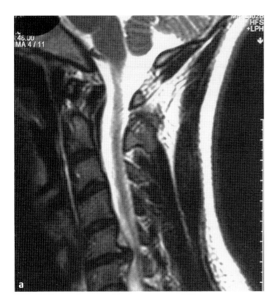
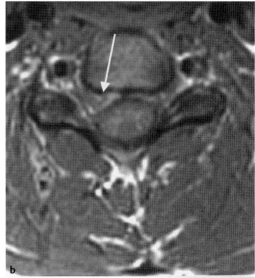

Fig. 3.4 (a, b) The sagittal and axial MRI of the 25-year-old patient (see also Fig. 3.1a, b) show a large disk prolapse at intervertebral level C5–C6 right with foraminal components. The patient had sensory loss and pain in dermatome C6. (Images provided courtesy of Dr. W. Küker, Dept. of Neuroradiology, Univ. Hospital Tübingen, Germany.)

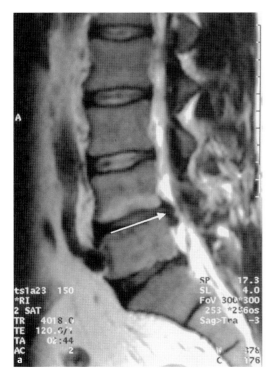
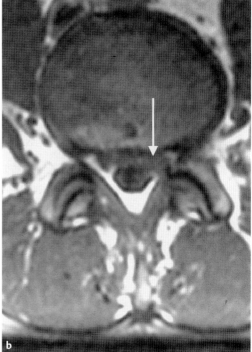

Fig. 3.5 (a, b) Imaging of a 41-year-old patient with compression of root L5 left, paresis of grade 3, and pain in the left L5 dermatome. The sagittal and axial MRI show a disk prolapse extending into the recessus at the intervertebral level L4–L5 left. (Images provided courtesy of Dr. W. Küker, Dept. of Neuroradiology, Univ. Hospital Tübingen, Germany.)

nerve roots running through the dural sac can be visualized. The specific advantage of myelography is the possibility of conducting a dynamic examination of the patient not only reclining (as in CT and MRI) but also in seated or standing position. This characteristic determines the most important indications for conducting this examination, such as suspicion of instability of the spine, spondylolisthesis, and spinal canal stenoses that may not be readily detected in recumbent position.

If a disk prolapse can be shown by CT or MRI and there is a clinical monoradicular syndrome relevant to this finding, most surgeons do not require preoperative myelography. However, the proce-dure is helpful if the symptoms of disk disease are clearly position dependent (since then there may be a mobile component), if more than one root is affected clinically, or if the clinical and neuroradiological findings do not correspond.

As already mentioned, supplementary computed tomography (myelo-CT) can be performed after myelography (**Fig. 3.6a, b**). Finally, the indication for myelography should be checked if a cerebrospinal fluid examination is required for differential diagnosis, especially if there is suspicion of inflammatory neuropathy (e.g., neuroborreliosis) or a malignancy with tumor cell dissemination within the subarachnoid space.

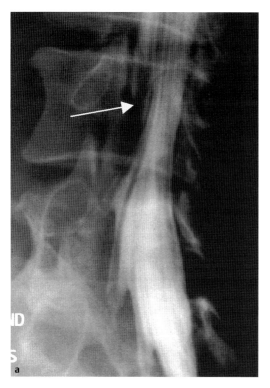
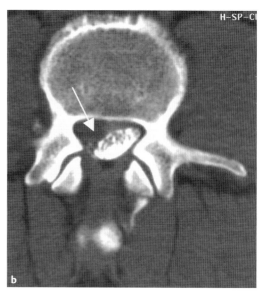

Fig. 3.6 Imaging findings in a 47-year-old patient with compression of the right L4 root, grade 4 paresis of the knee extensor, and sensory disorders, as well as pain in dermatome L4 right. **(a)** Lumbar myelography, lateral oblique view. After introduction of 20 ml contrast medium into the dural tube by means of a lumbar puncture at intervertebral level L3–L4, the lower portion of the dural tube is easily recognized in the radiograph. The spinal cord ends at vertebral levels T12–L1. Thus the caudal fibers can be seen as dark structures that emerge through the intervertebral foramina and are there surrounded by the root sac, filled with cerebrospinal fluid and thus visualized thanks to contrast. At the level of L4, there is an open space, resulting from a disk prolapse, which constricts the dural tube and compresses the L4 nerve root (arrow). **(b)** CT after myelography at L4. The dural tube contains contrast medium and is light; the caudal fibers can be recognized as rounded structures. The disk prolapse (arrow) pushes the dural tube to the left and back. (Images provided courtesy of Dr. W. Küker, Dept. of Neuroradiology, Univ. Hospital, Tübingen, Germany.)

Diskography

Diskography is an examination method that is rarely used in neurological and neurosurgical hospitals but does find application in some orthopaedic hospitals. In this process, contrast medium is introduced into the affected disk. Diskography offers the possibility of visualizing the internal structure of the disk. The procedure is not essential for clinical routine. However, it could be suitable for verifying the pathogenic hypotheses as to the cause of clinical symptoms in disk disease.

During the examination the disk is tested for pain sensitivity. Injection of the contrast medium raises the pressure in the nucleus pulposus. Some authors believe that pain is only elicited when the pressure stress and the chemical stimulus extend to the outer third of the anulus fibrosus (Moneta et al 1994), but this only happens if the inner fibers of the anulus fibrosus are damaged. In a healthy disk, its inner, denser, uninnervated layers prevent an expansion of chemical or mechanical stimuli out to its exterior layers.

3.2.6   Pharmacological Therapy

The objective of pharmacological therapy of patients with disk prolapses is first and foremost the reduction of pain, inflammation, and muscle tension. The standard pharmacological therapy in the acute phase is treatment with nonsteroidal anti-inflammatory drugs (NSAIDs), for example, diclofenac, and muscle relaxants, including benzodiazepines like diazepam (Deyo and Phillips 1996; Van Tulder et al 1997; Cherkin et al 1998). The usefulness of therapy with muscle relaxants has not been confirmed by controlled studies.

There are a few retrospective and uncontrolled studies of medication for patients with nonspecific back pain (Van Tulder et al 1997; Cherkin et al 1998). The authors concluded that the disease pictures had to be more closely defined and the usefulness of the various approaches to pharmacological therapy had to be evaluated.

NSAIDs are useful in the treatment of acute disk disease because they relieve pain and suppress inflammatory processes that are associated with root compression and contribute to swelling. In addition, the field of pain therapy has accepted the hypothesis that adequate early analgesia is important for the prevention of chronification of pain (Zenz and Jurna 2001). Supplementary administration of opiates is rarely necessary; if they are used, it is only for a few days. A systematic review showed that paracetamol is ineffective for reducing pain and disability in individuals with low back pain (Machado et al 2015).

Some patients experiencing pain respond well to supplementary oral administration of low corticosteroid doses. Short-term administration of these drugs over a period of a few days (e.g., 100 mg of methylprednisolone daily) is appropriate for the control of postoperative, frequently night-time pain that is most likely the result of postoperative scar formation. The frequently used local injections of steroids near the spinal canal are not necessary.

The controversial discussion of the pathogenesis of locally elevated muscle tone and the usefulness of treating it with medication is presented in Chapter 2 General Principles. We have reported that physical therapy treatment of lumbar disk prolapse following the strategies outlined here (Brötz et al 2003) is probably more successful without than with concurrent administration of muscle relaxants (Brötz et al 2010). In the chronic phase, pharmaceutical treatment tends toward drugs used in the treatment of depression and epilepsy. Orientation is provided by the overview presented in **Table 3.2**.

Table 3.2 Pharmacological treatment

Drug group	Drug	Dosage (single dose, mg)	Doses per day	Duration of treat-ment	Indication/ Disease phase	Contraindications	Side-effects
Nonopioid analgesics							
Nonsteroidal anti-inflammatory drugs (NSAIDs)	Acetylsalicylic acid	500–1,000	2–3	Days	Acute	Gastrointestinal ulcers, asthma	Gastrointestinal symptoms, increased bleeding
	Diclofenac	25–50	2–3	Days	Acute	Gastrointestinal ulcers	Gastrointestinal symptoms
	Ibuprofen	200–800	2–3	Days	Acute		
	Naproxen	250–500	2	Days	Acute		
	Indomethacin	50–75	2–3	Days		Kidney damage	Kidney damage, gastrointestinal symp-toms
Other	Paracetamol	500–1,000	2–4	Days	Acute	Kidney damage	
Opioids							
	Morphine	20–100/day	2–3	Days	Acute		Nausea, constipation, urinary retention
	Fentanyl	25–100 µg/h		Days	Acute		Nausea, constipation, urinary retention
	Buprenorphine	0.2–1.2/day	2–3	Days	Acute		Nausea, constipation, urinary retention
	Tramadol	50–100	2–4	Days	Acute		Nausea, constipation, urinary retention

▲ (continued)

Table 3.2 Pharmacological treatment (*continued*)

Drug group	Drug	Dosage (single dose, mg)	Doses per day	Duration of treatment	Indication/ Disease phase	Contraindications	Side-effects
Coanalgesics							
Corticosteroids	Methylprednisolone	25–50	2–4	Days	Acute	Gastrointestinal ulcers, diabetes mellitus	Gastrointestinal symptoms, osteoporosis, depression, many others
Antidepressants	Amitriptyline	25–75	1–3	Weeks–months	Chronic	Arrhythmia Voiding disorders Glaucoma	Vertigo, weight gain
	Clomipramine	25–75	1–3	Weeks–months	Chronic	Heart arrhythmia Bladder emptying disorders Glaucoma	Vertigo, weight gain
Anticonvulsants	Gabapentin	600–900	2–4	Weeks–months	Chronic		
	Pregabalin	75–150	2–3	Weeks–months	Chronic		
	Carbamazepine	200–400	2–4	Weeks–months	Chronic		Vertigo, unsteady gait, allergy

3.2.7 Surgical vs. Conservative Treatment

Establishing an indication for surgical treatment of lumbar, thoracic, and cervical disk prolapse is a controversial topic that can only be presented here as a broad overview. There are no controlled studies comparing surgical and conservative treatments performed according to modern quality criteria. In any case, there should be an effort toward interdisciplinary agreement (e.g., as part of a joint case conference) in which the surgical disciplines of neurosurgery and orthopaedics as well as neuroradiology as a diagnostic and neurology as a diagnostic and therapeutic discipline are represented.

The following rules of thumb for establishing an indication can be formulated and will find relatively broad agreement:

- High-grade pareses developing within less than 24 hours as well as bladder or bowel dysfunction are an urgent indication for surgery.
- The longer a neurological deficit exists, the lower is the probability that it will resolve as a result of surgery.
- The failure of conservative treatment, even in the absence of neurological deficits (isolated pain syndrome), is a relative indication for surgery.

- In all indications for surgery, there must be a careful investigation of whether the symptoms or neurological deficits can indeed be ascribed to the diagnosis indicated by imaging.

Finally, it must be taken into account that the success of surgical treatment depends on both the surgeon's expertise and on the surgical technique and that these factors make cohort comparison of patients who received surgery and those who did not difficult unless a well-defined prospective treatment protocol was followed. Thus the surgical procedure is competing not only with a variety of conservative treatment procedures but also with a variety of surgical (especially allegedly minimally invasive) procedures that may not always be appropriate for patients with neurologically urgent indications for surgery.

Postoperative pain syndrome caused by scar formation and resulting persistent root pain is among possible complications, particularly in surgery for prolapsed lumbar disks. This complication has probably become less frequent since the introduction of microsurgical techniques: local bleeding contributed significantly to excessive postoperative scarring while microscopic techniques permit less traumatic surgery.

According to McKenzie (1981, 1986, 1990), McKenzie and May (2003), and Maitland (1986, 1994), determining the most appropriate physical therapy for patients with back and neck pain requires a mechanical diagnosis that notes changes in symptoms caused by movement. On the basis of the disease history, the visible, external signs (such as incorrect spinal posture or limping), and the reaction of symptoms to repeated end-range spinal movements, a *working hypothesis* about the cause of symptoms can be established and specific therapy can be initiated.

Findings are documented before and after every treatment session, allowing the therapist and the patient to monitor progress. The diagnosis and the treatment that it calls for are regularly reviewed. After five treatment sessions, symptoms should be seen to improve. If this is not the case, additional diagnostic workup must be discussed with the treating physician and, if necessary, the treatment strategy must be changed.

For instance, chronified pain syndrome or psychosomatic disorders cannot readily be treated by mechanical therapy based on symptoms and should be treated differently from primarily mechanical disorders (Hildebrandt et al 1996; Waddell 1998; Hasenbring et al 1999; Zieglgänsberger 2002).

Diagnosis and documentation applicable to all sections of the spine are explained in this chapter. The special characteristics of the lumbar, thoracic, and cervical spine as well as the diagnostic assessment forms are found in the corresponding Chapters 6 to 8.

4.1   Medical History

The history of the disease and the patient's occupation lead to conclusions about the cause of the symptoms and the possible chances of healing. Disk prolapses occur most frequently between the ages of 25 and 55. The patient's answers to questions about *occupation* and *hobbies* and the associated postures and movements provide valuable information about the everyday stress on the spine.

Typical *trigger factors* for disk prolapses are extended periods of sitting, driving, stooping, turning, lifting, pulling, and pushing. The patient is not always aware of a trigger. Symptoms that appear suddenly can be assumed to have mechanical causes. If the patient reports a stealthy onset of the disease, a nonmechanical cause for the symptoms must be considered (see Chapter 3 Medical Diagnosis and Treatment).

The duration of the *disability* period can give some indication of the prognosis. The longer a patient has been disabled with back pain, the lower the probability that they will be able to return to daily work.

> **Examples**
>
> - In a UK study, the likelihood of returning to the original workplace after 6 months of disability fell to 50% (Waddell 1996).
> - In a study in Norway, 42% of patients who were disabled after 6 months had still not returned to their workplaces after 12 months (Hagen and Thune 1998).

Duration of the current episode is commonly defined as the time since the patient has been suffering uninterruptedly (with no single pain-free day) from the symptoms that prompted them to come for physical therapy. On the basis of this duration, the symptoms can be classified as acute (up to 6 weeks), subacute (6–12 weeks) or chronic (longer than 12 weeks; see Chapter 2 General Principles). Evaluation of the goals achieved during therapy and the prognosis for expected duration of therapy depend on the duration of the complaint. Usually, the longer the disease persists, the more difficult and lengthy the treatment and the smaller the increments toward healing.

The achievable end result is also better in patients with acute symptoms. A paresis that has only lasted for a few days often regresses with successful treatment, but if it has persisted unchanged for 1 year it is unlikely to resolve. The fact that the correlation between duration of the problem and probability of improvement applies both to physical therapy interventions and to the spontaneous course of such problems makes it difficult to determine whether the cause of improvement in symptoms is physical therapy or the passage of time. This is also true for surgical interventions.

The *development* of symptoms and *previous therapy* provide information as to whether the healing process has already begun. If the patient reports that their symptoms are steadily getting worse, the possibility of neoplastic disease must be considered. Such deterioration in patients with disk damage can also be promoted by inappropriate conduct such as lifting heavy objects, gardening, sitting for long periods, or incorrect treatment strategies.

The physical therapist must inquire about the type, duration, and effect of *medications* the patient has taken. Some conclusions about the nature of the disease can be based on the efficacy of medications. For instance, if anti-inflammatory agents and corticosteroids have relieved pain, the disease is presumably associated with an inflammatory process. Even prolapsed disks are frequently associated with an inflammatory reaction. On the other hand, corticosteroid treatment also provides symptomatic relief for many tumor patients.

The *previous history* and the course of earlier episodes provide valuable information for the assessment of a current episode. Problems that occur and disappear with changing physical stress indicate a mechanical event. Symptoms that set in slowly and without apparent cause can also have other, nonmechanical, causes.

Usually disk damage has a history that has lasted for years. Patients often complain of back and neck pain that they have suffered at more or less regular intervals. The patient must be asked about the effects of the treatment administered in each case. This information may be able to influence treatment planning. Inefficacious and damaging measures must be discontinued or avoided, respectively. The goal of treatment should be to enable the patient to avoid recurrence of symptoms.

Patients are asked when they feel better and when they feel worse. The questioning should take into account different times of day and specific postures and activities. Symptoms that are not made better or worse by any particular movement are presumably not of a mechanical nature.

Individuals who suffer disk damage usually experience increased pain in the morning, at rest, while sitting, or stooping. To determine the susceptibility of the symptoms to mechanical factors (*irritability* according to Maitland 1994), the patient is asked how long it takes in a specific position or movement for the symptoms to intensify, and how long it takes until these symptoms return to their original level under the influence of a better position or movement.

An increase in pain caused by *coughing, sneezing,* or *straining* is considered to be evidence of a disk prolapse. It is not clear whether the associated increase in intra-abdominal pressure also increases the pressure in the disk or whether flexion of the spine increases mechanical irritation.

A history of *trauma* or an *operation* can be associated with the current symptoms and constitutes a contraindication for mechanical examination and treatment.

Patients with disk damage move less but they usually have a normal appetite; consequently they are more likely to gain than to lose weight. An *undesired weight loss* could point to a tumor or other medical condition. If, in addition, a general feeling of unwellness and weakness is reported, the possibility of a malignancy should be discussed with the treating physician.

4.2   Diagnosis by Observation

Loss of lordosis and *lateral shift of the spine* are typical for patients with disk damage. In contrast to idiopathic scoliosis, in shift, there is generally no observable countercurve. This means that in lumbar and thoracic shift, the shoulder girdle is displaced to one side in relation to the pelvis (**Fig. 4.1a–d**).

In cervical shift, the head is displaced to one side with respect to the shoulder girdle. The direction of shift is labeled according to the displacement of the cranial section of the body. Thus in a right lumbar shift, the shoulder girdle is displaced to the right with respect to the pelvis. In most cases, but not always, shift is observed away from the side affected by disk damage.

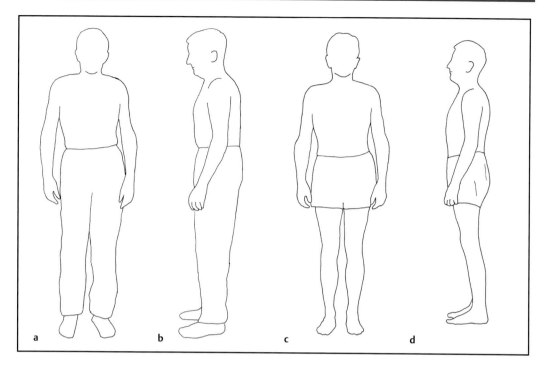

Fig. 4.1 Shift and loss of lordosis. The patient has a prolapsed disk at intervertebral level L5–S1 left.
(a, b) The patient is in the acute phase of the disease with a shift to the right and loss of lordosis in the lumbar spine.
(c, d) The same patient after successful physical therapy.

Loss of lordosis in patients with lumbar disk damage can be recognized from the position of the pelvis (the symphysis and lower arch of the ribs are closer together than the neutral position) or from a forward inclination of the upper body (**Fig. 4.1**).

In patients with cervical disk damage, the head is often pushed forward (protraction) or drooping (see Chapter 8, **Fig. 8.3**).

It has been assumed that the accumulation of disk tissue on the affected side causes the contralateral shift and the loss of lordosis (McKenzie 1981, 1986, 1990), but this is not an explanation for a shift to the affected side.

Persistence of a shift after surgical removal of disk tissue also casts doubt on this mechanism. Waddell (1998) interpreted the incorrect posture as the effect of a muscle spasm (see Chapter 2 General Principles). Presumably the shift is caused by reduction of compression on the affected nerve root.

In addition to the incorrect position of the spine, *limping* in the affected leg can often be observed, especially with pain radiating into the leg. It must be determined here whether the stride length or the stance phase are shortened. A shortened stride length indicates nerve extension pain. A shortened stance phase can potentially be explained by increased pressure in the disk and thus on the nerve root.

In evaluating the success of therapy, the distance that can be walked without an increase in symptoms is a helpful measure.

Patients with cervical disk damage often hold *the affected arm bent close to the body* to avoid nerve extension pain.

4.3 Movement Tests of the Spine

In addition to the classical techniques for examination by physicians (see Chapter 3 Medical Diagnosis and Treatment), movement tests of the spine provide information as to whether the current symptoms are triggered by disk damage. Disk damage and the resulting symptoms are mechanical in nature. For this reason, the symptoms usually change in a specific way during repetitive spinal movements. On the basis of such specific changes, the diagnosis of disk damage becomes likely. In addition, it is easy to determine prospectively whether and by what movements the symptoms can be improved through mechanical physical therapy. The reliability of diagnoses established by means of the examinations described by McKenzie (1981, 1986, 1990) is high (see also Fritz et al 2000; Razmjou et al 2000; Kilpikoski et al 2002).

Before starting the movement tests, the information from the medical history and the visual examination is considered in order to determine a preferred direction of motion and the irritability of the symptoms. This indicates the order of test movements and the intensity of testing.

4.3.1 Order of Test Movements

The goal is to establish the most certain diagnosis possible with the use of a small number of test movements (see 4.6.1 Typical Changes in Symptoms of Disk Damage). At the same time, the therapist must find a movement that the patient can practice themselves to improve their symptoms. Intensifying the symptoms must be avoided. As soon as a test movement has been found that produces the desired effect (see 4.6 Diagnosis) of centralizing radiating pain or reducing central pain, further testing is no longer necessary.

The medical history and visual examination provide information that indicates beneficial movement directions and movements that aggravate the symptoms. In this exploration, the following factors must be borne in mind:
- The strain of activities of daily living.
- Trigger factors.

- The patient's own observations of movements that improve or aggravate their condition.
- Spontaneous posture and movement patterns.

Basic Principles for Specific Test Movements

Reduction of Symptoms Expected Through Extension of the Spine
- Bending in everyday activities as trigger and exacerbating movement.
- Aggravation through sitting, standing up from sitting, and after sitting.
- Improvement in prone position or when walking.
- Loss of lordosis visible.

Reduction of Symptoms Expected Through Rotation of the Spine
- Unilateral symptoms.
- Pronounced shift.

Reduction of Symptoms Expected Through Flexion of the Spine
- Extension in everyday activities as trigger and exacerbating movement.
- Aggravation in standing position and walking.
- Improvement while sitting.
- Pronounced lordosis visible.

4.3.2 Intensity of the Movement Test

The extent to which symptoms are affected by mechanical maneuvers has been termed *irritability* by Maitland (1986, 1994) and is evaluated according to the following criteria:
- Are the symptoms constant or intermittent?
- How rapidly can the symptoms be triggered or intensified?
- How intense are the symptoms (pain scale 0–10; sensitivity: reduced—numb, muscle function 5–0)?
- How long does it take for the symptoms to return to the original level?

An *intensive examination* includes several test movements in *one* session with at least 10 repe-

Examples

- In the case of *intermittent pain* that increases from 1/10 to 4/10 after 30 minutes of sitting and falls back to 1/10 after 5 minutes of walking, the mechanical examination can be intensive.
- In the case of *constant pain* that increases from 5/10 to 9/10 after 1 minute of walking and only falls back to the original level after 15 minutes of lying down, the mechanical examination is conducted with the utmost care.

titions over the full range of motion. A transient increase in symptoms is considered acceptable.

A *careful examination* includes only one position or a small number of test movements with two to five repetitions over the full range of motion. Intensification of the symptoms must be avoided.

4.3.3 Changes in Symptoms During the Test Movements

Before the test movements the patient is asked about the following characteristics of their current symptoms:
- Painful area (section of the spine, radiation into a dermatome).
- Pain intensity (0–10).
- Type of sensory disorder (slightly reduced, tingling, fuzzy, numb).
- Area of the sensory disorder (draw the boundaries on the patient or enter on a documentation form; **Fig. 6.1b**; **Fig. 7.1b**; **Fig. 8.1b**).

Next, the following objective examination parameters are determined:
- Muscle strength (see Chapters 6–8; 6.3.1, 7.3.1, 8.3.1).
- Spinal mobility (see Chapters 6–8; 6.3.3, 7.3.3, 8.3.3).
- Nerve tension test (see Chapters 6–8; 6.3.2, 7.3.2, 8.3.2).

After examination by the physical therapist, the patient is asked to perform specific spinal movements with several repetitions, to the extent possible, and the behavior of the symptoms *during the movements* is described.

After the test movements all symptoms are reviewed and documented again:
- Painful area.
- Pain intensity.
- Type of sensory disorder.
- Area of sensory disorder.
- Muscle strength.
- Spinal mobility.
- Signs of nerve extension.

4.4 Examination of Nerve-gliding Capacity

Nerve tension tests are part of every standard examination in disorders of the lumbar spine. The *Lasègue sign* (*straight leg raise*, SLR) is evidence of disorders in the lumbosacral plexus and nerve roots L5 and S1, whereas the *inverted Lasègue sign* (*prone knee bend*, PKB) examines tension of the femoral nerve and nerve roots L1–L4.

The nerve tension test of the upper extremity (*upper limb tension test*, ULTT) and the global nerve tension test (*slump*) are not yet generally accepted (see Chapters 7 and 8).

Lasègue described the painful effect of knee extension and hip flexion in patients with sciatica in 1864. Clinical studies showed an increase of sciatica upon additional dorsal extension of the ankle or flexion of the neck or lifting of the unaffected leg (Fajersztajn 1901; Woodhall and Hayes 1950; Breig and Troup 1979; Troup 1981).

Woodhall and Hayes (1950) ascribed the pain response when lifting the unaffected leg to the lateral tension on the affected nerve root that results when the contralateral leg is lifted.

Breig (1960, 1978), Breig and Marions (1963), and Breig and Troup (1979) conducted several studies on the effect of movements on the dura mater and the sacral nerves on patients who had just died, and gave a convincing demonstration of nerve extension in movements that trigger pain clinically (see Chapters 2 and 12). In nerve tension tests, according to these studies, the nerve roots are not only subjected to increased tension but are additionally pressed against the prolapsed disk and thus extended.

Clinical and biomechanical studies showed comparable results for tension tests of the upper sacral and cervical roots (Breig 1978; Elvey 1997; Butler 1998; Hall and Elvey 1999; Van der Heide 2000; Kleinrensink et al 2000; Nadler et al 2001).

Monitoring these parameters is of great importance since in cases of disk damage, the limited capacity for nerve gliding is likely responsible for much of the patient's discomfort.

4.4.1 Administration of the Nerve Tension Test

- The starting position must be standardized.
- The individual components of the movement can be performed in different order. For test results to be comparable, the order must be uniform.
- The individual components of the test movement are performed one after the other and the nerve roots or nerves are moved and held at end-range position.
- The movements are passive and slow.
- The movement is stopped when the patient complains of pain or sensory disturbance, makes a clear evasive movement, or offers resistance. This can represent the normal end of the range or be evoked by reflex muscle activity that can be considered a protective mechanism (protective spasm) (Maitland 1986, 1994; Elvey 1997; Butler 1998).

4.4.2 Evaluation of Results of the Nerve Tension Test

The test is evaluated as positive in the following cases:
- The symptoms familiar to the patient are reproduced or intensified.
- A clear positional response can be seen (e.g., neck extension).
- A distinct side difference occurs.

4.4.3 Pain on Approximation

Sometimes patients report pain from movements of the extremities that should lead to reduced extension (approximation) of the nerves affected by a disk prolapse. If pains that are predominantly elicited by approximating movements of the extremities persist and if they are felt in the spine or along the peripheral nerves, test movements that are the opposite of the nerve tension test should be performed.

4.5 General Instructions for Filling out Diagnostic Assessment Forms

Special directions for documentation of findings are located, together with the diagnostic assessment forms in the relevant chapters on the lumbar, thoracic, and cervical spine (Chapters 6–8: **Fig. 6.1**; **Fig. 7.1**; **Fig. 8.1**). In the following a few specifics about the diagnostic assessment form will be given.

Diagnostic Assessment Form Page 1

Suspected Diagnosis at First Visit
The diagnosis given on the prescription or the physician's orders can be either a suspected or a definite diagnosis. It can agree with or differ from the diagnosis established on the basis of the test movements. Often the prescription or the order only classify the symptoms as a syndrome (e.g., lumbago).

Trigger Factors
Triggers responsible for numerous cases of disk damage are: sitting for long periods of time, long drives, helping someone move, gardening, renovation, and lifting heavy objects.

Not all patients can name a trigger factor. If the symptoms occur in the morning, activities on the day before may have been the trigger.

Previous Treatment of the Current Episode
The previous therapeutic measures are circled and comments may be added.

Medications
- *Benzodiazepines* are muscle relaxants. The most frequently used drug is diazepam.
- *Nonsteroidal anti-inflammatory drugs* (NSAIDs) are pain relievers that are not based on steroids (cortisone) and also have an anti-inflammatory effect.
- *Steroids* (cortisone drugs) are highly efficacious inflammation inhibitors used in noninfectious inflammations.

Medical History

The medical history should answer the following questions:

- How often and at what intervals has the patient already had back or radiating symptoms?
- Were they symptom free in the meantime?
- What were the triggers of the earlier episodes?
- What treatment was helpful or harmful at that time?

Physical Therapy Diagnosis

Although the diagnosis will only be established after a complete physical therapy examination, it is helpful for a better overview to note it on the first page of the diagnostic assessment form.

Examples

- (Mechanically) reducible disk problems.
- Problems that cannot be modified mechanically.
- Problems that are predominantly psychosocial.

The hypothesis that the patient's problems are dominated by psychosocial factors can be supported in observations like the following: constantly changing descriptions of pain, demonstrative reaction to pain, extremely jerky evasive movements, or movements in directions that were earlier described as painful (see Chapter 11 Psychosocial Risk Factors).

Justification for the Diagnosis

This question calls for a summary of the aspects leading to the diagnosis or hypothesis. The evaluation may change in the course of treatment. In that case, it is useful to be able to review the arguments.

Diagnostic Assessment Form Page 2

Body Diagram

- All current and transitory symptoms are entered.
- Constant pain is marked with c. This means that the patient is never free of pain, not even for 1 hour.
- Intermittent pains are marked with an i.

- Pains are entered with a broken line and sensory disorders with a dotted line.
- Alternatively, pains can be marked red and sensory disorders blue.

Diagnostic Assessment Form Page 3

Upper Section (Better/Worse)

- The applicable findings are circled.
- What is sometimes applicable is underlined.
- The time until occurrence of aggravation or improvement is noted over the corresponding finding.

Reaction to Repeated End-range Movements

This part is only answered *after* documentation of the findings on Diagnostic Assessment Form Page 4: Control Diagnosis.

Initial Status

Before the test movements, all parameters should be recorded:

- At this moment, from where to where does the pain extend?
- In which position (supine, prone, standing)?
- How intense is the pain (pain scale 0–10)?

Order of Tests

The sequence of tests is selected in an order that is most frequently relevant to patients with disk damage. If they are performed in a different order, this should be documented (1, 2, 3, etc.), since it may be that after one test a new initial status may result for the next one.

Documentation

- Column 1: the test movements are listed.
- Column 2: the patient's reaction during the movement is noted.
- Column 3: the behavior of the symptoms after the movement is noted.

The spelling is given over each column; the meaning of the abbreviations is explained in the legend. Working with abbreviations and signs saves space and time.

In addition to documentation with signs, the precise extent and intensity of the pain after test movements should be noted. In patients with positive nerve tension signs it is useful to test these after every test movement and also to note this finding in the third column. In this way, the examiner obtains a precise picture of changes in symptoms during test movements and is able to compare findings from different days.

This way of gathering data facilitates changing examiners or therapists if necessary.

Diagnostic Assessment Form Page 4: Control Diagnosis

This page is used to document progress in every therapy unit.

Pain
Pain is recorded with the *visual analog scale* (VAS) or the *numeric analog scale* (NAS) (0 = no pain, 10 = strongest pain imaginable). The patient can place an X at the appropriate point on the scale (visual scale) or is asked for a number (numerical scale).

In all four pain assessments, the location of the pain at the time in question and the activity during which the pain exhibited this degree of intensity are recorded. The pain is recorded before and after physical therapy—if possible under a stress, that is, in standing position. Documentation of the minimal pain in the last 24 hours gives information as to whether the pain is constant (i.e., never 0/10) or intermittent (**Fig. 4.2**).

Pain Radiation
This is measured in centimeters from the affected spinal segment along the course of the pain as far as the distal boundary of the radiation (even if no pain is felt in the spine).

If the patient indicates pain in two discrete locations within one dermatome (e.g., buttocks and outer side of the calf to the outer ankle) the pain radiation is measured from segment L5–S1 to the outer ankle.

Sensory Disorder
The area covered by the disorder is outlined on the patient's skin with a ballpoint pen. Lateral, upper, and lower boundaries are individually tested by drawing the finger over them. In the control examination on the next day, the change in the sensory disorder can be determined and, if applicable, the distal or proximal displacement of the boundary can be noted.

Muscle Function Test
This test is necessary when there is suspicion of nerve root compression causing muscle weakness. The evaluation during testing of the segment-indicating muscle associated with the affected spinal section (see Chapter 2 General Principles) is based on the following scale:
- 0: no visible or palpable muscle tension.
- 1: visible or palpable muscle tension without significant motion.
- 2: full range of motion without gravity.
- 3: full range of motion against gravity.

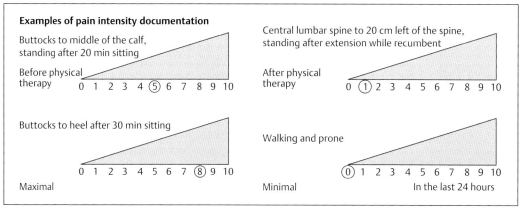

Examples of pain intensity documentation

Buttocks to middle of the calf, standing after 20 min sitting

Before physical therapy   0 1 2 3 4 ⑤ 6 7 8 9 10

Buttocks to heel after 30 min sitting

0 1 2 3 4 5 6 7 ⑧ 9 10

Maximal

Central lumbar spine to 20 cm left of the spine, standing after extension while recumbent

After physical therapy   0 ① 2 3 4 5 6 7 8 9 10

Walking and prone

⓪ 1 2 3 4 5 6 7 8 9 10

Minimal   In the last 24 hours

Fig. 4.2 Documentation of pain intensity.

- 4: full range of motion against moderate resistance over the range and at the end.
- 5: five times full range of motion against strong resistance over the range and at the end.

When force development is limited or if the full range of motion is not achieved, it is necessary to test for pain inhibition and mechanical limitation of movement in order to avoid false positive results.

Signs of Nerve Extension

These are classified as conspicuous or inconspicuous. To monitor progress, it is useful to record additional information in case of a positive nerve tension test. The extent of the movement that causes onset of the nerve extension pain is estimated or (when possible) measured.

The location of the pain is recorded. When the unaffected side is being tested, the patient is asked about crossover pain on the affected side.

Mobility

The mobility of the spine is assessed. In lumbar and thoracic disk damage, the measurement of the finger to floor distance in flexion is a useful parameter. In addition, shift is described (see Chapters 6–8).

4.6 Diagnosis

The most important criterion for assuming that a problem is caused by disk damage is the pain behavior during the examination. When the spine is moved, radiating pain can be shifted toward the spine (centralization) or spread out further toward the foot or hand (peripheralization; **Fig. 4.3a–d**).

Centralization of the radiating pain is considered a predictor of successful progress under conservative treatment (Donelson, Silva et al 1990; Donelson, Grant et al 1990; Long 1995; Sufka et al 1998; Werneke et al 1999; Brötz et al 2001, 2003; Brötz, Burkard, Weller 2010).

In patients with disk prolapses who experience no central back pain but only radiating pain from the buttocks to individual toes or from the shoulder to individual fingers, there is often no centralization to the midline of the spine. It can happen that the distal pain disappears and still, at

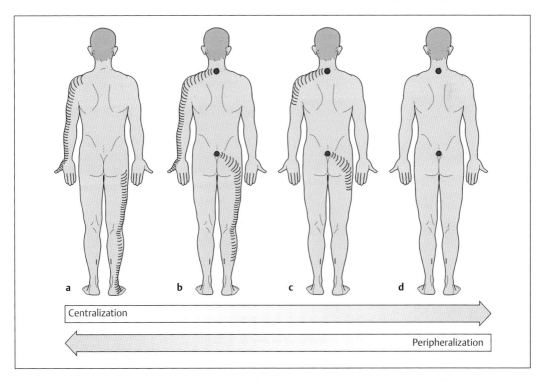

Fig. 4.3 Centralization (the change in pain radiation) runs from (a) to (d) and peripheralization runs in the opposite direction.

the same time, there is no back pain. For instance, sometimes the pain centralizes as far as the buttocks and then disappears without transitional back pain.

This gives rise to the following definitions for centralization and peripheralization:

📬 **Definition of Centralization:** The distal spread of the radiating or radicular pain disappears *during* the spinal movement. At the same time central pain, more toward or in the center of the affected spinal segment, can arise or increase. This change remains *after* the movements.

📬 **Definition of Peripheralization:** The direction of development is opposite to that of centralization.

To determine whether the change persists after the movements, it is necessary to assess the pain radiation in the same position before and after the movements (e.g., supine with extended legs).

The stability of the centralization must also be determined. If the test movement was performed in recumbent position, it is necessary to check whether the centralization persists under loading (standing and walking). Also to be determined is the maximal pain radiation in the course of 24 hours.

📬 **Note:** *Persistence of centralization* is determined under the three following conditions:
- Immediately after movement.
- Under loading.
- Over the course of 24 hours.

Contrary to pain radiation, sensory disorder decreases with improvement of symptoms from proximal to distal. This means that the proximal boundary of the sensory disorder peripheralizes to more distal parts of the dermatome. Residual sensory disorders are thus usually found in the tips of the fingers or toes.

📬 **Note:** If the pain radiates on a given day at least once for longer than 30 minutes, over exactly the same distance as on the first day of treatment and if this radiation reaches as far as the knee or the elbow, the possibility of surgery should be considered because continuation of physical therapy in such patients leads to a very slow permanent resolution of the problems.

4.6.1 Typical Changes in Symptoms of Disk Damage

Mechanically Reducible Disk Problems

- After repeated movement (usually 10 times) in the beneficial direction, the pain is shifted *rapidly during the movements* from distal toward the spine until it finally decreases.
- At the same time, spinal mobility improves.
- The improvement persists after the repeated movements.
- In the nerve tension test, the pain is experienced later than before the movements.
- Sensory disorders and muscle weakness normally improve over days, not during the exercise.

The mechanism of action of mechanical physical therapy is conceived of as follows. Optimal movement exerts pressure at the point to which the gelatinous nucleus is displaced. The nucleus moves away from the pressure, pressure on the nerve root is relieved, and the radicular pain disappears. It is not known whether in some patients this maneuver not only leads to a return of the disk material but also to partial sequestration of the disk prolapse.

In the nerve tension test, the nerve can glide better, so that the movement can continue to be performed without pain. The limitation of movement through accumulation of gelatinous mass at the edge of the vertebral body is decreased. At the same time, spinal mobility improves. When unfavorable movements are repeated the opposite changes are observed. Consequently, these movements must be avoided.

Mechanically Nonreducible Disk Problems

- In response to repeated movements, the pain *shifts rapidly during the movements* more outward, toward the extremities, and finally increases. In this type of change, the test movement should not be repeated more than five times.

- No movement can be found that centralizes the pain.
- At the same time, spinal mobility generally becomes worse.
- The worsening persists after the repeated movements.
- In the nerve tension test, the pain is experienced earlier than before the movements.
- The test movements should not be performed in such a way that sensory disorders and muscle weakness increase.

Disk Disease that is Not Classified as a Prolapse

Donelsen et al (1997) showed that centralization and peripheralization of pain are significantly correlated with tears in the anulus fibrosus (see Chapter 12 Selected Studies on the Topic of Spinal Disorders). The inhibition of movement can often be considerable, whereas pain radiation only extends as far as lateral to the spine or to the first large joint (e.g., hip, shoulder).

Patients with nonspecific pain, whose radiological diagnosis shows no disk prolapse, can still have treatable disk disease.

If the test movements evoke the same changes in symptoms as in a confirmed disk prolapse it can be assumed, even without radiological diagnosis, that disk disease is present.

If no radiating pain is reported, the suspected diagnosis of disk damage can be established on the basis of the following parameters:

- The pain changes during movement, but not in location, only in intensity (McKenzie 1981, 1986, 1990; Donelson et al 1997; McKenzie and May 2003).
- Spinal mobility also changes during movement.
- These changes persist after the movements.
- The nerve extension sign is often negative from the beginning.
- There are no neurological deficits.

4.6.2 Establishing the Diagnosis

After the complete physical therapy examination, a working diagnosis can be established. For this purpose, those aspects that speak for and against a specific diagnosis must be considered.

The working diagnosis of *disk disease* can be established on the basis of **Tables 4.1** and **4.2**.

To advise the patient and plan the treatment, an estimate of treatment success is necessary. For this purpose, an answer is required as to whether *the symptoms are reducible by means of physical therapy* (**Table 4.3**).

On the basis of the repeated spinal test movements, alternative diagnoses may be made (**Table 4.4**). Under certain circumstances, further examinations could be suggested or specific treatments could be introduced. These are different from the therapy strategies for patients with disk disease.

Table 4.1 Is it a mechanical problem?

Yes	No
• History of intermittent neck or back pain • Sudden onset of symptoms • Trigger factor known or not • Good overall condition • Changes in symptoms during movement • Intermittent or constant symptoms • Symptoms match known anatomical facts (dermatomes, myotomes)	• Insidious onset of the disease • No trigger factor known • General feeling of malaise • Weight loss • No changes in symptoms during movement • Constant symptoms • Symptoms do not match anatomy (dermatomes, myotomes, discrepancies between straight leg raise and sitting with extended legs). These characteristics indicate a chronified pain syndrome or influence of psychosocial factors

Table 4.2 In case of a mechanical problem: are there signs that indicate disk disease?

Yes	No
• Pain centralized or peripheralized on spinal movement • Limitation of movement • Spinal mobility changes with pain • The changes persist after the movements • Signs of nerve extension can be positive or negative	• The location of the pain does not change during spinal movement • Mobility can be free or limited • Spinal mobility remains the same during test movements • After the movement test, there is no change • Signs of nerve extension can be negative or positive

Table 4.3 Can the symptoms be reduced by physical therapy?

Yes	No
• Upon repeated movement the pain shifts more from outside toward the spine and finally decreases • At the same time, spinal mobility improves • The improvement persists after the repeated movements • In the nerve tension test, the pain is experienced later than before the movements	• In repeated movement the pain shifts distally toward the extremities and finally increases • No movement can be found that centralizes the pain • The mobility of the spine becomes worse • The aggravation persists after the repeated movements • In the nerve tension test, the pain is experienced earlier than before the movements

Table 4.4 Simplified representation of the classification of various findings from the medical history and diagnostic tests by specific diagnoses

Diagnosis	Trigger factors	Medical history	Location of pain	Limitation of motion	Constant or intermittent pain	Pain behavior during the movement test	Pain behavior after the movement test	Nerve tension test	Physical therapy
Disk disease and disk prolapse	Sudden onset of intense pain, usually on flexion of the spine or in the morning	Fluctuating pain for years	Central or radiating to a dermatome	Present, in one or more directions	Intermittent or constant	Pain during and at the end of the movement Centralization or peripheralization with spinal pain increase or decrease	Change persists, reduced or intensified, centralized or peripheralized	Negative or positive Positive with disk prolapse	Therapy according to the method described here Avoidance of movement in painful directions Rapid improvement during treatment
Instability, facet pain	Static stress standing, extension of spine, e.g., lower arm support	Played many sports in childhood and youth, especially sports requiring extreme spinal movements (e.g., gymnastics, ballet)	Local spine or radiating to a dermatome	None in hypermobile instability; may be present in segmental instability	Intermittent	Increase with extension, reduction with flexion	No change	Negative	Stabilization, strengthening
Spinal or foraminal stenosis	Walking, standing spinal extension	Increasing problems for years	Radiating to one or more extremities, possibly leg problems with cervical stenosis	Can be present or absent	Intermittent	Intensified by extension, improved by flexion	No change	Negative or positive	Exercises in flexion, stabilization

▲ *(continued)*

Table 4.4 Simplified representation of the classification of various findings from the medical history and diagnostic tests by specific diagnoses (*continued*)

Diagnosis	Trigger factors	Medical history	Location of pain	Limitation of motion	Constant or intermittent pain	Pain behavior during the movement test	Pain behavior after the movement test	Nerve tension test	Physical therapy
Chronified pain syndrome	Fluctuating, always changing triggers	For more than 3 months, usually years	Pain in many body areas, often not dermatome related	Can be present or absent	Constant	Fluctuating changes, usually aggravates all movements	Fluctuating changes, usually aggravates all movements	Negative or positive	Multiple patient activation in spite of pain Possibly in combination with behavioral therapy
Psychosocial factors	Fluctuating, always changing triggers	For days to years	Diffuse pain in many body areas Fluctuating reports	Can be present or absent	Constant or intermittent	Fluctuating changes, usually aggravates all movements Demonstrative statement of pain	Fluctuating changes, usually aggravates all movements	Negative or positive Clear signs: discrepancy between SLR and sitting with extended legs	After consultation with treating physician Possibly not affected by physical therapy
Tumor	None	Problems increasing for last months General malaise Possible history of tumor disease	Can be diffuse or unambiguously classified with an anatomical structure	Can be present or absent	Constant	No effect	No change	Negative or positive	No improvement through physical therapy

5 Therapy

5.1 Overview

Internationally, the clinical guidelines for the treatment of back pain are largely in agreement. Comparison of 11 guidelines from 11 countries, in English, German, or Danish, showed a high degree of consistency in diagnostic classification and diagnostic and therapeutic measures (Koes et al 2001). In many case series and a small number of controlled studies, the disease course in patients with back and neck pain and pain radiating into the extremities was examined. Only some of these studies exclusively included patients with radiologically confirmed disk prolapse (Weber 1983; Saal and Saal 1989; Saal et al 1990; Bush et al 1992; Zentner et al 1997; Vroomen et al 2000; Atlas et al 2001; Weinstein et al 2006a, 2006b).

In other studies, the inclusion criteria were only defined clinically (Weber 1994; Faas et al 1995; Indahl et al 1995; Malmivaara et al 1995; Stankovic and Johnell 1995; Cherkin et al 1998; Seferlis et al 1998; Mannion et al 1999; Kjellman and Oberg 2002; Petersen et al 2002). The disease course was studied both for patients with acute and chronic problems. The objective of the studies was usually the differentiation of efficacious and inefficacious treatment measures as well as preparation of cost–benefit analyses.

In this process, the first question concerned the spontaneous course of the disease without specific therapeutic measures. The concept of *spontaneous course* has to be taken relatively since the great majority of patients had adopted specific measures, with or without seeking professional advice, to obtain relief from their suffering.

In a double-blind, placebo-controlled study of the effect of the nonsteroidal anti-inflammatory compound piroxicam, involving 208 patients with prominent acute lumbar radicular symptoms and signs, Weber et al (1993) recommended bed rest for 1 week and then slowly increasing activity, unaccompanied by physical therapy. For pain relief, additional paracetamol was used as needed. After 4 weeks, the authors observed marked improvement of leg and back pain in 70% of patients and 60% of patients were able to work. However, even after 1 year, 30% were still physically challenged at work and in their activities of daily living. The results for the piroxicam group corresponded to those of the control group.

In a randomized study, Indahl et al (1995) investigated 975 patients with back pain and pain radiating to the legs, some of whom had neuroradiologically confirmed disk prolapse. The first group received detailed information about the mechanics of the spine, disk damage, and possible inflammation. They were encouraged to move the spine as normally as possible, without any fear. There was no further treatment. The second group received no instruction of this kind and served as the control group. The lead investigators of the study did not participate in the treatment. The control patients were treated by measures considered standard care in Norway. The first group showed a significantly improved reduction in the disability period. After 200 days, only 30% of patients, compared to 60% in the control group, were unable to work.

These results indicate that relatively simple and low-cost education strategies can lead to an improved prognosis or at least decreased cost.

Reviewing the available evidence, Deyo and Phillips (1996) concluded that about 80% of patients with nonspecific back pain improved, independently of specific treatments.

Nevertheless, because of long-term medical treatment and sickness-related disability, back pain represents a considerable burden on the healthcare system. In comparison to the spontaneous course without specific treatment, the operational goals of physical therapy could thus be defined as reduction of the disability period, a lower rate of long-term impairment, and a lower recurrence rate. According to these criteria, numerous therapeutic approaches exhibited no evidence of efficacy.

Massage

Although massage is frequently prescribed for back and neck pain (Chrubasik et al 1998), there are very few randomized studies that investigate its efficacy. In a systematic literature search, Furlan et al (2002) found eight randomized studies that compared the effect of massage, both classic and acupuncture based, with other treatments. The authors concluded that massage can be helpful for patients with subacute and chronic back pain, especially in combination with exercise and information. Conversely, whether the exercises and information alone would be less efficacious than any such treatment with additional massage remains unclear. It is possible that passive massage treatment may even have a negative effect on the patient's own activities. Moreover, if the hypothesis is correct that in disk damage, the tension of back extensors is a protective mechanism (see Chapter 2 General Principles), then a treatment form that decreases muscle tension would be contraindicated for patients with disk damage.

Balneotherapy

This form of therapy is usually prescribed and studied in combination with physical therapy (Gerber et al 1993; Chrubasik et al 1998; Strauss-Blasche et al 2000; Toepfer et al 2002). The therapeutic usefulness of heat application for short periods (e.g., fango packs), as used for pain syndromes in various European countries (Chrubasik et al 1998), is unclear.

Bed Rest

In the literature and according to international guidelines for the treatment of back pain, there is agreement that bed rest lasting longer than 4 days should be avoided (Deyo 1986; Deyo and Phillips 1996; Van Tulder et al 1997, 2006; Waddell et al 1997; Waddell 1998; Koes et al 2001 van Tulder et al 2006).

Physical Therapy

There are a few retrospective, prospective, and randomized studies of physical therapy.

Comparative Studies of Surgical and Conservative Treatment

In 1983, a prospective, randomized, two-arm study revealed that patients with lumbar disk prolapse receiving conservative treatment (n = 66) had significantly worse results after 1 year regarding ability to work, neurological deficits, pain, and lumbar spine mobility than a group receiving surgical treatment (n = 60), in which an open surgical technique with fenestration was used (Weber 1983). After 4 and 10 years, however, there were no longer any significant differences between the two patient groups. The average duration of recovery after discharge from the hospital was shorter in the group treated by conservative means (7 weeks) than in the surgical group (11 weeks).

Since the strategies of both conservative treatment and surgical techniques have undergone significant development in the last 20 years, these results cannot easily be applied to the current situation. For instance, a large multicenter study including 472 patients from 11 states in the United States compared surgical and conservative treatment of prolapsed disks (Weinstein et al 2006a, 2006b). The attempt to randomize patients for a treatment strategy failed. Half of the patients who were to be treated surgically were not operated on and 30% of the patients randomized for conservative therapy received an operation. No significant differences in the parameters measured—pain, function, satisfaction, self-perceived improvement, and ability to work—were observed between the groups. This study yielded no reliable information about the superiority of one treatment strategy over the other.

Like Weber's study (1983), this more recent study also did not specify the conservative treatment but left it up to each therapist (usual care). Only 44% of the conservatively treated patients received physical therapy. Although the surgical patients reported more impairment from pain and less ability to work, they were more satisfied with the symptoms and the healthcare than the patients who received conservative treatment.

Comparative Studies of Conservative Procedures

Saal and Saal (1989) retrospectively reported good results for ability to work, pain intensity, and use of the healthcare system by patients with lumbar disk prolapse (n = 64) who received a broad range of physical therapy procedures, but there was no control group.

Bush et al (1992), in a prospective single-arm clinical and radiological study, examined 165 patients with lumbar root compression syndrome who had been treated with epidural steroid injections. After one year, 86% of patients exhibited satisfactory improvement of the clinical symptoms. Neuroradiologically confirmed reduction of a disk prolapse was seen in 64 of 84 patients; 14% of the patients had been treated surgically.

In a randomized study of patients with acute back pain, Malmivaara et al (1995) compared the results of a group I (n = 67) of patients who received 2 days of bed rest, a group II (n = 52) of patients who performed 10 spine extensions every hour, and a control group III (n = 67) of patients who went about their normal activities. Patients in control group III exhibited significantly better results for pain duration and intensity, spinal mobility in flexion, and ability to work than the other two groups. This suggests that the stereotypical practice of spinal extension in patients with acute nonspecific back pain is as useless as strict bed rest.

Faas et al (1995) compared the results in patients with acute back pain randomized into the following three groups: group I (n = 122) was informed about measures for back care usual in the Netherlands and treated with analgesics (control group); group II (n = 119) was treated twice a week with low doses of ultrasound (placebo treatment); and group III (n = 122) did daily prescribed spinal flexion exercises. There was no significant difference among the three groups with respect to duration of disability. This leads to the conclusion that the usual spinal flexion exercises do not represent a useful strategy for patients with acute nonspecific back pain.

A prospective randomized study reported that patients who had been treated for acute back pain with physical therapy according to the McKenzie Method® suffered fewer recurrences and used fewer sick leave days in the 5 years after treatment than a control group of patients who took part in back school (Stankovic and Johnell 1995).

In a randomized study in the United States, Cherkin et al (1998) compared the success and costs of chiropractic and physical therapy according to the McKenzie Method® (1981, 1986), with no specific treatment, for patients with back pain. Chiropractic and physical therapy produced only minimally better, nonsignificant results but costed significantly more.

In a prospective, randomized clinical study, the results of general exercise, physical therapy according to the McKenzie Method®, and a control group were compared (Kjellman and Oberg 2002). Seventy patients with neck pain were included in the study and examined after 3 weeks, 6 months, and 12 months. All three groups showed the same degree of improvement in pain intensity and impairment. A significant improvement in the *Distress and Risk Assessment Method Scores* was only seen in the group treated according to the McKenzie Method®, together with a slight, insignificantly lower utilization of the healthcare system (ibid.).

Long et al (2004) asked the provocative question of whether the type of physical therapy exercise affects the treatment results. A symptom-oriented mechanical study of 312 patients looked for a preferred direction of motion that centralized and reduced pain. One patient group then exercised in the preferred direction and one in the nonpreferred direction, and a third group exercised without any specified direction of movement. In the group that moved in the preferred direction, the symptom improvement was significantly better than in the other two groups. This result confirms the therapeutic approach of using specifically directed movements.

The list of studies and results presented above points to the necessity of reviewing and documenting treatment successes in a critical manner. Detailed information about spinal mechanics, disk damage, or a possible inflammation, and the instruction to move the spine as normally as possible without anxiety, as well as physical therapy according to the McKenzie Method®, produced better results for individual target parameters in patients with nonspecific back or neck pain than nonspecific measures. Thus certain specific therapeutic systems may help certain patients. However, the question of which treatment will best help which patient most has not been answered by any of these studies.

Specific therapeutic methods must be investigated for their efficacy in a given disease. For this purpose it is necessary to establish a hypothesis as to the cause of the symptoms, by means of test movements of the spine, and then to implement a symptom-oriented treatment. Performing the usual exercises for symptoms not specified in detail cannot be helpful.

Neither Weber's (1983) study nor the multicenter study reported by Weinstein et al (2006a, 2006b) sanction a decision for or against surgery. This type of investigation should compare the results of a defined surgical technique, in which postoperative care and rehabilitation are also defined and monitored, with the results of a specific physical therapy approach. Only this kind of study will allow us to derive evidence-based conclusions and recommendations for management and follow-up.

Only effects that set in rapidly, that is, during or within days of treatment, can be ascribed with any degree of certainty to the therapy. In acute pain syndromes, improvement over the course of several weeks is more likely due to the natural course of things rather than to acute therapy, whereas in chronic pain that has persisted for longer than 3 months, slow improvement can still result from therapy.

Many authors have come to the conclusion that the risk of developing chronic pain and remaining permanently disabled increases with increasing duration of the disease (Waddell 1996, 1998; Diener and Leonhardt 1998; Hagen and Thune 1998; Hasenbring et al 1999; Loeser 1999; Werneke et al 1999; Tölle and Berthele 2001; Zieglgänsberger 2002). This underscores the need to aim for rapid resolution of the symptoms.

In patients whose problems were caused by disk damage or prolapse, symptoms change rapidly during spinal movement (see Chapter 4 Diagnosis in Physical Therapy). These changes can be ascribed to the treatment with a certain degree of plausibility.

5.2   Course of Treatment

In the following, we will describe our BASE PT approach of physical therapy for disk damage. The basis of the method is repeated spinal movements and movement of the extremities with the goal of mobilizing nerve tracts and activating local stabilizing muscles. The treatment includes measures specifically designed for treatment of paresis. In addition, it contains detailed instructions for training in mobility, strength, coordination, and fitness, so that the patient can be brought to a normal capacity level. Milestones for function and improvement time are defined. Recommendations for further treatment *after* a disk operation (see Chapters 5.7, 6.6, 7.6, 8.6) are also based on BASE PT.

Our own prospective single-arm studies (Brötz et al 2003; Brötz, Burkard, et al 2010) of the concept described here suggest that it is efficacious for patients with lumbar disk prolapse. There is also positive clinical experience for the cervical and thoracic spine (Brötz et al unpublished), but there

are also no studies comparing this approach with other treatment methods.

5.2.1   Psychosocial Aspects

The psychological aspects of the healing process can be divided into three stages (for an overview see Grawe 2000). The attention of a physician or physical therapist as well as the application of specific measures or prescription of a medication can encourage confidence in help and hope for healing. At first this promotes nonspecific improvement in the patient's well-being. This can be classified as a placebo effect (Montgomery and Kirsch 1997; Cherkin et al 1998; Amanzio and Benedetti 1999; De Pascalis et al 2002; Hrobjartsson 2002; Kaptchuk 2002; Moyad 2002; Walach and Sadaghiani 2002), which, by definition, is independent of the actual mode of action of the administered treatment.

Confidence is an important requirement for the healing process, which can be subdivided into the following three phases:

Phase 1
- The patient should be supported in assuming a positive disease course and this brings about nonspecific improvement.

Phase 2
- The signs and symptoms of the disease improve.
- Mobility, strength, sensory function, coordination, and condition also improve.
- The degree of impairment decreases.

Phase 3
- Improvement stabilizes.
- Psychosocial adaptation leads to resumption of all activities of daily living, sometimes including work or previous activities.

The therapist plays a role in preventing the patient from becoming stuck in one of the first two phases. The placebo effect can cause the patient to continue participating in a nonefficacious treatment without moving closer to the goal of re-entry into normal life (Deyo and Phillips 1996). This danger is particularly present in passive forms of therapy in which the patient exercises neither control nor responsibility for action. By now, there is widespread consensus that patients with disk disease should usually receive detailed patient education and co-operate actively in their own healing (Saal and Saal 1989; Waddell 1996, 1998; Cherkin 1996, 1998; Chrubasik et al 1998; Koes et al 2001).

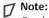

Note:
Psychosocial adaptation includes:

- Improvement of well-being.
- Improvement of function.
- Stabilization and normal psychological and social integration.

5.2.2   Functional Aspects

In cases of disk damage, the following four stages can be defined in the period before restoration of normal functioning:

Acute Phase

Symptoms change in direct association with movements and changes in capacity. For instance, with beneficial movements, the pain is centralized and reduced, whereas with harmful movements it is peripheralized and intensified.

Only individual exercises that specifically centralize and reduce pain are practiced, and harmful movements are systematically avoided.

Stabilization

This phase of healing is marked by the fact that the symptoms resulting from movements and stresses that peripheralize and intensify pain in the acute phase are no longer immediately produced and intensified. Medications can be reduced or discontinued.

Movements of the extremities supplement the therapeutic exercises with the goal of preserving or improving nerve-gliding capacity. Rotational movements of the spine in both directions are added.

Restoration of Original Functioning

When the patient is largely and sustainably symptom free, symmetrical pain-free mobility of the spine and the extremities is tested in all directions and, if necessary, practiced. Spinal flexion frequently improves through end-range movement

in rotation, so that flexion itself need not be explicitly practiced.

Posture and movement checks with activation of local stabilizing muscles are practiced and trained. Maximal strength and speed strength of extremity and trunk muscles are also trained. Weak muscles must be kept in the best trophic condition possible, with the help of physical therapy (Sunderland 1979). This can be done by activating the muscles to the best possible extent.

At the same time, free mobility must be maintained for joints that cannot perform end-range movement because of muscle paresis, thus helping to avoid muscle contractures. First, simple movements are used, such as climbing stairs, knee bends, walking on tiptoe, walking on heels, single-axis end-range arm and hand movements as well as extension in prone position. Later, complex movement sequences such as running or juggling are added to improve coordination and fitness.

Special movements related to the patient's activities of daily living are practiced, so that the load is distributed over the active and passive support apparatus of the spine and extremities. Exercises that the patient can practice on their own at home are preferable to work with training equipment, which should be largely dispensed with.

Normal Everyday Capacity and Prevention

With increasing capacity, the patient gains the confidence to resume activities of daily living, including their work. In activities of daily living, the practice effort must be reduced to a realistic level, individualized for the patient's circumstances.

As a minimal preventive measure, the entire spine should be regularly extended to the limit of motion, repeatedly before getting up and in the course of the day, and during the day it should be regularly actively straightened. The ideal pattern would be 15-minute exercise units, performed morning, noon, and night, that cover all the points mentioned.

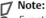

Note:
Functional change includes:

- Acute pain with rapid changes.
- Stabilization with less or no pain and without rapid aggravation under stress.
- Restoration of original functioning.
- Everyday activity with preventive exercises at normal capacity.

5.2.3   Temporal Aspects

The course of healing over time depends on the extent of damage and the efficiency of the wound healing process that can be impaired by medicines (e.g., corticosteroids) or independent concomitant diseases (e.g., diabetes mellitus). This affects the duration of disability, which also depends on the type and possibility of individual accommodation at work. To avoid aggravation of the patient's symptoms by unfavorable activities (e.g., sitting, bending), the physical therapy should begin immediately upon onset of symptoms.

Acute Phase

The acute inflammatory phase lasts approximately 5 days after any tissue injury (see Chapter 2 General Principles). During this time, if therapy is successful, there should be distinct improvement in all symptoms and maximal pain radiation should be reduced (centralization). Because of the rapid change in symptoms and thus in the exercises identified as helpful, the first five therapy sessions should take place on 5 consecutive days. The treatment time is between 30 and 60 minutes.

Stabilization

The treatment effects usually stabilize in 7 to 10 days. At this time, it should be possible to reduce the morning dose of analgesics without increase of pain, and finally discontinue them altogether. The treatments can be reduced to two therapy sessions per week.

Restoration of Original Capacity

Load increase is used to restore function. The frequency of treatments can be reduced to one session a week or every 2 weeks. The goal is increasing load and ability to work after 2 to 6 weeks.

Normal Everyday Stress and Prevention

A check-up and consultation about everyday training should occur approximately 8 weeks after the start of treatment. After a disk prolapse with neurological deficit, regeneration to extensive or complete reduction of paresis and sensory disorders may take up to 1 year.

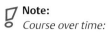 **Note:**
Course over time:

- Within 5 days: pronounced improvement of all symptoms and centralization of pain.
- Week 2 to 3: discontinuation of medications and increasing tolerance of stress.
- Week 2 to 6: good load capacity, able to work.
- Within 1 year: complete capacity, complete or extensive resolution of neurological deficits.

For patients with a prolapsed disk, radicular pain, and neurological deficits, for whom physical therapy has not been successful after five sessions, treatment with corticosteroids to decrease swelling and inflammation, or surgery, should be considered (see Chapters 3.3, 3.4).

5.3   Basic Procedure in Physical Therapy for Patients with Disk Damage

The procedure is the same for all sections of the spine. The special characteristics of the cervical, thoracic, and lumbar spine are found in the corresponding Chapters 6 to 8.

5.3.1   Findings and Documentation

In every therapy session, the control findings (see Chapter 4 Diagnosis in Physical Therapy and the diagnostic assessment forms in Chapters 6–8) are recorded and all relevant subjective (symptoms) and objective values (signs) are documented. The test movements of the spine are repeated and evaluated as in the diagnosis. In contrast to the diagnosis in the first therapy session, in which there is no further testing if the test movement leads to centralization of the pain, in the following therapy sessions all spinal movements are tested. Movements that intensify the pain and peripheralize it are not tested to the end range of motion and are not repeated.

Documentation includes the movements tested and the changes in pain and mobility of the spine and nervous system. After each test movement, the painful area, pain intensity, and signs of nerve extension are examined and documented.

The therapeutic movements and instructions to the patient for self-training are determined on the basis of these findings. Documentation of the findings at each therapy session makes the course of treatment clear to the therapist, the physician, and the patient.

5.3.2 Testing and Practicing the Therapeutic Movements

Usually the movement tests permit identification of at least one movement that improves the symptoms. This is the movement that the patient should repeat on their own every hour, usually 10 times in immediate succession, with the greatest range of motion possible. If the patient is given more than one movement at the same time as a new strategy it cannot be determined which exercise improves or aggravates the symptoms. The patient is instructed to observe the symptoms while practicing on their own as carefully as during the therapy session.

At least in the first two therapy sessions, only movements are used that the patient carries out on their own. This makes clear to them that they can and should contribute to their healing through their own efforts. Only in exceptional cases are passive spinal movements added after the third therapy session to intensify the pain-reducing effect. Passive movements of the extremities intended to improve nerve-gliding capacity may be necessary after the acute phase.

The therapeutically useful movements change in the course of healing. For instance, at first one-sided movements are necessary but later they are replaced with symmetrical movements or supplemented with additional movements. For this reason, to begin with, therapy should be administered for *at least 5 days in a row*. Only one exercise is changed at a time so that it is clear whether the change has a good or an unfavorable effect on the symptoms. For the same reason, neither medications nor everyday activities, such as returning to work, should be changed at the same time as the exercises.

Activities of daily living are practiced in addition to the therapeutic movements. In every case this includes lying and turning in bed, getting up and lying down, sitting erect, and standing up from the toilet. Depending on how pronounced the patient's symptoms are, this is followed by posture training in standing position and walking as well as training for optimal posture and movement at the workplace. Walking is used as a therapeutic movement as soon as possible. Awkward posture and movements must be discussed with the patient in detail. Usually, sitting and all bending of the spine should be temporarily avoided.

5.3.3 Instructing and Informing the Patient

Patients have a great desire for information (Indahl et al 1995; Deyo and Phillips 1996; Waddell 1996; Cherkin et al 1998; Burton et al 1999). For this reason, a patient should be informed by the physician or physical therapist about the anatomy of the spine, the position of disks and nerves, the mechanism of disk damage, and the injury and healing of the fibrous ring (see Chapter 2 General Principles). At the same time, it is important to explain to the patient that therapy is determined by the clinical signs and symptoms and that most theoretical explanations of the therapy for disk disease are hypothetical rather than being confirmed by adequate studies. Most of all, patients are informed of the probable duration of the disease, the importance of active participation in the treatment, and the necessity to adapt lifestyle to prevent recurrence.

Since the situation is often challenging and complicated, patients frequently ask the same questions. The therapist should devote sufficient time to informing the patient so well that they reliably do the assigned exercises and stick to the rules for their activities.

In the therapy described here, willingness to comply is largely independent of education, social status, age, or gender. However, adequate spoken communication is essential.

🗍 **Note:**
  1. Instructions for the patient:

- Take on your share of the responsibility for your recovery!
- Observe all your symptoms precisely, before, during, and after the repeated movements.
- Judge whether the symptoms get better or worse, or whether they stay the same.
- If your symptoms get worse when you do the assigned exercises, stop that exercise. Under no

circumstances should the pain shift further to the periphery and into the leg or the arm.

- A transient increase in back or neck pain with simultaneous decrease of pain in the arm or leg should be considered an improvement.
- Perform the assigned number of repetitions of the beneficial movement at the assigned intervals. In most cases, 10 repetitions per hour have been proven to be a useful rate.
- Consistently avoid postures and movements that are uncomfortable for you.

2. Three aspects of every therapy session:
- Documentation of subjective, objective, and quantifiable findings.
- Testing and practicing the therapeutic movements.
- Instructing and informing the patient.

5.4 Mechanical Effect of the Therapy on the Disk Injury

Many longitudinal neuroradiological studies show that disk prolapses can lose volume over the course of several months (Bush et al 1992; Maigne et al 1992; Maigne and Deligne 1994; Slavin et al 2001; Henmi et al 2002; Reyentovich and Abdu 2002). Either magnetic resonance imaging (MRI) or computed tomography (CT) have been used for confirmation (see Chapter 3 Medical Diagnosis and Treatment). In the studies cited, only those patients were examined with MRI or CT whose symptoms had improved as a result of various conservative treatments. The relationship between the size of the disk prolapse and the clinical symptoms and signs thus remains unclear (Bush et al 1992; Weber 1994; Komori et al 2002; Brötz et al 2008). In addition, the mechanisms leading to clinical changes during mechanical therapy are unknown.

McKenzie (1986) suspected that pressure on the disk at the injured anulus fibrosus can reduce the displacement of the disk. Other authors discuss dehydration, shift within the intervertebral space, or resorption through inflammation as the cause of changes in the appearance of prolapsed disks on CT or MRI (Bush et al 1992; Maigne et al 1992; Maigne and Deligne 1994; Ikeda et al 1996; Slavin et al 2001; Henmi et al 2002).

To study the question of the mechanical effects of repeated end-range spinal movements on the prolapsed disk tissue and the irritated nerve root in patients with lumbar disk prolapse and the

corresponding nerve root irritation syndrome, we studied 11 patients by means of MRI. Before the first physical therapy session and 3 to 7 days later, on average, on the fifth day, a control MRI was performed. The expansion and water content of the disk tissue were determined and the patients' symptoms at the various measurement times were documented. In all 11 patients, the symptoms showed pronounced improvement or had disappeared entirely. However, the MRI images showed no changes (Brötz et al 2008). The hypothesis that the specific movements move the disk tissue away from the nerve roots was thus not confirmed.

From the mechanisms leading to disk damage and from clinical observations, we conclude that extension of the affected section of the spine is usually a useful therapeutic movement (see Chapters 6–8). It is imaginable that the extension produces pressure on the dorsal section of the disk, pushing the displaced gel mass forward (McKenzie 1986; Adams, May et al 2000) and thus reducing symptoms.

Since presumably the gel mass only moves very slowly, it is necessary to perform the therapeutic movements repeatedly and to the limit of the range. In a disk prolapse, shift into the original position seems unlikely. It remains undecided whether these ideas apply to all patients in whom the movements lead to reduction of symptoms.

It is possible that movement in a preferred, centralizing direction achieves dehydration of the prolapsed disk through pressure. Moreover, better blood circulation at the point of disk damage could accelerate biochemical processes and reduce the concentration of pain mediators.

In acute lumbar disk prolapse, restored capacity for end-range extension of the spine can be considered proof of successful healing (Kopp et al 1986; Alexander et al 1992; Brötz et al 2001, 2003, 2010). Correspondingly, avoiding flexion can contribute to pain relief in chronic back pain (Snook et al 1998).

Although repeated end-range extension of the spine centralizes and reduces pain in most patients it is not useful to prescribe this movement automatically as a therapy for all patients with disk damage, since, in case of disk prolapse, the swollen nerve root can be compressed in the intervertebral foramen. In an *intraforaminal* disk prolapse, in which the disk tissue is also occupying space, treatment is particularly difficult. Movements that exercise beneficial pressure in the affected area

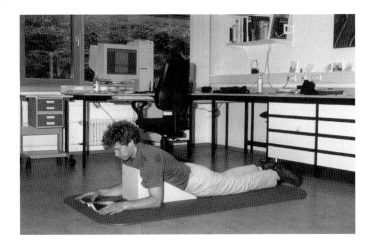

Fig. 5.1 Prone position supported with a reading wedge.

(extension, rotation, lateral flexion to the affected side) can also lead to a further narrowing of the intervertebral foramen and additional compression of the nerve root. In consequence, the movements must be of such moderate intensity that while working effectively for shift of the disk they do not harm the nerve root.

Only the mechanical diagnostic tests lead to temporarily beneficial movements. In the acute phase, if symptoms radiate only to one side or when a shift is present, the first requirement is often asymmetrical rotation or lateral flexion or shift correction (see Chapter 6 Lumbar Spine). In some patients with lumbar disk damage the pain is first centralized by means of spinal flexion in recumbent position. Although the mechanism of this improvement is puzzling, therapeutic movements should be selected on the basis of symptoms.

The ability to extend the spine is used as a control parameter in cases of acute and chronic cervical, thoracic, and lumbar pain. As soon as extension is possible without increase of pain, it is practiced as a therapeutic movement. It may then replace previously assigned asymmetrical or flexion movements.

During stabilization and restoration of normal function, pain-free end-range spinal mobility in extension, rotation, lateral flexion, translation, and flexion is tested and, if necessary, practiced (see Chapters 6–8).

Reading Wedge
Lying relaxed in prone position with a slightly raised upper body is a beneficial change from the usual everyday forward-bending position. As soon as the patient can lie in prone position without increased pain, they should spend as much time as possible in this position.

The prone position supported by a reading wedge is very beneficial for reading and working (**Fig. 5.1**). The best measurements for the foam wedge are a density of 35 (the measure of hardness), 26 cm high, 32 cm wide, and 50 cm long. Wedges of this kind are not available commercially but must be ordered directly from foam manufacturers. If the wedge is ordered by the treating physician some health insurance providers will cover its cost.

The wedge is used with hospitalized and ambulatory patients with a prolapsed disk, both during acute treatment and thereafter, to prevent neck and back pain or another disk prolapse. After disk surgery, this unstressed position is also useful for working and for regaining the ability to extend the spine.

5.5 Mobilization of the Nervous System

Nerve extension was described as a useful strategy in the treatment of neurological disorders as early as the 19th century, especially in tuberculosis, tabes dorsalis (locomotor ataxia), and sciatica (Sugar 1990). In France and England, surgical interventions were performed in which the nerve was laid bare and extended directly. This treatment was chiefly applied to the sciatic nerve and the brachial plexus. The diseases to be treated in this way ranged from pain syndrome to tetanus, epilepsy, and peripheral pareses to ataxia (Cavafy 1881; Marshall 1883).

However, the diagnoses and classification of symptoms with specific diseases as performed in that time cannot be evaluated with today's methods and understanding. For instance, we can only speculate which types of ataxia were treated this way.

Cavafy (1881) described 17 patients with ataxia who were treated with surgical nerve extension. Some of these patients also had severe pain. It is reported that in some of them improvement of pain and ataxia were observed. To extend the sciatic nerve, the surgeon exposed the nerve at the level of the gluteal fold, held it with a hook or a finger and pulled it forcefully. Hanging up the leg by the exposed nerve was also described. The surgery was performed under chloroform anesthesia or some unidentified local anesthesia. The results of the treatment ranged from impressive improvement (neuralgia) to fatal outcome (tetanus; see Cavafy 1881; Symington 1882; Marshall 1883).

Today the idea is to mobilize nerves rather than to extend them. In cases of disk damage but also in neurological diseases such as Guillain-Barré syndrome and subarachnoid bleeding, movement of the extremities and the spine elicits pain. Presumably this pain, at least in the case of disk damage, is caused by limitation of nerve gliding. For this reason, restoration of nerve-gliding capacity with the help of specific movements is a plausible treatment strategy.

Every movement also involves the movement of neural structures. In a massage, the nerves running through the muscles are moved. Mobilization of the spine also has a mechanical effect on the nerve roots and the central nervous system. With every step, the sacral plexus is lengthened in the free-leg phase and shortened in the engaged leg.

The *gliding* and *tension techniques* have been chiefly used for targeted mobilization of the nervous system (Maitland 1986, 1994; Butler 1998).

Gliding Techniques

Movements of the extremities or the spine are performed in such a way that nerves or nerve roots to be treated are never under complete tension. While a nerve is being extended over a joint, it may be relaxed over the neighboring joint. The movement patterns are taken from the nerve tension tests (straight leg raise, prone knee bend, upper limb tension test, slump; see Chapters 6–8).

Tension Techniques

Movements of the extremities or the spine are performed in such a way that one or more nerves are under maximal tension. The nerve tension tests can be used as movement patterns.

5.5.1 Progressive Steps in Treatment Intensity

The patient is asked to report immediately any changes in symptoms caused by the treatment. The treatment method and intensity are determined by the type and irritability of the symptoms (see Chapter 4 Diagnosis in Physical Therapy). The relevant points here are pain intensity, location, and quality of sensory disorders as well as mobility.

To justify continuation of treatment, pain intensity should be decreasing as a result of physical therapy. Onset or increase of sensory disorders should be avoided. As the sensory disturbance decreases, the proximal border of the disorder shifts distally. Improvement of the quality usually moves from numb to fuzzy, tingling, slightly reduced sensation, to complete recovery. Worsening usually progresses in the opposite order. The range of motion achieved in the nerve tension test without an increase in symptoms provides information about the change in mobility.

Pain caused by nerve mobilization techniques often sets in *several hours after the exercises.* For this reason, therapy must be initiated carefully, with little tension and few repetitions (at first, three repetitions of a movement three times a day). Movements of the extremities are performed fluidly and slowly, without remaining in the painful position. Resistance, evasive movements, and reflex muscle tension must be taken into consideration. Passive movements are more effective and gentler than active movements.

During treatment, the physical therapist moves the patient's arms or legs and the patient tries to relax. Then the patient is taught to do the exercises on their own. Mobilization of the unaffected extremity often has a positive effect on the symptoms. Just as a nerve extension pain can be triggered in the affected extremity by moving the unaffected extremity (see Chapter 4 Diagnosis in Physical Therapy), the right amount of movement in the unaffected extremity can also have a positive effect on the affected side. This effect can be explained by the tension on the affected nerve root that arises when the unaffected extremity is moved.

In a very irritable situation, treatment takes place far away from the suspected trigger of the symptoms (e.g., dorsal extension of the ankle joint in the case of lumbar disk prolapse) so that no additional symptoms are triggered. As soon as the symptoms only occur as a result of intensive movement and then rapidly disappear, the movement can also take place in the anatomical area of the suspected triggering structures.

The next step of the treatment is to increase the number of repetitions. Then the movement is performed with more tension, and the pain or sensory disorder triggered at the end of the movement is tolerated. All symptoms elicited by therapy should disappear immediately after the therapeutic movement is ended.

5.6 Assessment of the Therapy and Evaluation of a Possible Change of Treatment Strategy

To keep the period of the patient's discomfort as short as possible and to avoid the chronification of pain, it should be determined after the fifth therapy session whether the result of treatment is satisfactory or whether a change seems indicated. If necessary, the diagnosis should be reviewed. In case of chronic, therapy-resistant pain, not only surgery but also treatment of psychosocial aspects of the disease should be considered (see Chapter 11 Psychosocial Risk Factors).

Target Parameters that Should Be Achieved by Physical Therapy after 5 Days

The goals listed below are accepted as evaluation criteria in clinical practice. The decision as to whether the progress of therapy is satisfactory also depends on the personality and expectations of the patient. Sometimes satisfaction does not correlate with objectivizable parameters. Patients who are almost free of symptoms can be dissatis-

fied because they still feel they have a disability. On the other hand, some patients are satisfied with a noticeable improvement although they have not yet reached their goal. Patience and the willingness to tolerate disability and pain for a certain length of time while collaborating actively in one's own recovery are necessary for the success of conservative therapy.

Note:
Target parameters after 5 days:

- Centralization of radiating pain (measured in centimeters on day 1 and day 5, distance on the skin from the point of the most distal pain projection to the affected spinal segment) by at least 20%.
- Pain reduction: reduction of the maximal pain in the last 24 hours on the visual or numeric analog scale (VAS) by at least 50%.
- Improved nerve extension signs: the straight leg raise test can be measured in centimeters and should achieve an increase of 50%.
- Reduction of pain duration (in hours) per day by 50%.
- Change or peripheralization of sensory disorders by at least 5 cm.
- Muscle function test (MFT): improvement of possible loss of strength level by one category (see Chapters 3 and 4).

Summary:
Progress and Goal Setting of the Physical Therapy Treatment Plan

- A detailed physical therapy diagnosis is made before the therapeutic exercises are begun.
- Therapy begins immediately after the onset of acute symptoms so that the patient is not subjected to a waiting period.
- The first five therapy sessions are conducted on 5 successive days.
- The duration of the sessions depends on individual need; a period of 30 to 60 minutes is usually appropriate.
- A diagnosis is documented at every therapy session and the effect of the exercises is monitored according to specific target parameters.
- Useless and damaging procedures are not repeated.
- The patient is instructed to collaborate in the healing process actively and responsibly.
- The patient is guided from the acute phase through stabilization and restoration of function to reintegration into normal daily living.
- The total number of necessary therapy sessions depends on the severity of the symptoms and individual tendency to healing.

- After termination of the treatment, the patient should be able to work, perform activities of daily living without limitations, and be satisfied.
- The patient should be able to exercise independently and prevent relapses.
- The patient should no longer need to call on the healthcare system.

5.7   Indications for Surgery

There is controversy in the literature about the indications for disk prolapse surgery as the most appropriate treatment. There is also a difference of opinion about the best time to decide for or against an operation.

According to international consensus, surgery is indicated for the following neurological disorders (Weber 1983; Bush et al 1992; AWMF 2012; Vroomen et al 2000; Witt and Stöhr 2003):
- Bladder and bowel disorders.
- Saddle anesthesia.
- Disorders in the legs in case of prolapsed disk in the cervical and thoracic spine.
- Sudden onset of paralysis or high-grade paresis.
- Therapy-resistant pain.

In patients with radicular pain, paresis, or sensory disorders, it is possible to determine after five therapy sessions whether there has been satisfactory improvement in the symptoms or whether the patient should be advised to have an operation (Brötz et al 2003; Brötz, Burkard, et al 2010). In the United States, many authors recommend 6 to 12 weeks of conservative therapy before disk surgery (Weber 1983; Saal and Saal 1989; Cherkin et al 1994; Postacchini et al 2002). In the Netherlands, most patients with nerve root compression only receive an operation after the disease has lasted for 4 to 6 weeks (Vroomen et al 2000).

Some literature also recommends several weeks of conservative therapy in patients with disk prolapse and radicular syndrome before a decision is made to operate (Witt and Stöhr 2003). The severity and duration of paresis are discussed as criteria (Weber 1983; Saal and Saal 1989, Saal et al 1990; Dubourg et al 2002; Postacchini et al 2002). There is no agreement about the extent to which imaging procedures can lead to an indication for surgery (Saal and Saal 1989; Bush et al 1992; Deyo and Phillips 1996).

Studies comparing the results of conservative versus operative treatment of disk prolapse were conducted (Weber 1983; Weinstein 2006a, 2006b; Peul 2007). However, precise data for the parameters discussed above are missing from this work.

Thus it is hardly possible to support the establishment of indications for surgery on scientifically controlled data. This can also be seen in the differing operation rates: in the United States, surgical treatment was twice as frequent as in most European countries and five times as frequent as in the United Kingdom (Deyo and Phillips 1996).

When the symptoms correlate with the disorders depicted by imaging, patients who expressly ask for surgery are operated on even when there is no urgent indication according to the above-mentioned criteria. However, the idea of some patients, that an operation will provide a rapid and sustainable solution to their problems without any further effort, is unrealistic (Jonsson and Stromqvist 1993; Johannsen et al 1994; Barlocher et al 2000; Nygaard et al 2000; Atlas et al 2001; Yorimitsu et al 2001).

Retrospectively, patients who do not benefit satisfactorily from conservative therapy have certain features in common. The following aspects decrease the probability of successful conservative therapy in patients with lumbar disk prolapses:
- Lumbar spinal canal stenosis (Saal and Saal 1989; see 5.1 Overview).
- Constantly reduced straight leg raise test (Bush et al 1992; see 5.1 Overview).
- Female gender (Bush et al 1992).
- Advanced age (Bush et al 1992).

5.8   Postoperative Therapy

There are many surgical procedures and this produces great variety in the extent and invasiveness and associated tissue injury. No specific postoperative therapy program has been defined and evaluated scientifically in a controlled fashion. Thus suggestions for the patient's postoperative conduct and physical therapy represent the individual opinions of the department's surgeons and physical therapists. They range from recommending normal movement and load from the first postoperative day to prescribing a corset or a cervical collar, both of which prevent any movement (Carragee et al 1996).

On the basis of a systematic literature review on the topic of rehabilitation after lumbar disk prolapse surgery, Ostelo et al (2007) came to the following results. There is no evidence for the need to limit activity, and an intensive training program is useful, especially when started 4 to 6 weeks after the operation. The authors found no evidence supporting or disputing the effect of starting an intensive training program immediately after the operation. Yet, a randomized study of active training immediately after the operation for a lumbar disk prolapse showed better results for the following criteria for patients (n = 29) who moved early and intensively than for patients (n = 31) who started with a less intensive program: in the straight leg raise test 3 weeks after the operation, pain intensity 6 and 12 weeks after the operation, spinal mobility 12 weeks after the operation, and satisfaction with the result of surgery 2 years postoperatively (Kjellby-Wendt and Styf 1998).

Carragee et al (1996), in a prospective, nonrandomized study in the United States, examined 50 consecutive patients with neuroradiologically confirmed disk prolapse with and without neurological deficits. All patients had undergone open microscopic disk surgery. They received no postoperative physical therapy but only the instruction to move and undergo spinal stress without limitation. The average duration of disability was only 1.7 weeks. Twenty-five percent of the employed patients returned to work on the next working day (operation on Friday, resumption of work on the following Monday). After an average of 3.8 years, two patients had reduced their workload and three patients took pain medication every day. The remaining patients who had been employed at the beginning of the study (n = 46) were able to pursue their work as usual.

The data collected by Carragee et al (1996) suggest that postoperative physical therapy is not necessary. However, other retrospective, prospective, and randomized studies of patients who had undergone open lumbar disk surgery showed a longer (41–260 days) postoperative period of disability, some with residual pain and relapses (Johannsen et al 1994; Kjellby-Wendt and Styf 1998; Atlas et al 2001; Yorimitsu et al 2001; Weinstein et al 2006a, 2006b).

For this reason, the subjective and quantifiable parameters of pain intensity, pain location, muscle strength, mobility, and nerve extension (see Chapter 4 Diagnosis in Physical Therapy) should be monitored postoperatively and the attempt should be made to treat deficits with physical therapy if appropriate.

The goals of physical therapy are the shortest possible disability time, prevention of chronification of pain persisting after surgery, as well as prevention of limitations in the activities of daily living and relapses.

As soon as the surgeon permits movement of the spine, these movements should be practiced. Spinal extension is an important target movement after surgery as well. At first, flexion should be avoided in order to prevent relapse and extension stress on the surgical scar and the nervous system.

After the acute phase, movements of the extremities are increased in order to prevent scarring of the nerve roots. This aspect of treatment is particularly important after the operation (Saal et al 1990; Jonsson and Stromqvist 1993; Brotchi et al 1999; Ross 1999; Spencer 1999; Vogelsang et al 1999; Krappel and Harland 2001).

The phases of wound healing must be borne in mind (see Chapter 2 General Principles). In the acute inflammatory phase, approximately the first 5 days, exercises must be performed carefully. It may be that there is still an active anesthetic effect, so that the patient feels no pain. During this period, there is a danger of overloading the newly operated spine, resulting in pain and disorders of wound healing.

These symptoms are frequently observed between the 5th and the 10th postoperative day. From the fifth postoperative day, stress in the form of intensive exercise and distance walked is increased. The course of therapy is then largely the same as for conservative treatment (see Chapters 6–8 for guidelines for the treatment of the individual regions of the spine).

6   Lumbar Spine

Pain syndromes occur most frequently in the lumbar spine. Consequently, the pathologies related to this region are the most studied. Disk damage in the lumbar spine is most frequent at the intervertebral levels L4–L5 and L5–S1.

> **Definition of Lumbago:** Back or low back pain. The pain is felt centrally in the spine.

> **Definition of Sciatica:** This refers to low back pain radiating to the buttocks, hips and/or the outer side of the legs, along the course of the sciatic nerve.

In this chapter, we will describe the physical examination and diagnostic tests for the lumbar spine, the evaluation criteria for establishing a physical therapy diagnosis, and the therapy for lumbar disk damage.

6.1   Diagnostic Assessment Form for the Lumbar Spine (Fig. 6.1a–d)

General guidelines for filling out the diagnostic assessment form are given in Chapter 4 Diagnosis in Physical Therapy. This includes information about the individual and the medical history (**Fig. 6.1a, c**), the body diagram (**Fig. 6.1b**), and documentation of pain and sensory disorder (**Fig. 6.1d**). For better understanding, some information from Chapter 4 and Chapter 5 Therapy will be repeated here.

> The diagnostic assessment form can be downloaded as a PDF file at www.mediacenter.thieme.com.

6.2   Diagnosis by Observation

Standing posture and gait sequence are evaluated in the physical examination.

Shift

In pathologies of the lumbar spine, shift is recognized by a lateral displacement of the shoulder girdle with respect to the pelvis (see Chapter 4, **Fig. 4.1**). The free space between the hanging arms and the trunk and pelvis as well as the distance of the hands from the thigh can serve as evaluation criteria. Upon left shift, the left arm is visibly further away from the trunk, hip, and thigh than the right.

Lumbar Lordosis

The normal convexity of the lumbar spine toward the abdomen is called lumbar lordosis; the individual variations are manifold. Nevertheless, it is possible to identify clear deviations from normal. Loss of the lumbar lordosis is typical for patients with disk damage (see Chapter 4, **Fig 4.1**). Patients look as though they are bending forward.

Limping

Limping is characterized by an asymmetrical gait. It has various forms and causes, and the following three aspects are considered:
- Stride length (free leg phase).
- Duration of engaged leg phase.
- Muscle function (e.g., missing push-off, paresis of dorsal foot flexor).

Usually there is a correlation between a shortened stride and a positive nerve extension sign (straight leg raise), which can be explained as pain provocation triggered by pull on the nerve root. This pain is not provoked in standing position.

A shortened engaged leg phase is normally correlated with a definite increase in symptoms under weight-bearing and can thus also be felt when the patient is standing symmetrically. Some patients exhibit both a shortened stride and shortened

Diagnostic assessment—lumbar spine a

Name: _____
Date: _____

Admission data
Therapist: _____

Referral diagnosis on registration: _____

Date of birth: _____

Occupation, hobby: _____

Posture, weight-bearing: _____

On sick leave since: _____

Causative factors: _____

Duration of current episodes: _____

Development: better/same/worse:
Prior treatment of current episode: physical therapy/fango/massage/sling table/
chiropractic/injections/medications/other
Medications: benzodiazepines/NSAIDs/steroids since: _____

Prior history: _____

Physical therapy diagnosis: _____

Justification of diagnosis: _____

Diagnostic assessment—lumbar spine b

Name: _____
Date: _____

Body diagram

Markings: ///// Pain ::::: Sensory disorder
Alternatively, pain is marked in red and sensory disorders are marked in blue

Diagnostic assessment—lumbar spine c

Name: _____
Date: _____
Better: Night/morning/daytime/evening/at rest/while moving/
stooping/stretching/sitting/lying down/standing/walking
Worse: Night/morning/daytime/evening/at rest/while moving
stooping/stretching/sitting/lying down/standing/walking
Coughing/sneezing/straining
Trauma: _____
Operation: _____
Unwanted weight loss   yes/no (_____ kg in _____ weeks)
Reaction to repeated, end-range movements
Starting situation: _____

| Moving | NT, CE, EL, PR, PE, NE,↑↓ | RI, RW, RNI, RNW |
	Change during movement	Change after movement
Prone, lower arm support		
1 × extension lying down		
5 × extension lying down		
1 × rotation lying down knee R		
5 × rotation lying down knee R		
1 × rotation lying down knee L		
5 × rotation lying down knee L		
1 × flexion lying down		
5 × flexion lying down		
1 × extension standing		
5 × extension standing		
1 × flexion standing		
5 × flexion standing		
Other:		

Diagnostic assessment—lumbar spine: follow-up d

Name: _____
Date: _____
Medications: benzodiazepines/NSAIDs/steroids   Shift: R   L
                                                  Limping: Yes no
Lordosis: normal/accentuated/reduced   Distance walked:
Pain: record area, activity or posture and intensity

0 1 2 3 4 5 6 7 8 9 10   0 1 2 3 4 5 6 7 8 9 10
Before PT   After PT

0 1 2 3 4 5 6 7 8 9 10   0 1 2 3 4 5 6 7 8 9 10
Maximal   Minimal   in the last 24 hours
Pain radiation in cm before PT _____ after PT _____
Sensory disorder
Area: _____
Characteristics: _____   better/same/worse
Muscle function test

	R	L			R	L
L3 adductors			Quadriceps			
L4 quadriceps			Tibialis anterior			
L5 extensor hallucis longus			Adductors			
S1 triceps surae			Adductors			

Signs of nerve extension

SLR right:		SLR left:	
PKB right:		PKB left:	

Mobility

Flexion	Extension	Rotation:	Shift/Translation
Finger to floor distance		Knee R	R
		Knee L	L

Fig. 6.1 (a–d) Diagnostic assessment form for the lumbar spine.
(NT = not tested; CE = centralized; EL = eliminated; PR = produced; PE = peripheralized; NE = no effect; ↑ = pain increases;
↓ = pain decreases; RI = remains improved; RW = remains worse; RNI = remains not improved; RNW = remains not worse;
R = right; L = left; PT = physical therapy; SLR = straight leg raise; PKB = prone knee bend.)

duration of the engaged leg phase. The effect of paresis on the gait will be described with the muscle function tests.

6.3 Diagnostic Tests

The diagnostic tests include muscle function and nerve tension tests as well as spinal test movements.

6.3.1 Muscle Function Tests

At the first examination of every patient, the segment-indicating muscles for nerve roots L4, L5, and S1 are tested. If there is a suspicion of compression of another root or a neuroradiologically diagnosed prolapsed disk at a different level, the corresponding segment-indicating muscles are also tested. The sides are compared by testing the individual normal range of motion and the individual normal strength.

Testing and Evaluation

Triceps Surae (S1)
- One-leg stand.
- The therapist supports the patient at the thoracic spine and sternum so that they do not lose their balance.
- The patient raises the heel from the floor (raising the body weight) as high as possible, with the knee extended.

Evaluation
- Full strength 5/5: full range of motion repeated five times.
- 4/5:
  – Heel raised fewer than five times.
  – Slight heel raise.
  – Ability to keep the heel off the floor when the lift was accomplished with additional push-off with the other leg.
- 3/5: examination in supine position: five times full range of motion in plantar flexion of the ankle against strong resistance over the range and at the end.

Note: The full strength of the triceps surae muscle cannot be tested with manual resistance, since the muscle is strong enough to lift the entire body weight against gravity. For this reason, an examiner of average strength is not able to challenge the muscle with the short lever of the foot.

- 2/5: examination in lateral recumbent position: full range of motion without gravity.
- 1/5: a contraction of the triceps surae can be detected by palpation of the tendon over the calcaneus and of the calf muscle.
- 0/5: no palpable contraction.

Gait with Paresis

Paresis of the plantar flexors causes decrease or disappearance of the push-off (forward movement of the body weight with the help of foot plantar flexion) at the end of the stance phase. The absence of the push-off phase shortens the stance phase on the affected side and the step length on the unaffected side.

Extensor Hallucis Longus (L5)
- Standing or supine.
- The patient raises the great toe with the ankle in midposition between dorsal extension and plantar flexion.
- The therapist applies resistance at the terminal joint.

Evaluation
- Full strength 5/5: five times full range of motion against strong resistance over the range and at the end.

Note: It is best to perform the full strength 5/5 test of the extensor hallucis longus simultaneously on both sides, so that mobility and strength can best be compared.

- 4/5: full range of motion against moderate resistance over the range and at the end.
- 3/5: full range of motion against gravity.
- 2/5: examination in lateral recumbent position: full range of motion without gravity.
- 1/5: a contraction of the extensor longus can be detected by palpation of the tendon over the dorsal side of the metatarsophalangeal joint and at the back of the foot.
- 0/5: no palpable contraction.

Gait with Paresis

An isolated toe extensor paresis usually does not alter the gait. In high-grade paresis, the gait resembles the gait in foot extensor paresis.

Tibialis Anterior (L4)

- Standing or supine.
- The patient raises the dorsum of the foot.
- The therapist applies resistance distally at the dorsum of the foot.

Evaluation

- Full strength 5/5: five times full range of motion against strong resistance over the range and at the end.

⬛ **Note:** Evaluation of full strength development of the tibialis anterior is only possible when the patient is standing.

- 4/5: full range of motion against moderate resistance over the range and at the end.
- 3/5: full range of motion against gravity.
- 2/5: examination in lateral recumbent position: full range of motion without gravity.
- 1/5: a contraction of the tibialis anterior can be detected by palpation of the tendon medially on the dorsal side of the ankle and of the lateral shin muscles.
- 0/5: no palpable contraction.

Test of Walking on the Heels

The heel walk test is quick to administer; in previously diagnosed paresis, it is a helpful parameter for monitoring progression or remission. To evaluate full strength, the dorsal foot extension test must be performed against resistance in the standing position.

Gait with Paresis

Paresis of the foot dorsiflexor is marked by repeated stumbling, shuffling, or excessive raising of the whole leg.

Quadriceps Femoris (L3, L4)

- Supine: the patient abducts the leg to be tested and bends the knee such that the thigh is lying on the bed and the lower leg is moved next to the edge of the bed, toward the floor.
- The patient extends the knee joint.

- The therapist applies resistance to extension of the knee joint at the ankle.

Evaluation

- Full strength 5/5: five times full range of motion against strong resistance over the range and at the end.
- 4/5: full range of motion against moderate resistance over the range and at the end.
- 3/5: full range of motion against gravity.
- 2/5: examination in lateral recumbent position: full range of motion without gravity.
- 1/5: a contraction of the quadriceps femoris can be detected by palpation of the tendon between the patella and the tibial tuberosity and of the muscles at the anterior aspect of the thigh.
- 0/5: no palpable contraction.

Test of the Function "Stepping onto a Chair"

This also tests the hip muscles.

⬛ **Note:** In an L3 root compression with hip flexors and adductor weakness, stepping onto a chair even with full strength in the thigh extensors is not possible without difficulty. Thus, if a patient cannot step onto a chair equally well with both legs, the quadriceps femoris and the hip muscles are tested individually.

Evaluation

Full strength 5/5: step onto the chair five times without gathering momentum.

Gait with Paresis

A knee extensor paresis can be seen in stair climbing. Exending the upper leg is achieved with a powerful push-off (momentum) with the lower, unaffected leg.

In high-grade paresis, it is impossible to climb stairs.

Adductor Magnus and Adductor Brevis (L3, L4)

- Lateral recumbent position: the leg to be tested is underneath.
- The therapist holds the upper leg in a slightly abducted position.
- The patient raises the lower leg with hip and knee joints extended and in adduction.
- The therapist applies resistance to the adduction at the knee joint.

Evaluation

- Full strength 5/5: five times full range of motion against strong resistance over the range and at the end.
- 4/5: full range of motion against moderate resistance over the range and at the end.
- 3/5: full range of motion against gravity.
- 2/5: examination in supine position: full range of motion without gravity.
- 1/5: contraction of the adductors can be felt by palpation of the muscles of the inner thigh.
- 0/5: no palpable contraction.

Gait with Paresis

With paresis of the adductors, the walking base is wide. When climbing stairs or stepping onto a chair, the leg cannot move securely and the knee deviates outward.

Iliopsoas (L2, L3)
- Supine.
- The patient bends the hip and knee joints.
- The therapist applies resistance to the hip flexion at the knee joint.

Evaluation

- Full strength 5/5: five times full range of motion against strong resistance over the range and at the end.
- 4/5: full range of motion against moderate resistance over the range and at the end.

> **Note:** In a case of confirmed or suspected disk damage and acute pain, the iliopsoas test can usually not be conducted to the limit of motion or with maximal resistance. End-range hip flexion triggers an associated movement of lumbar spine flexion. Where there is disk damage, flexion usually intensifies pain and testing should not be enforced. At the same time, the iliopsoas can exert tension via its attachment at the vertebral bodies and transverse processes of the lumbar vertebrae, thus causing pain.

- 3/5: full range of motion against gravity.
- 2/5: examination in lateral recumbent position: full range of motion without gravity.
- 1/5: a contraction of the iliopsoas can be detected by palpation of the tendon distal to the inguinal ligament and medial to the sartorius muscle.
- 0/5: no palpable contraction.

Gait with Paresis

In hip flexor paresis, the leg is moved forward in the swing phase by straightening the pelvis (flexion) and by ventral forward rotation of the affected side of the pelvis.

6.3.2   Nerve Tension Test of the Lower Extremity

> **Note**
> - Nerve tension tests are always conducted on both sides.
> - Where there is radiating pain, the unaffected leg is tested first.
> - Contralateral pain in which, during testing of the unaffected leg, the pain is intensified on the affected side, can be a sign of disk prolapse.

Raising the Extended Leg (Straight Leg Raise Test, Lasègue Sign)

This test tenses the following nerve roots and peripheral nerves:
- Nerve roots L5 and S1.
- Sciatic nerve.
- Sacral plexus.
- Tibial nerve.
- Peroneal nerve.

The pain of nerve extension can be felt in the lumbar spine and along the entire anatomic course of the peripheral nerves listed above (buttocks, middle of the posterior thigh, hollow of the knee, calf). A sensory disorder can be triggered or intensified in the area supplied by the affected nerve root, most frequently in the foot.

Instructions for the Patient
- I will raise your leg.
- Leave it quite loose.
- I will perform the movement slowly.
- You may feel pulling or pain.
- Please tell me when the movement becomes unpleasant. Then I will stop.

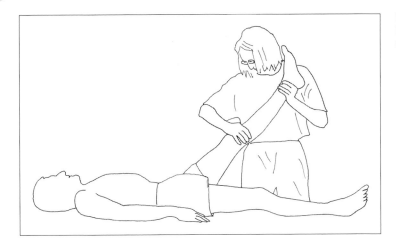

Fig. 6.2 Performing the straight leg raise test (SLR) or Lasègue sign.

- Please tell me if pain occurs or is intensified on the other side (in one-sided pain and during testing of the unaffected side).
- Please tell me where the pain sets in.

Implementation (Fig. 6.2)
- The patient is lying flat on their back.
- The spine is straight, without tilting to the side.
- No cushion under the body.
- The patient places their hands next to their body or on their stomach.
- The therapist moves the patient's knee into end-range extension (one hand above or below the intra-articular space of the knee, the other placed dorsally at the ankle).
- The therapist slowly raises the leg, which is in end-range knee joint extension, passively and straight up.
- No abduction or adduction, no inward or outward rotation of the hip joint.

Observations and Criteria for Stopping the Test Movement
- *Avoidance movements:*
  - Movement of the occiput toward the shoulder girdle.
  - Inclination of part or all of the spine toward the side being tested.
  - Ventral raising of the pelvis on the side being tested.
- *Resistance:* normal elastic end of movement.

- *Reflex muscle tension:*
  - Suddenly perceptible end of movement.
  - Jerky tension of the hip extensors and knee flexors.

The test is evaluated as *positive* in the following cases:
- The symptoms familiar to the patient are reproduced or intensified.
- A postural response is distinctly visible; for example, neck extension.
- A distinct side difference occurs.

The nerve plexuses and peripheral nerves into which nerve roots L5 and S1 run (lumbosacral plexus, sciatic nerve, tibial and peroneal nerves) pass through the ischiocrural muscles. When there is doubt in differentiating between a nerve extension pain and a muscle extension pain of the ischiocrural muscles, additional distinguishing tests (Breig and Troup 1979; see Chapter 12 Selected Studies on the Topic of Spinal Disorders) are performed.

Note
- On adduction and inward rotation of the hip, tension on nerve roots L5 and S1 and the lumbosacral plexus is increased. An increase of pain in the dorsal thigh while these additional movements are performed could also be interpreted as muscle extension pain in the ischiocrural muscles because of anatomical proximity.

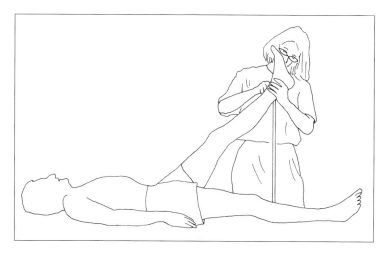

Fig. 6.3 Measuring the straight leg raise.

- Additional increase of pain during dorsal extension of the foot is more than likely due to nerve extension pain.
- An increase of pain in the leg during passive neck flexion can also not be interpreted as muscle extension pain but is probably the result of intensified tension on nervous system structures that is conducted by the dura mater to the nerve roots and the peripheral nerves.

Measuring the Straight Leg Raise Test (Fig. 6.3)

- The straight leg raise test is measured as the distance in centimeters between the outer malleolus and the table, using a rigid meter stick.
- Alternatively, a device that measures angles (inclinometer, goniometer, angle measuring device) can be applied to the extended leg.

Prone Knee Bend Test (PKB)

This nerve tension test tenses the following nerve roots and peripheral nerves:
- Nerve roots L1–L4.
- Lumbar plexus.
- Femoral nerve.

The pain of nerve extension can be felt in the lumbar spine and along the entire extent of the femoral nerve (groin, anterior thigh, inner calf). A sensory disorder can be triggered or intensified in the area supplied by the affected nerve root.

Administration and Measurement of the Prone Knee Bend Test (Fig. 6.4)

- The patient is lying on their stomach.
- The spine is straight, without tilting to the side.
- No cushion under the body.

Fig. 6.4 Prone knee bend test.

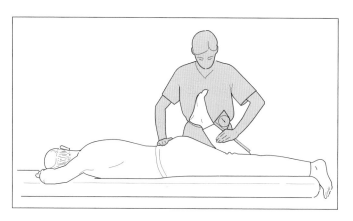

- The therapist slowly bends the patient's knee.
- At the same time, the therapist holds the patient's pelvis in place, with one hand on the sacrum to prevent a dorsal avoidance movement of the pelvis.
- The test is measured as the distance in centimeters between the heel and the sciatic tubercle, using a rigid meter stick.
- Alternatively, an inclinometer can be applied to the calf as it is raised.

Observations and Criteria for Stopping the Test Movement

- *Avoidance movements:*
  - Movement of the occiput toward the shoulder girdle.
  - Inclination of part or all of the spine toward the side being tested.
  - Dorsal raising of the pelvis on the side being tested.
- *Resistance:* normal elastic end of movement.
- *Reflex muscle tension:*
  - Suddenly perceptible end of movement.
  - Jerky tension of the hip flexors and knee extensors.

The test is evaluated as *positive* in the following cases:
- The symptoms familiar to the patient are reproduced or intensified.
- A postural response is distinctly visible, for example, neck extension.
- A distinct side difference occurs.

Differentiation between a nerve extension pain in the femoral nerve and a muscle extension pain in the quadriceps femoris (especially the rectus femoris) is difficult because of overlapping pain locations (groin, anterior thigh).

Note: Contralateral pain when the unaffected leg is bent, spinal pain, avoidance movement in the form of lateral tilt of the spine toward the side being tested (approximation within the nervous system), and distinct asymmetry of responses to the test are signs of nerve extension pain.

6.3.3   Test and Therapeutic Spinal Movements

In very irritable symptoms, that is, symptoms whose intensity is easily influenced, the tests should first be administered exclusively in recumbent position, without loading. If this does not yield sufficient diagnostic information, if the problems are not irritable, additional testing can be administered with loading, in standing position. If the problems are irritable, the pain usually increases under loading, so that test movements in standing position are not possible.

With the help of test movements, spinal mobility and the effect on the symptoms—especially pain—of repeated spinal movements are studied.

Evaluation of Mobility

Spinal mobility in flexion and extension is documented in the first therapy session. Rotational mobility is recorded as a test movement if the rotation test is considered useful. Translational mobility of the shoulder girdle with respect to the pelvis is tested if the patient exhibits a shift in their spontaneous posture or if there are therapy-resistant asymmetrical pains.

Spinal mobility can be evaluated without complicated measurement devices (for measures of free mobility see Chapter 6.5.8).

Observation of whether mobility is limited and whether mobility changes during exercise and in correlation with pain is decisive for diagnosis and treatment in the acute phase.

Flexion

The *finger to floor distance in spinal flexion* is a useful, measurable parameter for determining mobility. The factors that affect the finger to floor distance in spinal flexion include mobility of the lumbar spine, the hip joints, the nervous system, and the ischiocrural muscles as well as the relationship among arm, trunk, and leg length. The finger to floor distance in flexion is a measure of the patient's overall mobility. The measurement method must be standardized:
- The patient is standing.
- Their feet are parallel, one foot-width apart.
- The knee joints are extended and remain so during the movement.
- The patient is asked to bend forward as far as possible.
- The arms hang down vertically.
- As soon as the patient feels the accustomed pain or the pain increases, they should stop the movement.
- The distance of the index finger of the right hand from the floor is measured.

In addition to the finger to floor distance, the curvature of the lumbar spine is observed. A physiological flexion eliminates the lumbar lordosis and the silhouette of the spine forms a fluid line from the pelvis to the cervical spine (see **Fig. 6.33d**).

Extension

Spinal mobility in extension is tested with the patient in prone position or when they first prop themselves up from the prone position. The curvature of the lumbar spine is evaluated here as well (see **Fig. 6.28a**).

Repeated Test Movements

Since in disk damage extension of the affected region of the spine is usually a beneficial movement, it is tested first. If the symptoms are asymmetrical with shift or unilateral back or leg pain, asymmetrical test movements frequently lead to centralization and reduction of pain. For this reason, where symmetrical extension does not produce centralization, unilateral rotation, asymmetrical extension, or shift correction are tested in standing position.

The idea that movements can exert pressure on the injured region of the anulus fibrosus, forcing the gelatinous mass to medial or ventral, is a working hypothesis.

Note: Flexion is not tested unless all other test movements fail to produce centralization or reduction of pain.

The test movements should be passive for the affected section of the spine. This means that the patient is asked to relax the back, abdominal, and hip muscles as much as possible. This is quite possible for tests in recumbent position. If the patient is experiencing significant pain, the therapist can bear the weight of the leg and support the movement in rotation and flexion test movements.

Tempo and rhythm of the movements are slow but fluid. The patient should be able to stop the movement at any time. No momentum should be introduced.

The movements are performed with the greatest *range of motion* possible. If patients stop a movement, they are asked why. Possible reasons are pain, fear of pain, or limited range of motion.

The *intensity* of the test movements is always increased if a certain movement has a centralizing and reducing effect, but the pain has not disappeared completely.

The number of *repetitions* is between 2 and 10. If the pain is intensified or peripheralized by the movement test and remains at this intensity after the movement, the test is repeated twice at most. If the pain is intensified or peripheralized during the movements but returns to its original level and location after the movements, the test can be performed up to 10 times. If the pain is reduced or centralized, the test is performed 10 times.

The patient is asked before, during, and after the test movements where and at what intensity on the numerical analog scale (NAS) they are experiencing pain and whether anything changes in these perceptions. The therapist asks without introducing bias:

- Is your pain changing?
- Where does it hurt now?
- How intense is your pain now?

Note: Avoid leading questions (e.g., Is it getting better now? Does the pain go as far into your leg now?).

Almost every patient is able to assign a number to the pain intensity between 0 (no pain) and 10 (worst pain imaginable). The therapist should insist that the patient makes precise statements about their pain. Statements like "Now it's worse than before" or "It's OK" provide no useful information for planning further treatment.

If, for instance, the back pain has increased but the radiating leg pain has decreased or stopped, this might be more unpleasant for the patient but must be interpreted as an improvement of symptoms. This should be explained to the patient. Usually the patient can tolerate an increase of central pain if the positive aspect of centralization is explained to them.

In addition to documentation of the pain after every test movement, the signs of nerve extension (straight leg raise test, prone knee bend test) are measured and documented and the changes in spinal mobility are evaluated and documented as well. When all test movements have been completed, muscle strength and sensory disorders are tested for quality and location and documented.

Instructions for the Patient
- The test movements should be passive for the spine. Relax the back, abdominal, and hip muscles.
- Move as far as possible.

- Tell me how the intensity and range of your pain are changing.
- Stop the movement if the pain radiates further.

Extension Test

Prone Position (Fig. 6.5)
- Lie in a relaxed position on your stomach.
- Breathe calmly.

Support on Lower Arms (Fig. 6.6)
- Bend the elbows so that they are positioned directly under the shoulders (the way one reads a book at the beach).
- Remain in this position for about three breaths.
- Lie down again—stay loose.
- Repeat.

Hand Support, Extension while Recumbent (Fig. 6.7)
- Place hands under shoulders.
- Slowly extend elbows.
- Keep back and buttock muscles relaxed.
- Push up as far as possible.
- Lie down again—stay loose.
- Repeat.

Increasing Intensity
- At the end of the movement, hold and exhale deeply.
- Lie down again—stay loose.
- Repeat.

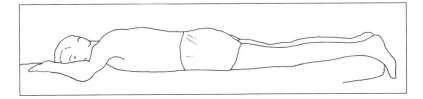

Fig. 6.5 Prone position.

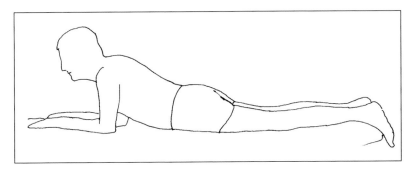

Fig. 6.6 Support on lower arms.

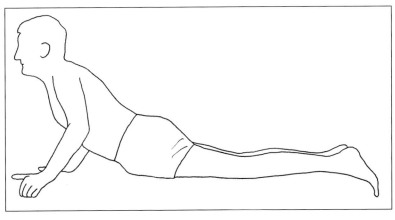

Fig. 6.7 Hand support, extension while recumbent.

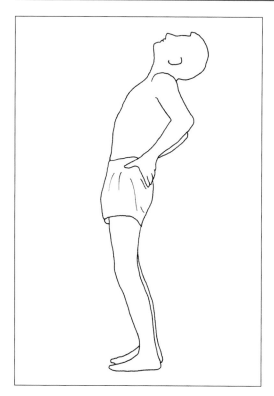

Fig. 6.8 Extension in standing position.

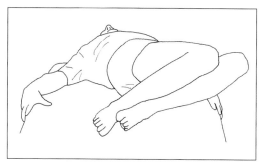

Fig. 6.9 Rotation while recumbent.

Extension in Standing Position (Fig. 6.8)
- Place hands on the back so that the fingertips point to the spine and the thumbs point to the side.
- Extend the back as far back as possible.
- Straighten up.
- Repeat.

Asymmetrical Tests

Rotation while Recumbent (Fig. 6.9)
Rotating the trunk to the unaffected side (both knees to the ipsilateral side) leads to centralization and reduction of pain more frequently than trunk rotation to the affected side (knees to contralateral side):
- Lie supine.
- Place feet next to each other on table.
- No space between the feet.
- Let both knees sink to the same side as far as possible so that the trunk is rotated.
- Return the knees to the middle.
- Repeat.

Simplifications
- For better relaxation of the muscles, the therapist bears the weight of the legs.
- Lateral recumbent position (see Chapter 7, **Fig. 7.6**):
  - Turn the upper body dorsally.
  - Return to the middle.
  - Repeat.

Asymmetrical Prone Position or Extension Recumbent
- Lie prone.
- Bend the leg on the affected side at hip and knee joints to the side, next to the body.
- Relax in recumbent position.

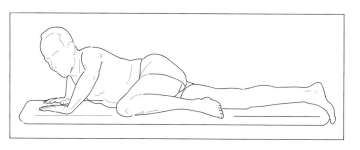

Fig. 6.10 Recumbent extension with knee/hip flexion.

Increasing Intensity

- Place hands at shoulder level.
- Extend the elbows in such a way that the shoulder girdle is slightly raised (the extent of the movement is much less in this position than in symmetrical extension in recumbent position).
- Lie down again—stay loose.
- Repeat.

Extension in Recumbent Position with Pelvis Pushed to the Side (Hips Off Center, Shift Correction in Recumbent Position)

- Prone position.
- Shift pelvis to the side to which the shoulder girdle is displaced in standing position (usually contralateral side). This causes an overcorrection of the shift, that is, a lateral shift of the shoulder girdle with respect to the pelvis in the opposite direction and thus creates ipsilateral lateral pressure on the disks.

Increasing Intensity

- Place hands at shoulder level.
- Extend the elbows so that the upper body is raised and the shifted body position is maintained.
- Lie down again—stay loose.
- Repeat.

Lateral Displacement of the Pelvis in Standing Position (Shift Correction) (Fig. 6.11)

- Standing.
- Stand with the side toward the wall at a distance of about two foot-widths.
- Place the feet directly next to each other.
- Lean the shoulder and upper arm of the side to which the shoulder girdle is displaced with respect to the pelvis against the wall.
- Bend the elbow on this side.
- Let the pelvis sink toward the wall.
- Move it back to the middle.
- Repeat.

Increasing Intensity 1

The further the feet are from the wall, the more intense the effect.

Increasing Intensity 2

- Place the free hand on your back.
- Extend the spine as far as possible (see **Fig. 6.27a**).

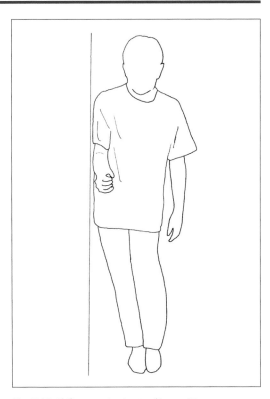

Fig. 6.11 Shift correction in standing position.

Flexion Test

Flexion while Recumbent (Fig. 6.12)

- Lie supine.
- Place one foot next to the other.
- Raise one leg after the other toward the abdomen. During this movement, bear the weight of the legs with the hands at the knees.
- Bend the legs as far as possible.
- Lower the legs as far as the hands can still hold them.
- Repeat.

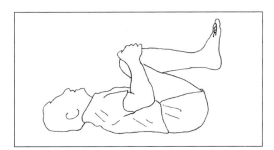

Fig. 6.12 Flexion in supine position.

Simplifications

For better relaxation of the muscles, the therapist bears the weight of the legs.

Flexion in Standing (Fig. 6.13)

- Standing.
- Place the feet two foot-widths apart.
- Bend the spine forward.
- The knees remain extended.
- Straighten up.
- Repeat.

6.4   Establishing the Diagnosis

All findings from the medical history, the visual examination, and the diagnostic tests are taken into account (see **Table 6.1**; for fundamental aspects, see Chapter 4 Diagnosis in Physical Therapy).

The diagnosis should be considered a working hypothesis. Through discussion with the treating physician, it may lead to undertaking further diagnostic or therapeutic measures.

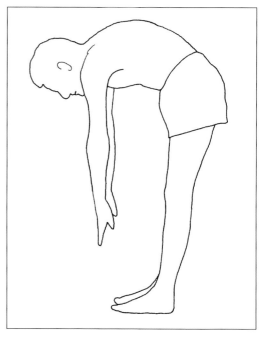

Fig. 6.13 Flexion in standing position.

Table 6.1 Simplified guide to interpreting changes in pain during test movements

Question	Answer	Conclusions
1. Can the problem be influenced mechanically by movement of the lumbar spine?	No	Tumor Inflammatory disease Disease of internal organs Hip disease More examinations **Note:** no mechanical therapy of the lumbar spine
	Yes	**Continue with question 2**
2. Does the same movement always trigger precisely the same pain reaction and does the pain return to its original form thereafter?	Yes	Adherent nerve roots **Note:** mechanical physical therapy Spinal or foraminal stenosis Instability, facet joint pain More examinations **Note:** In cases of stenosis: exercise spinal flexion, posture training In case of instability: stabilizing strength training
	No	**Continue with question 3**
3. Does the pain within one dermatome centralize or peripheralize or does central pain become better or worse from the same movement?	Yes	Disk damage Check for possible disk prolapse **Note:** mechanical physical therapy
	No	**Continue with question 4**

▶ (continued)

Table 6.1 Simplified guide to interpreting changes in pain during test movements (*continued*)

Question	Answer	Conclusions
4. Does the same movement produce differing pain reactions; is the pain immediately afterward the same as before or worse?	Yes	Chronified pain syndrome Psychosocial problem More examinations (see Chapter 11 Psychosocial Risk Factors) **Note:** In chronified pain syndrome: a variety of activations; nonspecific exercise programs, mechanical and strengthening In predominantly psychosocial problems: discuss physical therapy with the treating physician

Summary: Typical Findings in the Diagnosis of Disk Damage

- *Information in the medical history:*
  - Age: 20 to 55 years.
  - Duration: long or short (acute–chronic).
  - Sudden onset.
  - Trigger: stooping.
  - Changes in movement.
  - Constant or intermittent.
- *Character of the complaints:*
  - Pain in the lumbar spine.
  - Pain in the lumbar spine in combination with dermatome-related radiating pain.
  - Dermatome-related radiating pain without pain in the lumbar spine.
  - Dermatome-related sensory disorders.
  - Paresis, chiefly in individual segment-indicating muscles.
- *Visual examination:*
  - Kyphotic/shift deformation.
  - Limited movement.
  - Limping.
- *Behavior of symptoms upon repeated spinal movement:*
  - Rapid change during the movements.
  - The changes persist after the movements.
  - Centralization/peripheralization of the pain.
  - Improvement of mobility with decrease in pain and vice versa.
  - Nerve extension signs better/worse.
- Sensory perception and strength change from day to day, not within one therapy session.

Differential diagnoses (e.g., irritation of the sacroiliac joint, hip arthritis) require special differentiating tests. Findings that are typical in a diagnosis of *lumbar disk damage* cannot be found in these differential diagnoses. Repeated end-range movements of the lumbar spine barely have any effect on symptoms that are caused by irritation of the sacroiliac joint or by hip arthritis (for details of differential tests see the literature for manual diagnosis and treatment, for example the Maitland approach; Maitland 2000).

Disorders frequently associated with disk damage such as spinal and foraminal stenosis, spinal instability, facet joint pain, and an inflamed or fibrosed nerve root also cause certain stereotypical pain reactions (see Chapter 10 Diseases Occurring in Association with Prolapsed Disks).

In physical therapy using repeated spinal movements, the movements that may be beneficial for treatment of disk damage could provoke and intensify symptoms with a different cause (see Chapter 10). This makes successful conservative therapy in this kind of combined disease more difficult.

If the results of diagnostic tests indicate a prolapsed disk as the cause of the symptoms, a determination is made as to whether it is likely that the symptoms could be reducible. If the pain centralizes, there is a great likelihood that conservative treatment will be successful.

In some cases, no movement used in diagnostic testing centralizes or reduces the pain; on the contrary, every movement peripheralizes and intensifies every pain. With this kind of pain, the chances of successful conservative treatment are questionable. Nevertheless, it is reasonable not to make a decision for or against surgery as an alternative to conservative treatment until after five therapy sessions. The assessment of whether the problem can be reduced often changes in the course of treatment.

> **Note:** If signs and symptoms are identified during the physical therapy diagnosis that require immediate surgery (bladder and bowel disorders, saddle anesthesia, sudden paralysis or a high degree of paresis, unbearable pain), the treating physician should be consulted immediately.

6.5 Therapeutic Procedure with a Diagnosis of Disk Damage

Making a treatment plan begins with the question of how the patient will get to daily therapy. The patient's symptoms should not be exacerbated by the trip to therapy. If pain increases during standing, walking, and sitting, the patient may not be able to get to therapy on foot, by public transportation, or car. In such cases, a house call or hospitalization would be reasonable.

In neuroradiologically confirmed disk prolapse with radicular pain radiating to a leg, conservative treatment during a short hospitalization is promising (Brötz et al 2001, 2003, 2010). In this way, it is possible to ensure that the patient is moving appropriately, relieving pressure, and observing the hourly exercise session.

Usually the movement tests permit identification of at least *one specific* movement that improves the symptoms. The patients are asked to repeat the movement on their own every hour, usually 10 times in direct succession, with the greatest range of motion possible.

The therapeutically useful movements change in the course of healing. For instance, at the start one-sided movements are necessary but later they are replaced with symmetrical movements or supplemented with additional movements. For this reason, to begin with, therapy should be administered for *at least 5 consecutive days.*

Optimally, for patients with intense, acute pain, therapy should also be available Saturdays, Sundays, and holidays. If the first treatment occurred on Friday, there should be a telephone query on the following Saturday in any case, concerning the changes in symptoms. It must be determined whether the patient has interpreted the instructions correctly and observed their symptoms precisely. If the symptoms become worse, the exercises are discontinued.

Only *one* exercise for independent practice is changed at a time so that it is clear whether the change has a good or a bad effect on the symptoms. Neither medications nor everyday activities, such as returning to work, should be changed at the same time as the exercises.

Practicing unaccustomed movements can cause new complaints that have nothing to do with disk injuries. Thus, in practicing spinal extension, the thoracic spine is also extended. This unaccustomed movement can often cause diffuse pain in the thoracic spine. In most patients, repeated extensions in prone position cause sore pectoralis and elbow extensor muscles. The patient should be informed that these new complaints are to be expected and that they are a normal development and not dangerous.

Summary: Procedure in the Case of a Reducible Disk Problem

- *In the first 5 days:*
  - Acute pain with rapid changes.
  - The pain centralizes when the spine is moved and remains improved after the movements.
  - Well-being and signs such as the straight leg raise test and lumbar spine mobility improve.
- *Weeks 2 to 3:*
  - Medications should be discontinued.
  - The improvements in well-being and signs and symptoms stabilize with decreased to absent pain without rapid worsening on loading.
- *Weeks 3 to 6:* restoration of the original capacity and ability to work with normal psychosocial integration are the goal.
- *After 6 weeks:* activities of daily living, which include some preventive exercises, should be restored, with normal capacity to bear loads and stable psychosocial integration.
- *After 1 year:* complete capacity to bear loads, restoration of normal functioning, and complete or extensive reduction of neurological deficits can be expected.

6.5.1 Actively Performed Spinal Movements

Movements of the lumbar spine performed independently by the patient correspond to the previously described test movements. The sequence of exercises can deviate from the sequence of tests. For instance, at the beginning of treatment, asymmetrical movements lead to centralization and reduction of pain while symmetrical extension of the lumbar spine is only introduced after several days for further reduction and elimination of the pain.

In the following, the most frequently useful sequence of therapeutic movements is introduced for patients with lumbar disk prolapse and lumbar pain. The progressive steps of the individual movement directions are the same as those of the test movements.

Symmetrical Extension in Recumbent Position

Prone Position (see Fig. 6.5)
- Lie in a relaxed position on your stomach.
- Breathe calmly.

Support on Lower Arms (see Fig. 6.6)
- Bend the elbows so that they are positioned directly under the shoulders (the way one reads a book at the beach).
- Remain in this position for about three breaths.
- Lie down again—stay loose.
- Repeat 5 to 10 times.

Hand Support, Extension in Prone Position (see Fig. 6.7)
- Place hands under shoulders.
- Slowly extend elbows.
- Keep back and buttock muscles relaxed.
- Push up as far as possible.
- Lie down again—stay loose.
- Repeat 10 times.

Increasing Intensity
- At the end of the movement, hold briefly and exhale deeply.
- Lie down again—stay loose.
- Repeat 10 times.

Symmetrical Extension in Standing Position

Extension in Standing Position (see Fig. 6.8)
- Place hands on the back so that the fingertips point to the spine and the thumbs point to the side.
- Extend the back as far backward as possible.
- Straighten up.
- Repeat 10 times.

Asymmetrical Rotation

Rotation in Recumbent Position

⬦ **Note:** Rotating the trunk to the unaffected side (knees to the ipsilateral side) leads to centralization and reduction of pain more frequently than trunk rotation to the affected side (knees to contralateral side).

Lateral Recumbent Position (see Chapter 7, Fig. 7.6)
- Lie in lateral recumbent position (on the affected side).
- Turn the upper body dorsally.
- Return to the middle.
- Repeat up to 10 times.

Supine Position (see Fig. 6.9)
- Lie supine.
- Place one foot next to the other.
- No space between the feet.
- Let both knees sink to the side as far as possible so that the trunk is rotated.
- Return the knees to the middle.
- Repeat up to 10 times.

Asymmetrical Extension in Recumbent Position

Variation 1: Asymmetrical Extension with Knee and Hip Flexion on the Affected Side (see Fig. 6.10)

Prone Position
- Prone position.
- Bend the leg on the affected side at hip and knee joints to the side, next to the body.
- Lie in relaxed position.

Hand Support
- Place hands at shoulder level.
- Extend the elbow so that the shoulder girdle is somewhat raised.
- Lie down again—stay loose.
- Repeat 10 times.

⬦ **Note:** The range of the motion in asymmetrical extension in recumbent position is significantly smaller than in symmetrical extension in recumbent position.

Variation 2: Extension in Recumbent Position with Pelvis Shifted to Side

Prone Position
- Prone position.
- Shift pelvis to the side to which the shoulder girdle is displaced in standing position (usually

contralateral side). This causes an overcorrection of the shift, that is, a relative lateral displacement of the shoulder girdle with respect to the pelvis in the direction opposite to the shift that can be seen in the standing position. Moreover, this produces ipsilateral lateral pressure, that is, on the side to which the disk has shifted.

Hand Support, Extension in Prone Position

- Place hands at shoulder level.
- Extend the elbows so that the upper body is raised and the shifted body position is maintained.
- Lie down again—stay loose.
- Repeat 10 times.

Asymmetrical Extension in Standing Position

Lateral Displacement of the Pelvis in Standing Position (Shift Correction) (see Fig. 6.11)

- Stand.
- Stand with the side toward the wall at a distance of about two foot-widths.
- The feet are directly next to each other.
- Lean the shoulder and upper arm on the side to which the shoulder girdle is displaced with respect to the pelvis against the wall.
- Bend the elbow on this side.
- Let the pelvis sink toward the wall.
- Move it back to the middle.
- Repeat 10 times.

1. Increasing Intensity

The further the feet are from the wall, the more intense is the effect.

2. Increasing Intensity

- Place the hand away from the wall on the back.
- Extend the spine as far as possible.
- Move it back to the middle.
- Repeat 10 times.

In rare cases, flexion in the first therapy sessions leads to centralization and reduction of pain in patients with disk damage. For this reason, this exercise must be mentioned. Even if flexion is identified as a useful therapeutic movement, the prone position and other progressive steps of symmetrical extension should be checked every day. As soon as rotation or the prone position is possible without increase or peripheralization of pain, flexion is replaced by rotation or extension in recumbent position.

Flexion in Recumbent Position (see Fig. 6.12)

- Lie supine.
- Place one foot next to the other.
- Raise one leg after the other toward the abdomen, bearing the weight of the legs with the hands at the knees, as much as possible.
- Bend the legs as much as possible.
- Lower the legs again as far as the hands can still hold them.
- Repeat up to 10 times.

6.5.2　Spinal Movements Passively Performed on the Patient by the Therapist

In exceptional cases, to intensify the symptom-reducing effects of active movements, passive spinal movements are added from the third therapy session onward. They are classified as *manual therapies* or treatment with the hands. These treatments are divided into *mobilization* and *manipulation*. These two techniques are defined differently in the literature by various authors.

Definitions of Mobilization

- Passive movements performed with a rhythm and range such that the patient can stop them at any time (Maitland 1984, 1994).
- Passive, usually repeated movements at slow speed and gradually increasing amplitude (Bischoff 1994; Sachse 1995).
- Passive movement at low speed within or at the limit of passive mobility (Koes et al 1996).
- One or more movements at a low speed and varying amplitudes within the limit of passive mobility (Hurwitz et al 2002).

Definitions of Manipulation

- 1. Passive movement. 2. Rapid movement with small amplitude that is not necessarily extended to the end of the range of motion. This movement cannot be stopped by the patient (Maitland 1986).

- Pulsed passive movement performed with little force at high speed and low amplitude (Bischoff 1994; Sachse 1995).
- Pulsed movement at high speed, going beyond the passive (limited) range of motion (Koes et al 1996).
- A controlled, pulsed movement performed at high speed and low amplitude (Hurwitz et al 2002).

Summary: Most Important Aspects of the Varying Definitions

- Mobilization: active or passive movement at a low speed within or at the limit of passive mobility. The movement can be interrupted by both the therapist and the patient.
- Manipulation: pulsed passive movement at high speed within or beyond the limit of passive mobility. This movement cannot be interrupted by the patient. Because of the speed it cannot be well controlled by the therapist so that there is a risk of pain and, in rare cases, of structural damage.

The efficacy of spinal manipulation in patients with acute or chronic back pain has not been documented. Some patients do seem to benefit from it but the few existing studies on this topic do not define manipulation (Koes et al 1996). The effect of manipulation in patients with disk prolapse has not been systematically studied.

> **Note:** Since passive thrusting movements are also associated with the danger of a negative effect or tissue injury, this type of manipulative movement, especially in patients with prolapsed disks, is not advisable.

Passive mobilization techniques are only performed here once a direction of movement has been found that centralizes and reduces the pain. The passive movement is oriented in the same direction as the centralizing movement performed by the patient themselves and is intended to intensify the reducing effect of the latter.

Mobilization Techniques

As in the movements performed by the patient themselves, the patient is asked to report any change of symptoms immediately. Passive mobilization is done slowly, rhythmically, and with large amplitude. The number of repetitions is between 5 and 15, depending on the effect.

Patients with pain caused by intervertebral disk damage find it beneficial to carry out extension and rotation mobilization in the prone position with the same rhythm as their breathing. For this reason, pressure is usually applied when the patient is exhaling and released when they are inhaling. Other movements are performed more slowly, without attention to the respiratory rhythm.

The behavior of the symptoms and the range of passive movement determine the amplitude of the mobilization movements. The movements are always returned to the original neutral position. The therapist maintains hand contact with the patient's back.

Instructions for the Patient

- I will move your spine passively.
- Leave it quite loose.
- I will perform the movements very slowly and fluidly.
- You can ask me to stop the movement at any time.
- Tell me how the intensity and location of your pain are changing.

The treatment table is adjusted so that the therapist can maintain the spine in extension. In extension mobilization (**Fig. 6.14**), extension with positive pressure (**Fig. 6.15**), and rotational mobilization in prone position, this is a height at which the table reaches the upper third of the therapist's thigh. In rotational mobilization in supine position, the table is set to the level of the therapist's hip.

Extension Mobilization (Fig. 6.14)

- Prone position.
- The therapist stands next to the treatment table.
- The therapist places their hand closer to the foot of the table on the patient's back such that the therapist's pisiform bone is located approximately on the transverse process of the level to be treated.
- The therapist's other hand is positioned on the contralateral transverse process in such a way that the edges of the two little fingers make a right angle and the pisiform bones lie directly opposite at the level to be treated.
- In the patient's exhalation phase, the therapist exerts a slight, symmetrical pressure with both hands.

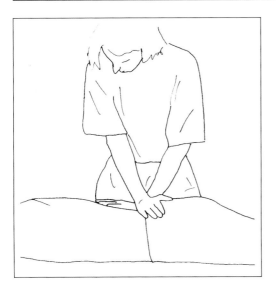

Fig. 6.14 Extension mobilization.

- In the inhalation phase, the therapist releases the pressure without breaking hand contact with the back.
- Repeat approximately 10 times with increasing intensity.
- The neighboring segments are also treated.

Extension in Recumbent Position with Positive Pressure (Fig. 6.15)

- The therapist positions their hands as in extension mobilization and exerts pressure.
- The patient supports themselves on their hands.

- The therapist maintains the pressure and moves their hands and trunk in such a way that the direction of pressure on the patient's spine remains approximately the same.
- The patient returns to prone position.
- The therapist relaxes the pressure.
- Repeat.

Rotation Mobilization

Bilateral Rotation Mobilization in Prone Position

- Prone position.
- The therapist stands next to the treatment table.
- The therapist places their hand closer to the foot of the table on the patient's back such that the therapist's pisiform bone is located approximately on the transverse process of the level to be treated.
- Their other hand is positioned on the contralateral transverse process in such a way that the edges of the two little fingers make a right angle and the pisiform bones lie directly opposite each other at the level to be treated.
- In the patient's exhalation phase, the therapist exerts a slight, asymmetrical pressure with one hand.
- In the inhalation phase, the therapist releases the pressure without breaking hand contact with the back.
- In the next exhalation phase, the pressure is exerted on the other side of the spine.
- Repeat approximately 10 times with increasing intensity.
- The neighboring segments are also treated.

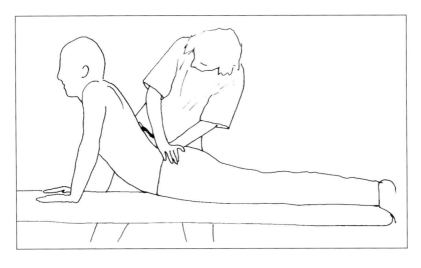

Fig. 6.15 Extension in recumbent position with positive pressure.

Unilateral Rotation Mobilization in Prone Position

- Prone position.
- The therapist stands next to the treatment table on the patient's side that is not to be treated.
- The therapist places one hand on the patient's back such that the therapist's pisiform bone is located approximately on the transverse process of the level to be treated on the contralateral side.
- The therapist places the other hand on the first one.
- In the patient's exhalation phase, the therapist exerts a slight pressure with both hands.
- In the inhalation phase, the therapist releases the pressure without breaking hand contact with the back.
- Repeat approximately 10 times with increasing intensity.
- The neighboring segments are also treated.

Rotation Mobilization in Supine Position (Fig. 6.16)

- Supine position, close to the treatment table edge to which the knees are to be moved.
- The therapist stands on this side, looking at the patient's face.
- The therapist's leg that is closer to the table is positioned forward, the other leg further back (stride position).

- The patient places their feet on the bench one next to the other.
- The therapist lifts both the patient's legs and positions the dorsal aspect of the feet/lower leg in the therapist's groin.
- With one hand the therapist immobilizes the patient's thorax, and with the other moves the knees toward the ground.
- This position is held for a moment.
- Return to the neutral position.
- Repeat.

6.5.3 Passive Leg Movements for Mobilization of the Nervous System

A central emphasis of the treatment concept described here is the patient's independence. If it is possible to reduce the symptoms by means of active measures, passive measures are not employed.

With regard to pain reduction and increasing the range of motion of the affected extremities, passive movements are only more effective than active movements for patients with lumbar and cervical disk prolapse. Consequently, the first point to be tested during physical therapy is the effect of passive mobilization techniques of the nervous system. If passive movements of the legs reduce symptoms and if after therapy the nerve

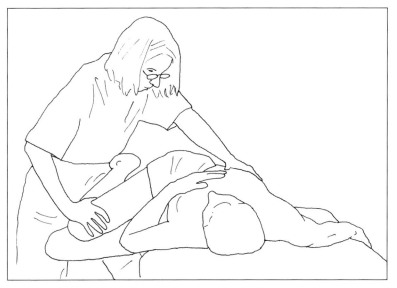

Fig. 6.16 Rotation mobilization in supine position.

tension tests show a greater range of motion than before, they are performed again. In addition, the patient is instructed in appropriate self-training (see 6.5.4 Leg Movements Performed by the Patient for Mobilization of the Nervous System).

The patient is asked to report immediately the changes in symptoms caused by the treatment. The treatment method and intensity are determined by the type and irritability of the symptoms (see Chapter 4 Diagnosis in Physical Therapy). In a very irritable situation, treatment takes place at some distance from the trigger of the symptoms, for instance, dorsal extension of the ankle joint to treat lumbar disk prolapse.

In principle, the unaffected extremity is moved first, without the triggering of additional symptoms. As soon as the symptoms only occur as a result of intensive movement and then rapidly disappear, the movement can also take place in the anatomical area where the symptoms are felt.

The next increase of intensity in the treatment is to increase the number of repetitions. Then the movement is performed with more tension, and the pain or sensory disorder triggered at the end of the movement is accepted.

Note: All symptoms elicited by the therapy should disappear immediately after the therapeutic movement is ended. *Pain* caused by nerve mobilization techniques often sets in *several hours after the exercises.* For this reason, a movement is begun carefully, with low tension, and is not repeated more than three times. Movements of the extremities are performed fluidly and slowly, without remaining in the painful position. Resistance, evasive movements, and reflex muscle tension must be taken into consideration.

Progressive Steps of Passive Movements

Improvement of Mobility in the Straight Leg Raise Test

Step 1

- Supine.
- Dorsal extension of ankle.
- Plantar flexion of ankle.
- Repeat 3 to 10 times.

Step 2

- Supine.
- Hip flexion to 90° and maximal knee flexion.
- Hip and knee extension (the leg is lying on the table again).
- Repeat 3 to 10 times.

Step 3

- Supine.
- Maximal hip and knee flexion.
- Release hip flexion, extend knee.
- Repeat 3 to 10 times.

Step 4

- Supine.
- Maximal hip and knee flexion, dorsal ankle extension.
- Release hip flexion, extend knee, ankle in plantar flexion.
- Repeat 3 to 10 times.

Step 5

- Supine.
- Maximal hip and knee flexion, dorsal ankle extension.
- Release hip flexion, extend knee, maintain ankle in dorsal extension.
- Repeat 5 to 15 times.

Step 6

- Supine.
- Raise the extended leg as in straight leg raise test.
- Lay the leg down in neutral position.
- Repeat 5 to 15 times.

Step 7

- Supine.
- Raise the extended leg in adduction and inward hip rotation.
- Lay the leg down in neutral position.
- Repeat 5 to 15 times.

Improvement of Mobility in the Prone Knee Bend Test

Step 1

- Prone.
- Bend knee and fixate the pelvis such that no hip flexion is possible on the side being tested.

- Return the lower leg to neutral position.
- Repeat 3 to 10 times.

Step 2

- Prone.
- Bend knee and fixate the pelvis such that no hip flexion is possible on the side being tested.
- Keep the knee bent and extend hip joint.
- Return the thigh and lower leg to neutral position.
- Repeat 5 to 15 times.

6.5.4 Leg Movements Performed by the Patient for Mobilization of the Nervous System

If the passive leg movements have reduced symptoms, the patients are given instructions for self-training. The movements that they perform themselves should be associated with as little activity as possible in the leg and trunk muscles. For this reason, it is useful to use a towel or their own hands to bear the weight of the leg and support the movements (see Performance of Sliders below).

The patient is informed that the pain elicited by these exercises sometimes only occurs several hours later or on the day after the exercise. For this reason, it is advisable to begin carefully. At first, the movements are only practiced three times a day with three repetitions for each leg. The movement is first performed with the unaffected leg and then with the affected leg.

Sliders are the movements of the extremities intended to improve the slide capacity of the nerves and nerve roots.

Performance of Sliders (Fig. 6.17a, b)

- Supine position.
- One leg remains extended.
- Flex the other leg in hip and knee toward the abdomen.
- Support the thigh of this leg with a towel or the hands.
- Slowly extend the knee and lower the thigh slightly. Extend the knee until a pulling pain sets in at the back of the leg or the back.
- Immediately flex toward the abdomen again.
- Repeat.
- Change legs.

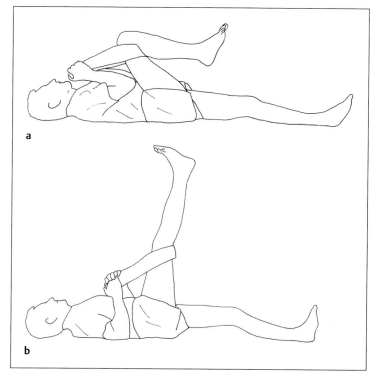

Fig. 6.17 (a, b) Leg movements as self-training for nerve mobilization (sliders).

6.5.5   Posture Correction

As soon as the patient's symptoms have improved and small loads no longer cause or intensify pain, the patient is informed about the advantages of upright posture. If appropriate, the spontaneous posture in walking and standing should be corrected accordingly.

In upright posture, head, shoulder girdle, pelvis, and feet are vertically aligned. The natural curvature of the spine is maintained. This provides even cushioning of a load. The muscles are oriented in their optimal direction of pull and can perform their function with the least effort possible.

When an individual imagines balancing a heavy load on their head, the body automatically moves into an upright position. Muscles of the abdomen and back work together in harmony. Arms and legs can be moved without effort.

Note: Strengthening trunk muscles and lifting posture correction are not advisable until the rehabilitation phase (see Chapter 9 Rehabilitation and Prevention).

6.5.6   Acute Phase

In the acute phase, many patients experience increased pain in standing position and walking, while lying down relieves pain. In that case, the patient should spend a great deal of time lying down. However, strict *bed rest* is usually not helpful because after long periods of lying down, this position too will intensify pain. The phase in which the patient lies in bed almost without interruption should not last longer than 2 to 3 days.

In successful conservative treatment, the distance the patient can walk without enhanced pain increases from day to day, so that the prescription of bed rest is neither necessary nor useful.

Useful Guidelines for Conduct During the Acute Phase

Extending the spine is usually the efficacious direction of movement for the centralization and reduction of pain. If there is a pronounced lateral shift, lateral movements such as rotation or lateral correction in standing position or recumbent are needed before extension. The unfavorable direction of movement is usually spinal flexion.

For this reason, any stooping or flexion of the spine should be temporarily avoided. Since many normal movements in the activities of daily living are associated with stooping, modified forms of these movements, without forward bending, are taught. These activities are chiefly lying down, lying down in and getting up from bed, dressing and undressing, brushing teeth, eating, sitting down and standing up from the toilet, and in some cases, coughing and sneezing.

Lying

In recumbent position, the bed is placed in flat position and at most, a small head pillow is used. As soon as the patient can lie on their stomach without increased pain, they should spend a great deal of time in this position. Patients should only sleep on their stomach, if the neck is used to this sleeping position. The position should be varied occasionally, since movement usually contributes to pain relief.

Maintaining lumbar lordosis is best ensured in flat prone and supine position. In lateral position the head should be positioned in line with the extended back, so that flexion is avoided.

Turning

Turning or rolling from the prone to the supine position and vice versa takes place with extended lumbar spine flat on the bed. For some patients, the normal sequence of movements is to move from one position to the other via the sitting position.

Note: Turning via the sitting position should be avoided as much as possible since this change of position is associated with spinal flexion.

Change of Position

The change of position from *supine* to *sitting* is performed with extended spine via the lateral recumbent position. In learning this unnaturally stiff sequence of movements it helps most patients to imagine that they are moving as though they had swallowed a cane.

Normally, the change of position is less painful to one side than to the other. The preferred direction tends to be the side not affected by the disk damage so this direction should be tried first. If sitting up and lying down using this side is possible without an increase of pain, the patient should always make position changes toward this side for a short while.

Dressing and Undressing

Dressing and undressing (especially socks and shoes) are inevitably associated with flexion of the lumbar spine. Normally, one bends forward in a seated position in order to reach the feet with the hands. This movement should be modified in such a way that the foot that is being dressed is propped on the other thigh. In this process the spine can barely be kept extended or in lordosis because the flexion is transmitted by the hip joint to the pelvis and to the lumbar spine, but the degree of flexion can be minimized.

An alternative is to put on socks in supine position. Slip-on shoes are most suitable. If in spite of modified movements the patient feels increasing pain when putting on and taking off socks and shoes, they should accept help temporarily.

Tooth Brushing

In tooth brushing, strain on the lumbar spine can be reduced by standing with feet far apart and leaning the abdomen against the wash basin, a slight knee bend and support with the free hand. The spine is extended and only bent forward as far as necessary.

Sitting

Sitting is well known as a causative factor for disk prolapse. Even with successful efforts to maintain an erect posture, the lumbar spine is flexed more than in standing position. In addition, in radiating radicular pain while sitting, the irritated nerve in the region of the buttocks and the thigh, especially at the anterior edge of the sitting surface, is subjected to a pressure strain.

Sitting tends to produce and intensify pain in patients with lumbar disk prolapse. This is often only noticed when standing up. For this reason, all patients with lumbar disk damage should be advised to avoid sitting for the time being. If sitting is unavoidable (e.g., at work or while commuting to physical therapy) it is best to sit upright, with the support of a lumbar roll (see Chapter 9 Rehabilitation and Prevention).

Dining

For the time being, meals are taken while recumbent or standing, in order to avoid sitting. When eating in the lateral recumbent position, it is usually better to lie on the unaffected side.

Going to the Toilet

Since sitting on the toilet is unavoidable, the lumbar spine should be kept as extended as possible. When sitting down and standing up, the patient reduces strain on the spine by supporting themselves on the door handle or on their thigh.

Regular bowel movements can be supported by selected foods (e.g., dried fruit, flax seed) or by medications to reduce the time spent on the toilet to a minimum.

Coughing, Sneezing

Coughing and sneezing often intensify the pain of a prolapsed disk. The spinal flexion associated with coughing and sneezing is the likely cause for this increase of pain. For this reason the patient should support themselves while coughing or sneezing by pushing themselves up from the prone position or extending their spine in standing to avoid stooping.

Instructions for the Patient

- *Recumbent:*
  - Lower your bed to be completely flat and do not use more than one small pillow.
  - Alternate between flat prone and supine positions.
  - In lateral position the head should be positioned in line with the extended back so that flexion is avoided.
  - To change position, roll over the bed with a flat back so that the lumbar spine remains as straight as possible.
- *Standing up and lying down:*
  - Before changing position, extend the spine and keep it extended.
  - To change to sitting from the supine position, first go to the lateral recumbent position and vice versa.
- *Putting on and taking off socks and shoes:*
  - Place the foot being dressed on the thigh of the contralateral side.
  - Keep your spine as straight as possible.
  - Wear shoes that do not need to be tied.
- *Tooth brushing:*
  - Place your feet in a wide stance and lean on the wash basin.
  - Support yourself with one hand on the wash basin.

– Keep your spine extended with only a slight forward bend.

- *Sitting:* it is best to avoid sitting since you bend forward when you sit, which pushes the gelatinous mass of the disk backward toward the nerve root. In addition, the already irritated nerve at the buttocks and thigh is subjected to a pressure strain.
- *Eating:* for the most part, take your meals in lateral recumbent position or standing, in order to avoid sitting.
- *Sitting on the toilet, straining, standing up:*
  – Keep your lumbar spine as straight as possible.
  – Do not strain unnecessarily.
  – Stay erect in standing up from the toilet.
  – To stand up, support yourself on the door handle if necessary or on your thigh.
  – Take care to have regular bowel movements in order to minimize the time spent on the toilet.
- *Coughing, sneezing:*
  – When you have an urge to cough or sneeze, extend the lumbar spine as much as possible.
  – Consciously avoid stooping forward with the upper body, which is an automatic movement.

6.5.7   Stabilization

When the intensity of pain has been reduced, the patient has pain-free periods during the day, and movements and strains that in the acute phase peripheralized and intensified symptoms no longer immediately produce and intensify them. There is stabilization.

In addition to the spinal movements, passive movements and leg movements performed by the patients themselves to improve nerve-gliding capacity are tested and used for self-training (see Chapter 6.5.4).

In this phase, if appropriate, the patient's posture is corrected (see Chapters 6.5.5, 9.1, 9.2). The increase in muscle tension associated with erect posture that leads to an increase in pressure in the disks is now well tolerated.

Spinal rotation is practiced first with the knees to the affected side and usually on the following day with the knees to the unaffected side.

If the patient absolutely has to sit for their job, this is practiced (see Chapter 9 Rehabilitation and Prevention). Otherwise the patient continues to avoid sitting.

6.5.8   Restoration of Original Capacity

The capacity of the passive and active motor apparatus depends on mobility, strength, coordination, balance, and fitness. All these factors should be taken into account in an exercise program aimed at restoring the patient's capacity.

In the following, special exercises for patients with lumbar disk damage are described (for general considerations on rehabilitation and prevention of disk damage, see Chapter 9).

The degree of mobility that can be described as *free* depends on many individual factors. These include the relation between the length and width of the individual body parts as well as the firmness of connective tissue structures. In individuals with long legs and short arms, the finger to floor distance in flexion will be less than in people with the same spinal mobility and short legs and long arms.

In general, women are more mobile than men. There are no standard values for free mobility, but it is useful for therapists and patients to consult the target values given here for mobility. They are based on the observation of a series of healthy individuals and patients and seem to be achievable for many individuals.

▷ **Note:** A freely mobile joint is always free of pain. If pain is felt at the end of active mobility this can indicate mechanical impairment of the passive motor apparatus consisting of joint capsule, tendons, and ligaments, or it can indicate muscle contractures or impaired nerve mobility.

In rare cases, hypermobility occurs, in which the range of motion extends beyond the generally known range. Hypermobility of spine or legs is rarely seen in patients after a lumbar disk prolapse.

Free Mobility

Restoration of Extension

Hand Support: Extension while Recumbent (Fig. 6.18)
- Place hands under shoulders.
- Slowly extend elbows.
- Keep back and buttock muscles relaxed.

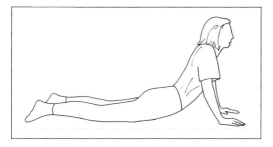

Fig. 6.18 Extension in recumbent position, free mobility.

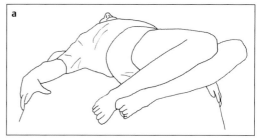

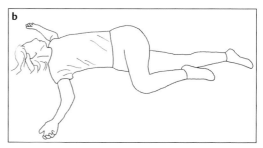

Fig. 6.19 (a, b) Rotation in recumbent position.

- Push up as far as possible.
- Lie down again—stay loose.
- Repeat 10 times.

Free mobility is achieved when the arms can be completely extended and symphysis of the pelvis remains on the ground, without pain in back or leg.

Restoration of Rotation

Rotation in Recumbent Position (Fig. 6.19a, b)
- Lie supine.
- Place feet next to each other.
- No space between the feet.
- Let both knees sink to the same side as far as possible so that the trunk is rotated.
- Return the knees to the middle.
- Change side.
- Repeat 10 to 15 times.

Note: Rotation to both sides in recumbent position should be equally possible. After a disk prolapse with a root compression syndrome, the rotation in which the knees are moved to the contralateral side usually produces nerve extension pain. This direction is then practiced with particular intensity in order to achieve free mobility of the nerve roots. At free mobility, both shoulders and the bottom leg can be brought to touch the ground without back or leg pain.

Restoration of Flexion

As the fibrous ring heals and at the point where the nerve root was compressed, a scar is formed that can lead to limited movement in the spine, the nerve root, and the peripheral nerves. For this reason, it is necessary to monitor flexion mobility at every therapy session and, if necessary, to practice it.

As soon as pain medication is stopped and the patient is largely free of pain for a week, flexion is practiced (if a limitation of movement in flexion is present). During this time, simultaneous additional increases in strain (e.g., resumption of work) should be avoided.

Since spinal flexion is the most frequent trigger for disk prolapse, this movement is practiced with special care. In order to prevent a pathological backward displacement of disk tissue, the spine is placed in end-range extension at least five times before and after every repeated exercise in flexion. Extension of the spine after repeated flexion is an important control parameter. If mobility in extension after flexion is just as pronounced as before, it can be assumed that the fibrous ring has healed and that no disk tissue was forced backward by the exercise.

Note: If extension is limited or blocked after flexion exercises, it is likely that disk tissue was once more displaced backward. In that case, flexion is an undesirable movement. If limited movement or pain in extension persists after flexion the practice of flexion is delayed for another 5 days.

Flexion in Recumbent Position

- First push upward from prone position five times (**Fig. 6.20a**).
- Supine position.
- Pull legs to abdomen (**Fig. 6.20b**).
- Lie down again.
- Repeat 10 times.
- At the end, also push upward from prone position five times (**Fig. 6.20c**).

Increasing Intensity

In flexion, also raise the buttocks.

Note: If flexion in recumbent position is possible for a week without symptoms, the intensity of the flexion may be increased.

When practicing seated with legs extended forward with extended knees, the spine is flexed and at the same time the nerves are extended so that at the end of the movement a pulling sensation may be felt in the back and the leg. If these symptoms disappear again after the movement, exercising can continue.

Flexion when Sitting with Legs Extended

- First push upward from prone position five times.
- Sit with legs extended.
- Knees extended.
- Bend upper body forward until a pulling sensation is felt in back or legs.
- Pull feet up (dorsal extension, the pulling sensation increases).
- Place chin on chest (the pulling becomes even more intense).
- Release—pause.
- Repeat 5 to 10 times.

- At the end, push upward from prone position five times.

Flexion in Standing

- First extend the spine five times in standing position (**Fig. 6.21a**).
- Knees are extended.
- Slowly bend upper body forward until a pulling sensation is felt in back or legs (**Fig. 6.21b**).
- Move chin toward the chest (the pulling increases).
- Straighten up one vertebra at a time.
- Repeat 5 to 10 times.
- At the end, also extend five times in standing position (**Fig. 6.21c**).

Note: Free mobility is achieved when you can achieve a finger to floor distance of 0 to 20 cm in standing flexion, without the onset of pain in back or legs.

Restoration of Free Nerve-gliding Ability

The progressive steps of the leg movements performed by the patient themselves in order to achieve free mobility of the legs and thus of the nerve roots and peripheral nerves are the same as the progressive steps of passive movements (see 6.5.3 Passive Leg Movements for Mobilization of the Nervous System—Progressive Steps of Passive Movements).

The exercises in supine position can be increased if the hip joint is flexed, adducted, and rotated inward.

Dorsal extension of the ankle can be used as an alternative or a supplement to increase the intensity of the movements described (see **Fig. 6.17a, b**) to improve nerve-gliding ability.

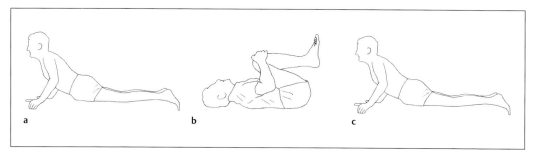

Fig. 6.20 Extension and flexion in recumbent position. **(a, c)** Extension. **(b)** Flexion.

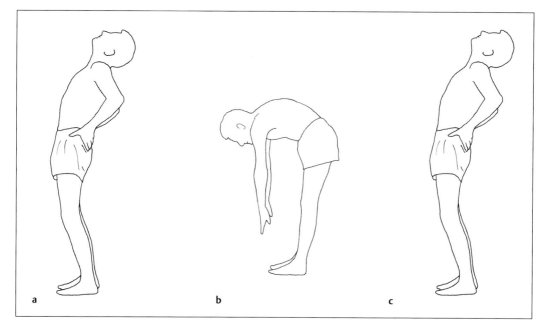

Fig. 6.21 Extension and flexion in standing position. **(a, c)** Extension. **(b)** Flexion.

Flexion in seated posture with legs extended and in standing position (see Restoration of Flexion above) are exercises that also improve nerve-gliding capacity.

Strengthening

In patients with lumbar disk prolapse, strengthening of paretic foot and leg muscles is emphasized. The most important measure is walking. As soon as the patient can walk without intensified pain, they should do this several times a day, with the distance walked increasing from day to day. Climbing stairs and walking over uneven ground are other ways of increasing intensity.

Special exercises are used to train individual muscles weakened by nerve root compression.

Strengthening the Foot Extensors (Triceps Surae)
- Walking on tiptoe.
- One-leg stand.

One-leg Stand on Toes (Fig. 6.22)
- One-leg stand.
- Alternatively raise and lower heel.

Note: The one-leg stand exercise is also used to improve balance.

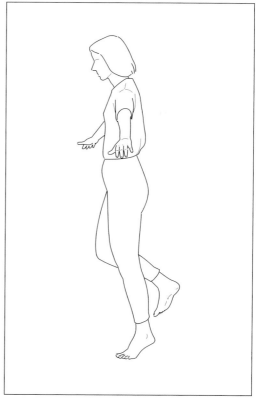

Fig. 6.22 One-leg stand on Toes.

Strengthening Foot and Great Toe Flexors

Strengthening the tibialis anterior and extensor hallucis longus.

Walking on the Heels

- Raise toes.
- Walk on heels.

Strengthening the Knee Extensors and Hip Muscles

Strengthening the quadriceps femoris, adductor magnus, and adductor brevis.

Knee Bends (Fig. 6.23)

- Keep upper body erect during the entire exercise.
- Slowly bend the knees.
- During deep knee bends the heels lift off the ground.
- Extend knees again.

Note: The knee bend exercise is also used to strengthen the trunk muscles and improve balance.

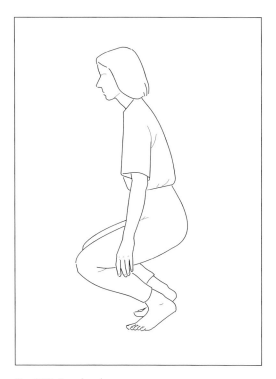

Fig. 6.23 Knee bends.

6.5.9 Rehabilitation, Activities of Daily Living, and Prevention

Reintegration into the activities of daily living is an important goal in the treatment of patients with disk prolapse. The physical therapy program is designed to allow previously working patients to resume their work after the shortest possible disability period. At the latest, this is the moment to practice upright, supported sitting (see Chapter 9 Rehabilitation and Prevention). Detailed instructions for the exercise of free, symmetrical mobility of all joints, coordination, balance, strength, and appropriate cardiovascular strain are found in Chapter 9.

In activities of daily living, the practice effort must be reduced to a realistic level that is individualized for the patient's circumstances. The ideal pattern would be 15-minute exercise units, performed morning, noon, and night, that cover the most important points of the individual training program. In addition, the patient should be given a few important suggestions for the conduct of everyday life.

Instructions for the Patient

- Improve your posture and straighten up more frequently than before.
- When sitting, support the forward lumbar curve with a small cushion or roll.
- In the morning before getting up and in the evening before falling asleep, lie on your stomach. Relax and read in prone position more often. A thick pillow or a reading wedge under your chest can be helpful.
- Check spinal mobility in *all* directions. Occasionally run through the entire training program.
- *Make a point of maintaining the mobility of the nerve root affected by the disk prolapse.*
- *Regularly extend your lumbar spine* when you have been sitting for a while or pursuing an activity in forward-bending position. Extend *before* the pain begins. Always compensate for one-sided strains.
- Do not make a habit of sparing yourself, because then the structures of the spine will become even less capable of dealing with strain. *Use it or lose it!*
- From time to time, treat yourself to a physical therapy session in order to analyze and treat bad

posture habits, limitations of movement, asymmetries, and lack of strength.

6.6   After an Operation

There are no scientifically studied and generally recognized postoperative therapy programs for any surgical treatment of a prolapsed disk. Therefore, if the therapist is planning to use the therapy concept described here, they should first obtain the agreement of the surgeon.

The *physical therapy examination* of patients operated on for a prolapsed disk is the same as described in Chapter 4 Diagnosis in Physical Therapy. The most complete physical therapy examination possible should be conducted before the operation (Chapter 4), so that postoperative changes can be documented. If this was missed, it should at least be done on the first postoperative day. Postoperative documentation is like documentation of conservative treatment (see Chapter 5 Therapy).

To ensure *uncomplicated wound healing* and *prevention of immediate recurrence,* the postoperative patient should observe the rules in 6.5.6 Acute Phase—Useful Guidelines for Conduct During the Acute Phase. If possible, the movement transitions should already be practiced with the patient before the operation.

For prevention of deep vein thrombosis, if the patient spends a great deal of time lying down after the operation, they must spend at least 1 minute per hour practicing dorsal extension and plantar flexion at the ankle during the first few days. In doing this, they should build up strong muscle tension (especially in the calf muscles) in order to facilitate venous return and prevent formation of a thrombus.

To *improve venous return,* as vascular training and to activate trunk muscles, isometric contraction exercises against a resistance are begun on the first postoperative day.

Simple Isometric Tension Exercises in Supine Position

Leg Exercise
- Supine position.
- Place feet to produce a 30° angle in hip joints.
- Raise toes as high as possible.
- The feet are braced against an imaginary resistance diagonally toward the ground and foot end (of bed). The legs do not move, the extensor muscles push, and the flexor muscles create the resistance.
- At the same time, the head is pushed toward the head of the bed.
- The muscle tension is transmitted to the trunk muscles and the spine is extended.
- The therapist checks whether abdominal and back muscle tension can be felt.
- Hold the tension for two breaths.
- Release. Relax for two breaths.
- Repeat 5 to 10 times.

Arm Exercise
- Supine position.
- Extend arms on the bed.
- Rotate shoulder joints outward.
- Press extended arms onto the bed.
- Push hands toward the foot of the bed.
- At the same time, push the head toward the head of the bed. The muscle tension is transmitted to the trunk muscles and the spine is extended.
- The therapist checks whether abdominal and back muscle tension can be felt.
- Hold the tension for two breaths.
- Release. Relax for two breaths.
- Repeat 5 to 10 times.

Pushing with Arms and Legs
- Combine the movements described above and perform them simultaneously.
- Hold the tension for two breaths.
- Release. Relax for two breaths.
- Repeat 5 to 10 times.

Note: The patient should repeat the isometric tension exercises 5 to 10 times every hour.

As additional thrombosis and pneumonia prophylaxis and vascular training, the patient should get up and walk as soon as possible. In most cases they will need help at first, since there could be postoperative circulation problems. If the disk operation proceeded without complications, the patient can sometimes already get up on the day of the operation or, at the latest, on the first postoperative day.

From the second postoperative day the isometric contraction exercises are supplemented with movement of the lumbar spine. Weight-free mobilization in extension and flexion is practiced in lateral recumbent position. The patient is instructed to perform the movements only in a range and with a force such that there is no pain and no pulling at the wound. Usually they can assume a prone position without difficulty, which they should do several times a day. The transition from supine to prone position is made with a straight spine (supine–lateral–prone).

From the third postoperative day physical therapy is conducted according to the same considerations and with the same therapeutic movements as the primary conservative treatment. The points of emphasis are determined by the findings. The therapy is symptom oriented. If the course of recovery is uncomplicated, one therapeutic movement can be added every day.

Possible Sequence of Exercises

- *First postoperative day:*
  - Isometric tension exercises.
  - Foot movements.
  - Standing up and walking.
  - Activities of daily living (see 6.5.6 Acute Phase—Useful Guidelines for Conduct During the Acute Phase).
- *Second postoperative day:*
  - Additional weight-free mobilization of the lumbar spine in extension and flexion in lateral recumbent position.
  - Prone position.
- *Third postoperative day:*
  - Continue or discontinue isometric exercises.
  - Increase distance and frequency of walking.
- *Fourth postoperative day:*
  - Every 2 hours extension in prone position with a small range of motion, five repetitions.
  - Increase walking again.
  - If applicable, strengthen weakened muscles and move the corresponding joints to end range.
  - **Note:** the ankle should be freely moveable even with extended knee joint in dorsal extension.
- *Fifth postoperative day:* possibly reduce medications but do not change any exercises at the same time.
- *Sixth postoperative day:*
  - Increase leg movements for nerve mobilization—three times three repetitions a day.
  - Continue or discontinue weight-free mobilization in lateral position.
  - Increase range of motion of extension in prone position.

- *Seventh postoperative day:* add rotation to affected side.
- *Eighth postoperative day:* add rotation to contralateral side.
- *Ninth postoperative day:*
  - Practice activities of daily living, such as sitting and lifting.
  - Increase strengthening exercises for the trunk muscles (see Chapter 9 Rehabilitation and Prevention).
- *Tenth postoperative day:*
  - The wound has healed to the point that the stitches can be removed.
  - Training (see Chapter 9) is conducted step by step.

Rehabilitation sessions at a facility are usually not necessary. An individual training program designed to suit the patient's signs and symptoms, which they can carry out independently, is preferable to group rehabilitation. It is the most efficient way to ensure rapid return to their social environment and the work process.

The duration of disability after surgery for a prolapsed disk, just like the duration of conservative treatment, depends on many factors and is not the same in every case (see Chapter 5 Therapy).

6.7   Case Study

A 28-year-old patient has a neuroradiologically diagnosed prolapsed disk at intervertebral level L5–S1 right, with nerve root compression S1 right (**Fig. 6.24**).

Admission Findings

In his medical history, the patient reported suffering repeatedly from back pain over a number of years. Playing soccer 2 days ago, he felt a sudden pain radiating from right of the spine into the right heel. He rated maximal pain intensity in the last 24 hours at 5/10 and the minimal at 0/10. Thus, the pain intensity varied and was most noticeable in the morning. The pain was triggered or intensified when he sat, stood up from a seated position, and when he rotated his spine.

It was possible to see a shift to the left and normal lumbar lordosis. In spinal flexion, the lumbar spine remained straight.

The patient had no sensory disorder and no weakness. The finger to floor distance in flexion

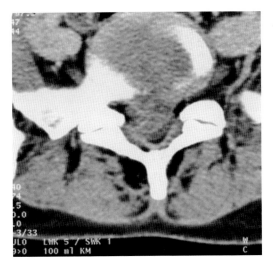

Fig. 6.24 Computed tomography of the prolapsed intervertebral disk L5–S1 right.

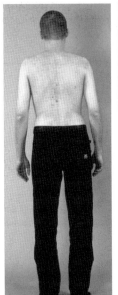

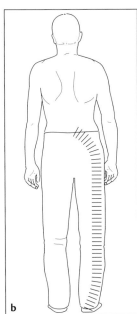

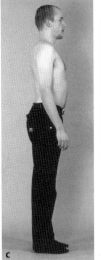

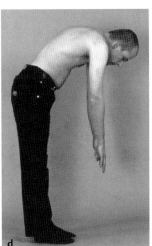

Fig. 6.25 (a–d) Findings on admission.

was 48 cm; the straight leg raise test on the right had a value of 80 cm (**Fig 6.25a–d**).

Movement Tests

With repeated end-range shift correction in standing position, the patient reported centralization of his pain up to the thigh (**Fig. 6.26a, b**). Central back pain was produced at the same time.

Additional extension caused centralization of the pain up to the buttocks (**Fig. 6.27a, b**). This improvement persisted after the movements.

Self-training

The patient performed the shift correction in standing position independently, 10 times per hour or, alternatively, extension in recumbent position with pelvis shifted to the left. He was asked to observe his symptoms and only continue if exercise caused the pain to shift toward the spine or decrease. He was told to discontinue the exercises if the pain radiated further to distal toward the foot or toes.

Control Finding after 4 Days
- Reduced shift.
- Central back pain, sometimes radiating diffusely as far as the buttocks.
- Maximal pain intensity: 3/10.
- Symmetrical extension in recumbent position finally reduced and eliminated the central pain

(**Fig. 6.28a, b**). It replaced the patient's asymmetrical self-training.

Further Training

In the days that followed, the training program was further intensified by adding leg movements to the spinal movements in order to improve the nerve-gliding capacity and prevent adhesion of the affected nerve roots (**Fig. 6.29a, b**).

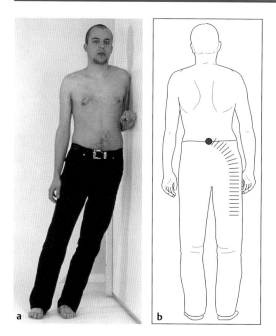

Fig. 6.26 (a, b) Shift correction in standing position.

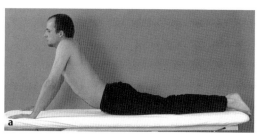

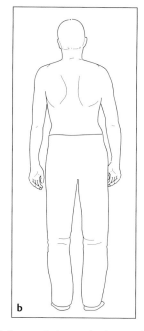

Fig. 6.28 (a) Symmetrical extension in recumbent position. **(b)** Pain after extension in recumbent position.

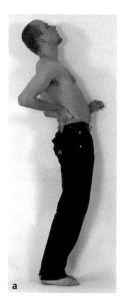

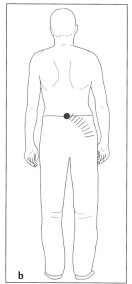

Fig. 6.27 (a, b) Shift correction in standing position with extension.

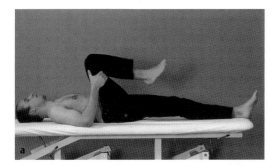

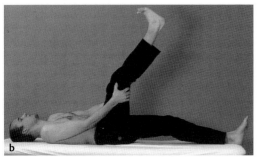

Fig. 6.29 (a, b) Intensification of the training program in the form of leg movements (sliders).

In the course of the next weeks, the patient received intensive training of spinal mobility in all directions.

Rotational mobilization (**Fig. 6.30**) was practiced first with the knees to the right and from the next day, also with knees to the left.

No symptoms were produced in flexion mobilization in recumbent position (**Fig. 6.31a–d**). After flexion, the spinal mobility in extension was free and also produced no symptoms.

Since mobility in flexion continued to be limited, flexion mobilization was practiced in standing position (**Fig. 6.32a–c**).

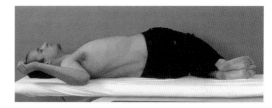

Fig. 6.30 Rotational mobilization.

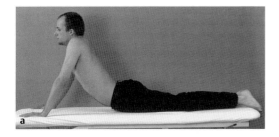

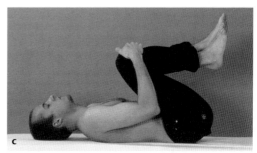

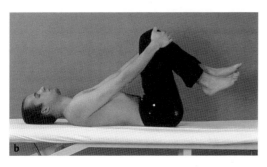

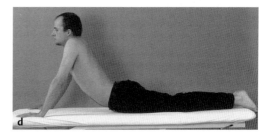

Fig. 6.31 (a–d) Flexion mobilization in recumbent position.

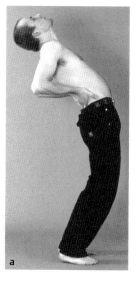
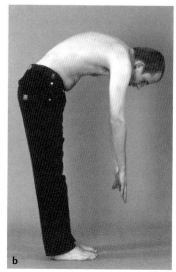
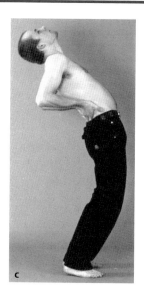

Fig. 6.32 (a–c) Flexion mobilization in standing position.

Findings 6 Weeks after the Start of Therapy

- No shift, normal lordosis.
- Curvature of the lumbar spine in flexion.
- Symptom free and satisfied.
- Able to work.
- Finger to floor distance in flexion: 30 cm.

- Straight leg raise test right: 96 cm.
- No weakness and no sensory disorder.

The visual examination of posture and capacity for flexion in the course of the illness are shown in **Fig. 6.33a–d**.

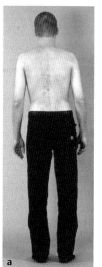
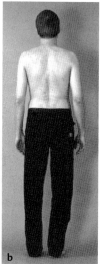
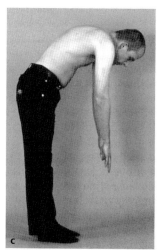
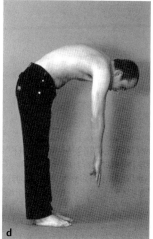

Fig. 6.33 Posture and ability to flex in the course of the illness. **(a, c)** On admission. **(b, d)** After 6 weeks.

Further Procedure

- Since mobility in flexion was still limited after 6 weeks, exercises continued.
- As a preventive measure, the patient was advised to practice extension in recumbent position in the morning, before rising, and in the evening after work.
- He was told to stand up from sitting frequently and perform repeated end-range spinal extension.

7 Thoracic Spine

Pain syndromes resulting from disk injury in the thoracic spine are rare, presumably because of the low degree of mobility in this section of the spinal column. Moreover, there is no direct transition here between mobile and stable sections. The literature concerning prolapse of thoracic disks is limited to description of individual cases and literature reviews (Whitcomb et al 1995; Morgan and Abood 1998; Turgut 2000; Wilke et al 2000; Miyaguchi et al 2001; Winter et al 2002). There are no studies describing the course of the disease in a large patient group.

The rate of surgical treatment for thoracic myelopathy in Japan was 5.1 per 1 million individuals a year. This corresponded to 9% of that reported for cervical myopathy during the same period. Nineteen percent of these patients were operated on for myelopathy associated with thoracic disk prolapse (Sato et al 1998).

The proportion of thoracic disk prolapses out of all disk prolapses is in the range of 0.2 to 5%, the annual incidence is 1 per million (Wilke et al 2000). In 35 consecutive patients with thoracic disk prolapses, intervertebral levels 6 to 7 and 7 to 8 were most frequently affected. Radicular syndromes were diagnosed in 18 patients, myelopathy in 23 patients (Levi et al 1999). Wilke et al (2000) proposed that 90% of patients with a diagnosed thoracic disk prolapse show signs of spinal cord compression.

Ventral herniation of the spinal cord resulting from tears in the dura mater was described in association with thoracic disk prolapse. The affected patients usually exhibited Brown-Séquard syndrome, a classical pattern of neurological deficits upon unilateral spinal cord injury characterized by ipsilateral weakness and loss of position sense with contralateral loss of pain and temperature sensation (Miyaguchi et al 2001). The nonspecific pain symptoms often associated with thoracic disk injury can lead to misdiagnoses such as esophagitis, nephritis, pancreatitis, gastrointestinal ulcers, or cardiopulmonary disease (Whitcomb et al 1995; Pal and Johnson 1997; Wilke et al 2000).

Because of its anatomical and mechanical similarity to the lumbar and cervical spines, it is reasonable for diagnosis and treatment of disk injury to the thoracic spine to proceed in the same way as for disk injury in the lumbar and cervical spines.

Upper Thoracic Spine

In disk damage and prolapse of the upper thoracic spine, poor posture similar to that in the cervical spine can be observed. Radicular symptoms often radiate to the shoulder blade and also into the upper arm when the T1 root is affected (Morgan and Abood 1998; Wilke et al 2000).

The nerve tension test in the upper extremities (upper limb tension test, ULTT) can be positive. Therapeutic movements for the treatment of disk problems in the cervical spine (usually extension) are conducted in such a way that if they are continued beyond the movement range of the cervical spine, they have an effect on the upper thoracic spine.

Lower Thoracic Spine

In case of disk injury and prolapse in the lower thoracic spine, poor posture associated with the lumbar spine can be observed. Radicular symptoms often radiate to the lumbar spine and pelvis.

The nerve tension test of the lower extremity (straight leg raise test; prone knee bend test) can be positive (Wilke et al 2000; Tokuhashi et al 2001). Therapeutic movements for the treatment of disk problems in the lumbar spine are conducted in such a way that if they are continued beyond the movement range of the lumbar spine, they have an effect on the lower thoracic spine.

The following sections describe the results of visual examinations and diagnostic tests for the thoracic spine, the evaluation criteria for establishing a physical therapy diagnosis, and the course of therapy for diagnosis of disk injury.

7.1 Diagnostic Assessment Form for the Thoracic Spine (Fig. 7.1a–d)

General points for filling out the diagnostic form are provided in Chapter 4 Diagnosis in Physical Therapy. They include personal information and medical history (**Fig. 7.1a, c**), body diagram (**Fig 7.1b**), and documentation of pain and sensory disorders (**Fig. 7.1d**). For a clearer understanding, some information from Chapter 4 and Chapter 5 Therapy is repeated here.

The diagnostic assessment form can be downloaded as a PDF at www.mediacenter.thieme.com.

7.2 Diagnosis by Observation

In the visual diagnosis, standing and sitting postures as well as gait are evaluated.

Shift

Depending on the area in which the disease is located, a shift in the thoracic spine can be observed corresponding to the evaluation criteria for cervical or lumbar shift. A lateral shift of the shoulder girdle with respect to the pelvis is evaluated on the basis of the free space between the hanging arms and the torso and pelvis as well as of the distance of the hands from the thighs.

A high-thoracic shift is characterized by a lateral displacement of the head with respect to the shoulder girdle. The chin and sternum are used as reference points to determine whether a shift is present.

Thoracic Kyphosis

Typically, patients with disk injury exhibit loss of lordosis in the affected section of the spine. In the thoracic spine, kyphosis is consistent with the natural curvature of the spine. It is therefore difficult to judge whether the patient's thoracic kyphosis is more pronounced than before the onset of their current condition.

Walking

Changes in gait are most likely to arise as the result of central paraparesis of the legs as a sign of an impending paraplegia resulting from spinal cord compression (Levi et al 1999; Wilke et al 2000; Miyaguchi et al 2001).

7.3 Diagnostic Tests

The diagnostic tests include nerve tension tests and test movements for the spine. Abnormalities of the motor system must be sought first of all in the legs, because these may be caused by spinal cord compression and usually require immediate surgical intervention.

7.3.1 Muscle Function Tests

There are no segment-indicating muscles for nerve root compression in the thoracic spine. If the medical history indicates muscle weakness, the abnormal muscles or muscle groups are tested.

Paresis of muscles supplied by a thoracic root does not cause a clinically discernible breathing disorder.

7.3.2 Nerve Tension Tests

Tension tests for the nerve roots of the thoracic spinal cord can only be conducted in very limited fashion. It may be possible to place the nerve roots of the upper thoracic spine (T1, T2) under tension with the upper extremity nerve tension test (see Chapter 8, 8.3.2 Nerve Tension Test of the Upper Extremity—Upper Limb Tension Test) and those of the lower thoracic spine (T10–T12) with the lower extremity nerve tension tests (see prone knee bend test and straight leg raise test in Chapter 6 Lumbar Spine).

Note:
- Nerve tension tests for the extremities are always performed on both sides.
- In case of radiating pain, the nonaffected side is tested first.
- Crossover pain, where testing the nonaffected side intensifies pain on the affected side, can be an indication of disk prolapse.

It is assumed that the nerve roots of the middle thoracic spine can only be placed under tension by spinal flexion (global nerve tension test [slump test], see below).

Note: Spinal flexion is not advisable in case of suspected or neuroradiologically confirmed disk prolapse because it could intensify shift of the nucleus

Diagnostic assessment—thoracic spine a
Name: _____
Date: _____

Admission data
Therapist: _____

Referral diagnosis on registration: _____

Date of birth: _____

Occupation, hobby: _____

Posture, weight-bearing: _____

On sick leave since: _____

Causative factors: _____

Duration of current episode: _____

Development: better/same/worse:
Prior treatment of current episode: physical therapy/fango/massage/sling table/
chiropractic/injections/medications/other
Medications: benzodiazepines/NSAIDs/steroids since: _____

Prior history: _____

Physical therapy diagnosis: _____

Justification of diagnosis: _____

Diagnostic assessment—thoracic spine b
Name: _____
Date: _____

Body diagram

Markings: ///// Pain ::::: Sensory disorder
Alternatively, pain is marked in red and sensory disorders are marked in blue

Diagnostic assessment—thoracic spine c
Name: _____
Date: _____

Better:	Night/morning/daytime/evening/at rest/while moving/ stooping/streching/sitting/lying down/standing/walking
Worse:	Night/morning/daytime/evening/at rest/while moving/ stooping/streching/sitting/lying down/standing/walking

Coughing/sneezing/straining
Trauma: _____
Operation: _____
Unwanted weight loss   yes/no (_____kg in _____ weeks)

Reaction to repeated, end-range movements
Starting situation: _____

Movement	NT, CE, EL, PR, PE,↑↓ RI, RW, RNI, RNW	
	Change during movement	Change after movement
Prone, lower arm support		
1 x extension lying down		
5 x extension lying down		
1 x rotation lying down knee R		
5 x rotation lying down knee R		
1 x rotation lying down knee L		
5 x rotation lying down knee L		
1 x flexion lying down		
5 x flexion lying down		
1 x extension standing		
5 x extension standing		
1 x flexion standing		
5 x flexion standing		
Other:		

Diagnostic assessment—thoracic spine: follow-up d
Name: _____
Date: _____
Medications: benzodiazepine/NSAIDs/steroids   Shift: R   L
                                                                              Limping: yes no
Lordosis: normal/accentuated/reduced   Distance walked:

Pain: record area, activity or posture and intensity

0 1 2 3 4 5 6 7 8 9 10   0 1 2 3 4 5 6 7 8 9 10
Before PT   After PT

0 1 2 3 4 5 6 7 8 9 10   0 1 2 3 4 5 6 7 8 9 10
Maximal   Minimal   in the last 24 hours

Pain radiation in cm before PT _____ after PT _____
Sensory disorder
Area: _____
Characteristics: _____ better/same/worse
Abnormalities in motor system

Signs of nerve extension

Slump knee extension right:	Slump knee extension left:
PKB right:	PKB left:
ULTT right:	ULTT left:

Mobility

Flexion	Extension	Rotation:	Shift/Translation
Finger to floor distance		Knee R	R
		Knee L	L

Fig. 7.1 (a–d) Diagnostic assessment form for the thoracic spine.
(NT = not tested; CE = centralized; EL = eliminated; PR = produced; PE = peripheralized; NE = no effect; ↑ = pain increases; ↓ = pain decreases; RI = remains improved; RW = remains worse; RNI = remains not improved; RNW = remains not worse; R = right; L = left; PT = physical therapy; PKB = prone knee bend; ULTT = upper limb tension test.)

pulposus toward the spinal cord. In this case, the nerve tension test should be omitted.

Global Nerve Tension Test (Slump Test)

The test exerts tension on the following neural structures:
- Meninges.
- Spinal cord.
- Nerve roots.
- Sacral plexus.
- Sciatic nerve.

The pain of nerve tension can be felt in the spine and in the entire area supplied by the nerve roots and nerves listed above.

Implementation (Fig. 7.2a–e)
- The patient sits at the edge of the treatment table, with their feet not touching the floor (**Fig. 7.2a**).

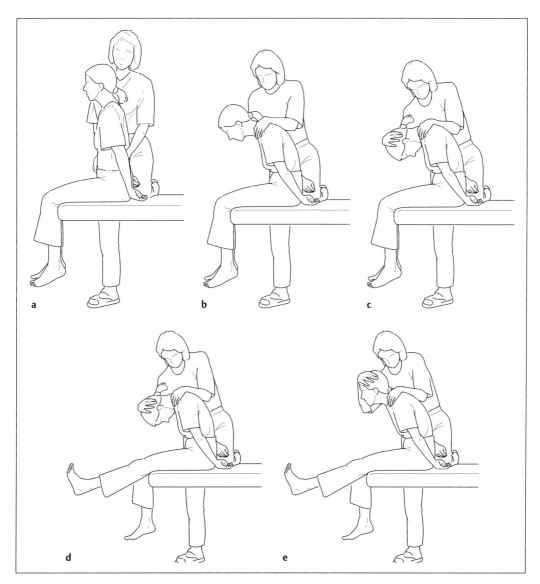

Fig. 7.2 (a–e) Slump test.

- Their hands are behind their back and their sacrum is vertical.
- The therapist holds the sacrum in place with their knee.
- The patient slumps forward (**Fig. 7.2b**; the spine is flexed, not the hip joint).
- The therapist increases the spinal flexion by pressing with their lower arm and hand on the patient's shoulder and thoracic spine.
- The patient bends the cervical spine (**Fig. 7.2c**).
- The therapist increases this flexion.
- The patient extends one knee joint (**Fig. 7.2d**).
- To increase the tension, the patient raises the dorsum of the foot (dorsal extension of the ankle).

Note: In the slump position with extended knee and dorsal extension of the ankle, the nervous system is under maximal tension.

- Relaxation of the nervous system by passive neck extension (**Fig. 7.2e**).
- Alternatively, plantar flexion in the ankle or knee flexion can be used to relax the nervous system.

Observations and Criteria for Stopping the Test Movement

- *Avoidance movements:*
  - Pelvic tilt.
  - Pushing the spine dorsally.
- *Resistance:* elastic termination of movement.
- *Reflex muscle tension:*
  - Suddenly palpable termination of movement.
  - Jerky tensing of the neck extensors.

The test is evaluated as *positive* in the following cases:

- The symptoms familiar to the patient are reproduced or intensified.
- A marked postural response is seen, for instance neck extension.
- There is a distinct side difference in range of motion of knee extension and pain is elicited.

To *differentiate* between nerve tension pain and pain from other causes, tension is reduced at a point some distance from the painful area, for instance, when there is pain in the lower thoracic spine, by reducing extension in the cervical spine.

Note:

- If the pain decreases, it was presumably caused by tension in the nervous system.
- If it remains unchanged, the cause of the pain is more likely to be found in a different structure.

7.3.3   Test and Therapeutic Spinal Movements

Whether to perform the tests first in recumbent or in seated position is determined by the effect on the symptoms of spinal weight loading caused by a vertical body position. In pain syndromes of the upper thoracic spine, the seated tests are preferable (as in the cervical spine). In pain syndromes of the middle and lower thoracic spine, the patient is tested in recumbent position (as in the lumbar spine).

The test movements should be passive for the affected section of the spine. This is only possible to a limited extent in the thoracic spine tests since the muscles that perform the movements partially attach to the thoracic spine and the ribs.

The test movements are used to investigate the mobility of the thoracic spine and the effect on the symptoms, particularly on the pain, of repeated movements of the spine.

Evaluation of Mobility

The mobility of the thoracic spine for flexion and extension is documented at the first therapy session. Rotational mobility is documented during the test movements as soon as rotation tests are considered useful. The translatory movement of the shoulder girdles with respect to the pelvis is tested if the patient's spontaneous posture shows a shift or therapy-resistant, asymmetrical pain.

Evaluation of thoracic spine mobility is particularly difficult because of its relative stiffness compared to the lumbar and cervical spine. Nevertheless, pronounced deviations from the generally normal range can be described. Limitation of motion and changes in mobility during exercises and in correlation with pain are decisive factors in diagnosis and treatment in the acute phase.

Repeated Test Movements

Since extension of the affected spinal level is usually beneficial in cases of disk damage, this is the first movement tested. If symptoms are asymmetrical with shift or unilateral back pain, asymmetrical test movements often result in centralization and reduction of pain. When extension of the thoracic spine does not produce centralization, the next step is to test one-sided rotation or shift correction in standing position.

The working hypothesis is the idea of using the movement to exert pressure on the injured area of the anulus fibrosus, thus pushing the displaced gelatinous mass medially or ventrally.

> **Note:** Flexion is only tested after all the other test movements fail to produce centralization or reduce pain.

Tempo and rhythm of the movement are slow but fluid. The patient must be able to stop the movement at any time. No impetus is applied.

The movements should be performed with the most extensive *range of motion* possible. If the patient stops a movement, they are asked why (e.g., pain, fear of pain, or limitation of movement).

The *intensity* of the test movements is always increased if a given movement has a centralizing and reducing effect but the pain has not yet disappeared completely.

The number of *repetitions* is between two and 10. If the pain is intensified by the movement tests or peripheralized, and remains unchanged in this form, and when there are signs of vegetative disorders or disorders in the legs, the tests are repeated no more than twice.

If the pain becomes more intense or is peripheralized during the movements and after the movements it returns to its original level and location, the test may be repeated up to 10 times. If the pain decreases or becomes centralized, the test is repeated 10 times.

The patient is asked before, during, and after the test movements where they feel the pain and at what level of intensity on the numerical analog scale (NAS), or whether the pain changes as a result of the movements:
- Is your pain changing?
- Where does it hurt now?
- How intense is your pain now?

> **Note:** Avoid leading questions such as: Is it getting better now?

Almost every patient is able to assign a number between 0 (no pain) and 10 (the worst pain imaginable) to the pain. The therapist should insist that the patient specifies how their pain is changing. Statements like "Now it's worse than before" provide no useful information for planning further treatment. For instance, if back pain has increased but the pain radiating to the ribs has decreased or disappeared, this may be more unpleasant for the patient but it is an indication that the symptoms are improving. This must be explained to the patient. The patient can usually tolerate an increase of central pain better if the positive side of centralization is explained to them.

For every test movement, not only the pain but also the change in spinal mobility is evaluated and documented.

Instructions for the Patient
- The test movements should be passive for the spine. Keep the back, shoulder, abdomen, and hips relaxed.
- Take every movement as far as possible.
- Tell me how the intensity and range of your pain change.
- Stop the movement if the pain radiates further.

Extension Test
Extension in Seated Position
- Seated.
- Move head backward with the chin positioned approximately parallel to the floor (see Chapter 8, **Fig. 8.6**).
- The back of your head is moved backward in a large arc so that your face points up to the ceiling.
- Return to the starting position.
- Repeat.

Prone Position (Fig. 7.3)
- Lie on your stomach in a relaxed position.
- Breathe calmly.

Support on Lower Arms (Fig. 7.4)
- Bend the elbows so that they are positioned directly under the shoulders (as though you were reading a book on the beach).

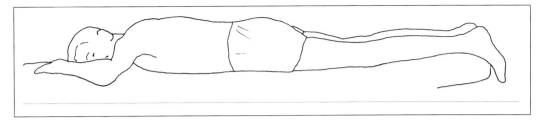

Fig. 7.3 Prone position.

- Remain in this position for about three breaths.
- Lie down again—stay loose.
- Repeat.

Hand Support, Extension while Recumbent (Fig. 7.5)

- Place your hands in front of your body.

📝 **Note:** The further forward the hands are placed in the "Hand Support, Extension while Recumbent" test, the higher up in the thoracic spine the extension; the further out toward the shoulders the hands are placed, the lower down the extension.
- Slowly extend elbows.
- Keep back and buttock muscles relaxed.

- Push up as far as possible.
- Lie down again—relax.
- Repeat.

Increasing Intensity

- At the end of the movement, hold briefly and exhale deeply.
- Lie down again—relax.
- Repeat.

Extension in Standing Position

- Place hands on the back at the level of the thoracic spine so that the fingertips point to the spine and the thumbs point to the side.

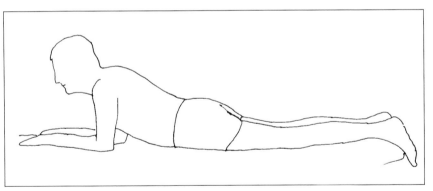

Fig. 7.4 Support on lower arms.

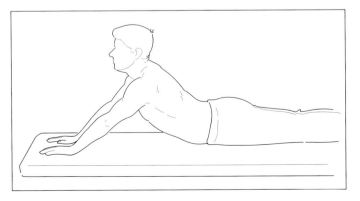

Fig. 7.5 Hand support, extension while recumbent.

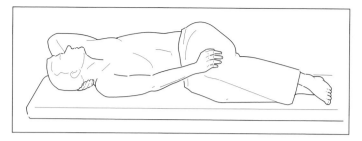

Fig. 7.6 Rotation in lateral recumbent position.

- Extend the back as far backward as possible.
- Straighten up.
- Repeat.

Asymmetrical Tests

Rotation while Recumbent, with Emphasis on Thoracic Spine (Fig. 7.6)

- Lateral recumbent position.
- Place the hand of the top arm onto the ribs.
- Turn the upper body and head dorsally.
- Return to the middle.
- Repeat.

Increasing Intensity

- Lateral recumbent position.
- Place the hand of the top arm behind your head.
- With the hand of the bottom arm hold the legs in position.
- Turn the upper body and head dorsally.
- Move the elbow of the top arm as far dorsal as possible.
- Return to the middle.
- Repeat.

Lateral Displacement of the Pelvis in Standing Position

- Standing.
- Stand with one side toward the wall at a distance of about two foot-widths (see Chapter 6, **Fig. 6.27**).
- Place the feet directly next to each other.
- *Symptoms in the lower thoracic spine:*
    - Lean the shoulder and upper arm of the side to which the shoulder girdle is displaced with respect to the pelvis against the wall.
    - Bend the elbow on this side.
- *Symptoms in the middle thoracic spine:* lean the arm of the side to which the shoulder girdle is displaced with respect to the pelvis against the wall at 90° elevation (flexion).
- Let the pelvis sink toward the wall.
- Move it back to the middle.
- Repeat.

Increasing Intensity 1

The further the feet are from the wall, the more intense the effect.

Increasing Intensity 2

- Support the hand not facing the wall on the back.
- Extend the spine as far as possible.

Flexion Test

Flexion in Seated Position (Fig. 7.7)

- Sitting.
- Slump.

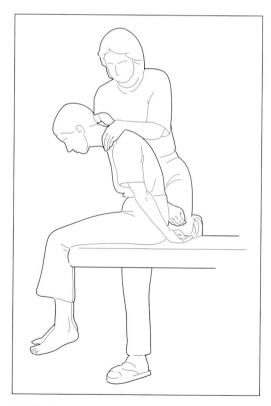

Fig. 7.7 Flexion in seated position.

- Straighten up.
- Repeat.

Flexion in Standing Position (Fig. 7.8)
- Standing.
- Place the feet two foot-widths apart.
- Bend the spine forward.
- The knees remain extended.
- Straighten up.
- Repeat.

7.4   Establishing the Diagnosis

All findings from the medical history, the visual examination, and the diagnostic tests are taken into account (see **Table 7.1**; for fundamental aspects, see Chapter 4 Diagnosis in Physical Therapy).

The diagnosis should be considered a working hypothesis. Through discussion with the treating physician, it may lead to undertaking further diagnostic or therapeutic procedures.

Summary: Typical Findings in the Diagnosis of Disk Damage

- *Information in the medical history:*
  - Age: 20 to 55 years.
  - Duration: long or short (acute–chronic).

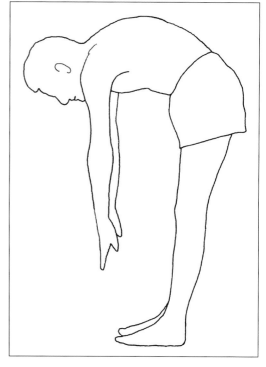

Fig. 7.8 Flexion in standing position.

Table 7.1 Simplified guide to interpreting changes in pain caused by test movements

Question	Answer	Conclusions
1. Can the problem be influenced mechanically by movement of the thoracic spine?	No	Tumor Inflammatory disease Disease of internal organs Further investigation **Note:** no mechanical therapy of the thoracic spine
	Yes	**Continue with question 2**
2. Does the same movement always trigger precisely the same pain reaction and does the pain return to its original form thereafter?	Yes	Shortened structures, nerve root adhesions **Note:** mechanical therapy Spinal or foraminal stenosis Instability, facet joint pain More examinations **Note:** In cases of stenosis: posture training, exercise spinal flexion In case of instability: stabilizing strength training
	No	**Continue with question 3**
3. Does the pain centralize or peripheralize within one dermatome?	Yes	Disk damage Check for possible disk prolapse **Note:** mechanical physical therapy
	No	**Continue with question 4**

▶ (continued)

Table 7.1 Simplified guide to interpreting changes in pain caused by test movements (*continued*)

Question	Answer	Conclusions
4. Does the same movement produce different pain reactions with pain that remains the same or increases after the movement?	Yes	Chronified pain syndrome Psychosocial problem More examinations (see Chapter 11 Psychosocial Risk Factors) **Note:** In chronified pain syndrome: varied activation; nonspecific exercise programs, mechanical and strengthening In predominantly psychosocial problems: discuss physical therapy with the treating physician

- Sudden onset.
- Trigger: stooping.
- Changes due to movement.
- Constant or intermittent.
- *Character of the complaints:*
  - Pain in the thoracic spine in combination with dermatome-related radiating pain.
  - Dermatome-related radiating pain without pain in the thoracic spine.
  - Dermatome-related sensory disorders.
- *Visual examination:*
  - Kyphotic/shift deformation.
  - Limited movement.
- *Behavior of symptoms upon repeated spinal movement:*
  - Rapid change during the movements.
  - Changes persist after the movements.
  - Centralization or peripheralization of the pain.
  - Improvement of mobility with decrease in pain and vice versa.
  - Nerve tension signs better or worse.
  - Sensory perception changes from day to day, not within one therapy session.

Differential diagnoses, for instance mechanical symptoms in rib mobility, require special differential tests; for details concerning differential tests see literature relating to manual diagnosis and therapy such as the Maitland concept (Maitland 2000).

Disorders frequently associated with disk damage such as spinal and foraminal stenosis, spinal instability, facet joint pain, shortened structures in the spinal column, and inflamed or fibrosed nerve roots also cause certain stereotypical pain reactions (see Chapter 10 Diseases Occurring in Association with Prolapsed Disks).

In the thoracic spine, the natural kyphosis and the associated lack of mobility in extension represent a special challenge in mechanical treatment of disk damage.

If the results of diagnostic tests indicate a disk prolapse as the cause of the symptoms, it needs to be determined whether the symptoms are potentially reducible. If the pain centralizes, there is a great likelihood that conservative treatment will be successful. However, there are no comprehensive clinical data to support this hypothesis.

In some cases, no movement used in diagnostic testing centralizes or reduces the pain; on the contrary, every movement peripheralizes and intensifies the pain. With this kind of pain, the chances of successful conservative treatment are low. Nevertheless, it is reasonable not to make a decision for or against surgery as an alternative to conservative treatment until after five therapy sessions. The assessment of whether the problem can be reduced often changes in the course of treatment.

Note: If signs and symptoms are identified during the physical therapy diagnosis that require immediate surgery (bladder and bowel disorders, saddle anesthesia, sudden paralysis or a high degree of paresis, unbearable pain), the treating physician should be consulted immediately.

7.5 Therapeutic Procedure with a Diagnosis of Disk Damage

Making a treatment plan begins with the question of how the patient will get to daily therapy. The difficulty of mastering the trip to therapy varies for patients with thoracic disk prolapse, depending on the level of the damage.

If the symptoms do not become worse in standing and walking, the patient can come to the physical therapist on foot or by public transportation. If the pain increases, the patients will not be able to do this either on foot, by public transportation, or in their own car. In such cases, a house call or hospitalization would be reasonable.

In neuroradiologically confirmed disk prolapse with radicular pain radiating to the ribs or an arm, conservative treatment, preferably during a short hospitalization, is promising (Brötz et al 2001, 2003; Brötz, Burkard, Weller 2010: Brötz Maschke, Burkard et al 2010). In this way, it is possible to ensure that the patient is moving appropriately, relieving pressure, and observing the hourly exercise session.

Usually the movement tests permit identification of at least *one specific* movement that improves the symptoms. This is the movement that the patient should repeat on their own every hour, usually 10 times in direct succession, with the greatest range of motion possible.

Summary: Procedure in the Case of a Reducible Disk Problem

- *In the first 5 days:*
  - Acute pain with rapid changes.
  - The pain centralizes when the spine is moved and remains improved after the movements.
  - Well-being and objective signs such as nerve tension tests and thoracic spine mobility improve.
- *Weeks 2 to 3:*
  - Medications should be tapered and then discontinued.
  - The improvements in well-being and signs and symptoms become stable, pain is decreased to absent, and there is no rapid worsening on capacity.
- *Weeks 3 to 6:* the goal is restoration of the original capacity and ability to work with normal psychosocial integration.
- *After 6 weeks:* activities of daily living, which includes some preventive exercises, should be restored with normal capacity and with stable psychosocial integration.

7.5.1   Actively Performed Spinal Movements

The movements of the thoracic spine that the patient performs independently as part of self-training correspond to the previously described test movements. The sequence of exercises can deviate from the sequence of tests. For instance, at the beginning of treatment, asymmetrical movements lead to centralization and reduction of pain while symmetrical extension of the thoracic spine is only introduced after several days for further reduction and elimination of the pain.

In the following, the most frequently useful sequence of *therapeutic movements* for patients with thoracic disk prolapse and unilateral radicular pain is introduced.

In disk prolapse of the *lower* thoracic spine the therapeutic procedure is approximately the same as for the lumbar spine and in disk prolapse of the *upper* thoracic spine the therapeutic procedure resembles that for cervical disk prolapse.

Asymmetrical Movements

Rotation in Lateral Recumbent Position
- Lateral recumbent position.
- Place the hand of the arm lying on top onto the ribs.
- Turn the upper body and head dorsally.
- Return to the middle.
- Repeat 10 times.

Increasing Intensity
- Lateral recumbent position.
- Place the hand of the arm lying on top behind your head.
- With the hand of the lower arm hold the legs in position.
- Turn the upper body and head dorsally.
- Move the elbow of the upper arm as far dorsally as possible.
- Return to the middle.
- Repeat 10 times.

Lateral Displacement of the Pelvis in Standing Position (Shift Correction)
- Standing.
- Stand sideways next to a wall at a distance of about two foot-widths.
- The feet are directly next to each other.
- Symptoms in the *lower* thoracic spine:
  - Lean the shoulder and upper arm on the side to which the shoulder girdle is displaced with respect to the pelvis against the wall.
  - Bend the elbow on this side.

- Symptoms in the *middle* thoracic spine:
- Lean the arm of the side to which the shoulder girdle is displaced with respect to the pelvis against the wall at 90° elevation (flexion).
  - Let the pelvis sink toward the wall.
  - Move back to the middle.
  - Repeat 10 times.

Increasing Intensity 1

The further the feet are from the wall, the more intense is the effect.

Increasing Intensity 2

- Support the hand not facing the wall on the back, at the level of disease.
- Extend the spine as far as possible.

Symmetrical Extension in Seated Position (Especially for the Upper Thoracic Spine)

Retraction and Extension
- Sitting.
- Move the head backward, positioning the chin parallel to the floor.
- Move the back of the head backward in a large arc until the face is pointing to the ceiling.
- Return to starting position.
- Repeat 10 times.

Symmetrical Extension in Recumbent Position (Especially for the Middle and Lower Thoracic Spine)

Prone Position
- Lie prone in a relaxed position.
- Breathe calmly.

Support on Lower Arms
- Bend the elbows so that they are positioned directly under the shoulders (the way one reads a book on the beach).
- Remain in this position for about three breaths.
- Lie down again—relax.
- Repeat 5 to 10 times.

Hand Support, Extension in Recumbent Position
- Place the hands in front of the body so that the extension particularly affects the thoracic spine section involved.
- Slowly extend the elbows.
- Keep back and buttock muscles relaxed.
- Push up as far as possible.
- Lie down again—relax.
- Repeat 10 times.

Increasing Intensity

- At the end of the movement, hold briefly and exhale deeply.
- Lie down again—relax.
- Repeat 10 times.

7.5.2 Spinal Movements Passively Performed on the Patient by the Therapist

In exceptional cases, to intensify the symptom-reducing effects of active movements, passive spinal movements are added from the third therapy session onward.

> **Definition of Mobilization:** Active or passive movement performed at a low speed within or at the limit of passive mobility. Therapist and patient can stop the movement at any time (see Chapter 6 Lumbar Spine).

> **Note:** Passive mobilization techniques are only performed if a direction of movement has been found that centralizes and reduces the pain. The passive movement is oriented in the same direction as the centralizing movement performed by the patient themselves. It is intended to intensify the reducing effect.

Mobilization Techniques

As in the movements performed by the patient themselves, the patient is asked to report any change of symptoms immediately. The movement is done slowly, rhythmically, and with large amplitude. The number of repetitions is between five and 15, depending on the effect.

Patients with pain caused by intervertebral disk damage find it beneficial when extension and rotation mobilization are carried out in the prone position with the same rhythm as their breathing. For this reason, pressure in extension is usually applied when the patient is exhaling and released when they are inhaling.

The other movements, extension in recumbent position with positive pressure and rotation mobilization in supine position, are performed more slowly and without attention to the respiratory rhythm.

The behavior of the symptoms and the range of passive movement determine the amplitude of movement. The movements are performed to end range and always return to the original neutral position, and the therapist's hands maintain contact with the patient's back.

Instructions for the Patient
- I will move your spine passively.
- Leave it quite loose.
- I will perform the movements very slowly and fluidly.
- You can ask me to stop the movement at any time.
- Please tell me how the intensity and location of your pain are changing.

The treatment table is adjusted so that the therapist can maintain their spine in extension. In extension mobilization, extension with positive pressure, and rotational mobilization in prone position, this is a height at which the table reaches the upper third of the therapist's thigh. In rotational mobilization in supine position, the table is set to the level of the therapist's hip.

Extension Mobilization (Fig. 7.9)
- Prone position.
- The therapist stands next to the treatment table.
- The therapist places their hand closer to the foot of the table on the patient's back such that the therapist's pisiform bone is located approximately on the transverse process of the level to be treated.
- The therapist's other hand is positioned on the contralateral transverse process in such a way that the edges of the two little fingers form a right angle and the pisiform bones lie directly opposite each other at the level to be treated.
- In the patient's exhalation phase, the therapist exerts slight, symmetrical pressure with both hands.

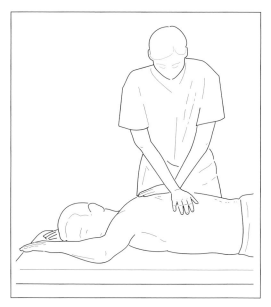

Fig. 7.9 Extension mobilization.

- In the inhalation phase, the therapist releases the pressure without losing hand contact with the back.
- Repeat approximately 10 times with increasing intensity.
- The neighboring segments are treated in the same way.

Extension in Recumbent Position with Positive Pressure
- The therapist positions their hands as in extension mobilization and exerts pressure.
- The patient supports themself on both hands (see Chapter 6, **Fig. 6.15**).
- The therapist maintains the pressure and moves their hands and trunk in such a way that the direction of pressure on the patient's spine remains approximately the same.
- The patient returns to prone position.
- The therapist relaxes the pressure.
- Repeat.

Rotation Mobilization

Bilateral Rotation Mobilization in Prone Position
- Prone position.
- The therapist stands next to the treatment table.

- The therapist places the hand closer to the foot of the table on the patient's back such that the therapist's pisiform bone is located approximately on the transverse process of the level to be treated.
- The therapist's other hand is positioned on the contralateral transverse process in such a way that the edges of the two little fingers form a right angle and the pisiform bones lie directly opposite each other at the level to be treated.
- In the patient's exhalation phase, the therapist exerts a slight, asymmetrical pressure with one hand.
- In the inhalation phase, the therapist releases the pressure without breaking hand contact with the back.
- In the next exhalation phase, the pressure is exerted on the other side of the spine.
- Repeat approximately 10 times with increasing intensity.
- The neighboring segments are treated in the same way.

Unilateral Rotation Mobilization in Prone Position

- Prone position.
- The therapist stands next to the treatment table on the side of the patient that is not to be treated.
- The therapist places one hand on the patient's back such that the therapist's pisiform bone is located approximately on the transverse process of the level to be treated on the contralateral side.
- The therapist places the other hand on the first one.
- In the patient's exhalation phase, the therapist exerts a slight pressure with both hands.
- In the inhalation phase, the therapist releases the pressure without breaking hand contact with the back.
- Repeat approximately 10 times with increasing intensity.
- The neighboring segments are treated in the same way.

Rotation Mobilization in Supine Position

- Supine position, close to the edge of the treatment table to which the knees are to be moved (see Chapter 6, **Fig. 6.16**).
- The therapist stands on this side, looking at the patient's face.

- The leg closer to the table is forward, the other leg further back (stride position).
- The patient places their feet on the bench one next to the other.
- The therapist lifts both the patient's legs and positions the dorsal aspect of the feet/lower leg in the therapist's groin.
- With one hand the therapist immobilizes the patient's thorax and with the other moves the knees toward the ground.
- This position is held for a moment.
- Return to the neutral position.
- Repeat.

7.5.3 Passive Leg or Arm Movements for Mobilization of the Nervous System

For mobilization of the nervous system, the effect of passive movements is tested first during physical therapy, since passive measures in this situation have proven to be more effective than active measures.

In disk damage of the *upper* thoracic spine, passive movements of the arms are performed first, in damage to the *lower* thoracic spine, the legs are moved first. In cases of disk damage to the *middle* thoracic spine, the effect of arm and leg movements on symptoms is tested.

Note: Movements of the thoracic spine in flexion, which also have a mobilizing effect on its nerve roots, are not performed because of the danger of displacing disk tissue toward the spinal cord.

If passive movements of the extremities reduce symptoms and if after therapy the nerve tension tests show a greater range of motion than before, they are performed repeatedly. In addition, the patient is instructed in appropriate self-training (see 7.5.4 Leg, Arm, and Spine Movements Performed by the Patient for Mobilization of the Nervous System).

The patient is asked to report immediately any changes in symptoms resulting from the treatment. The treatment method and intensity are determined by the type and irritability of the symptoms (see Chapter 4 Diagnosis in Physical Therapy). In a very irritable situation, treatment takes place at some distance from the trigger of the symptoms, for instance dorsal extension of the wrist in cases of *high* thoracic disk prolapse or dorsal extension of the ankle in *low* thoracic disk prolapse.

In principle, the extremity on the unaffected side is moved first; this should not trigger any additional symptoms. As soon as the symptoms only occur as a result of intensive movement and then rapidly disappear, the number of repetitions and the intensity of tension are increased. Pain at the end of the movement is tolerated.

Note: All symptoms elicited by the therapy should disappear immediately after the therapeutic movement is ended.

Progressive Steps of Passive Movements

Improvement of Mobility in the Upper Limb Tension Test (Especially for the Upper Thoracic Spine)

Step 1

- Supine position.
- The arms lie next to the body (neutral position).
- Dorsal extension of the wrist.
- Palmar flexion of the wrist.
- Repeat 3 to 5 times.

Step 2

- Supine position.
- 90° abduction of the upper arm.
- Elbow extension and palmar flexion in the wrist with neutral position of the lower arm.
- Elbow flexion and dorsal extension in the wrist with neutral position of the lower arm.
- Repeat 3 to 10 times.

Step 3

- Supine position.
- 90° abduction of the upper arm.
- Supination of the lower arm.
- Elbow extension and palmar flexion of the wrist.
- Elbow flexion and dorsal extension of the wrist.
- Repeat 3 to 10 times.

Step 4

- Supine position (see Chapter 8, **Fig. 8.18**).
- Shoulder depression.
- 90° abduction in shoulder joint.
- External rotation in shoulder joint.

- Supination of the lower arm.
- Elbow extension and palmar flexion of the wrist.
- Elbow flexion and dorsal extension of the wrist and finger extension.
- Repeat 3 to 10 times.

Step 5

- Supine position.
- Shoulder depression.
- 90° abduction in shoulder joint.
- Dorsal extension in wrist.
- Extension of fingers I to III.
- Abduction of the thumb.
- Supination of the lower arm.
- External rotation in shoulder joint.
- Elbow extension.
- Elbow flexion.
- Repeat 5 to 15 times.

Note: The movement to arrive at full mobility of the upper extremities is like the movement pattern for the upper limb tension test (see Chapter 8, **Fig. 8.2**).

Improvement of Mobility in the Straight Leg Raise Test

Step 1

- Supine position.
- Dorsal extension of ankle.
- Plantar flexion of ankle.
- Repeat 3 to 10 times.

Step 2

- Supine position.
- Hip flexion to 90° and maximal knee flexion.
- Hip and knee extension (the leg is lying on the table again).
- Repeat 3 to 10 times.

Step 3

- Supine position.
- Maximal hip and knee flexion.
- Release hip flexion, knee extension.
- Repeat 3 to 10 times.

Step 4

- Supine position.
- Maximal hip and knee flexion, dorsal ankle extension.

- Release hip flexion, knee extension, ankle in plantar flexion.
- Repeat 3 to 10 times.

Step 5

- Supine position.
- Maximal hip and knee flexion, dorsal ankle extension.
- Release hip flexion, knee extension, maintain ankle in dorsal extension.
- Repeat 5 to 15 times.

Step 6

- Supine position.
- Raising the extended leg as in straight leg raise test.
- Lay the leg down in neutral position.
- Repeat 5 to 15 times.

Step 7

- Supine position.
- Raise the extended leg in adduction and inward hip rotation.
- Lay the leg down in neutral position.
- Repeat 5 to 15 times.

Improvement of Mobility in the Prone Knee Bend Test (Especially for the Middle and Lower Thoracic Spine)

Step 1

- Prone position.
- Bend knee and fixate the pelvis such that no hip flexion is possible on the side being tested.
- Return the lower leg to neutral position.
- Repeat 3 to 10 times.

Step 2

- Prone position.
- Bend knee and fixate the pelvis such that no hip flexion is possible on the side being tested.
- Keep the knee bent and extend hip joint.
- Return the thigh and lower leg to neutral position.
- Repeat 5 to 15 times.

Improvement of Mobility in Slump Test

 Note

- The movements of the slump test are only performed repeatedly as an exercise when stabiliza-

tion has been achieved and pain and limitation of movement, persisting after the movements, are no longer triggered by flexion of the thoracic spine.
- This is only tested after restoration of thoracic spine mobility in extension and rotation.
- To improve mobility in the slump test, the entire movement sequence can be performed repeatedly (see **Fig. 7.2a–e**).
- To ensure that the end-range spinal flexion associated with the test does not displace the disk tissue dorsally, extension in prone position should be performed before and after the repeated movements.

7.5.4 Leg, Arm, and Spine Movements Performed by the Patient for Mobilization of the Nervous System

If the passive arm or leg movements have reduced symptoms, the patient is given instructions for self-training. First they practice with the extremities in which passive movements produced the greatest effect on their symptoms and on the nerve tension tests. It may be useful to exercise nerve-gliding capacity after stabilization, in arms, legs, and the movement sequence of the slump test.

The movements should involve as little muscle activity as possible. The patient is informed that the pain elicited by these exercises sometimes only occurs several hours after the exercise or on the next day. For this reason, it is advisable to begin carefully. At first, the movements are only practiced with each extremity three times a day with three repetitions. The movement is first performed with the unaffected side and then with the affected side.

Arm Movements as Self-training for Nerve Mobilization

- Standing erect (see Chapter 8, **Fig. 8.10a–c**).
- Stand sideways approximately one arm's length from a wall.
- 90° abduction and outward rotation in shoulder joint.
- Elbow extension.
- Supination of the lower arm.
- Place the hand on the wall with extended fingers.

- With the contralateral hand press the shoulder downward toward the tips of the toes.
- Tip head to the opposite side.
- Move back to the starting position.
- Repeat.

Leg Movements as Self-training for Nerve Mobilization

- Supine position (see Chapter 6, **Fig. 6.17a, b**).
- One leg remains extended.
- Flex the other leg in hip and knee toward the abdomen.
- Support the thigh of this leg with a towel or the hands.
- Slowly extend the knee of this leg and lower the thigh slightly. Extend the knee until a pulling pain sets in at the back of the leg or the back.
- Immediately flex toward the abdomen again.
- Repeat.

Movements of the Spine and Legs as Self-training for Nerve Mobilization

- Sitting position without the feet touching the floor (**Fig. 7.2a–e**).
- Hands behind the back with a straight sacrum.
- Slump forward (flex the spine, not the hip joints).
- Bend the cervical spine, move the chin toward the sternum.
- Extend one knee.
- Pull up the dorsum of the foot on this side (dorsal extension in ankle).
- Return to the upright seated position.
- Repeat.

7.5.5   Posture Correction

As soon as it is possible to assume an upright position without increased symptoms, the patient with thoracic disk damage is informed about the advantages of upright posture. This can take place as soon as the first therapy session (as for cervical disk damage) or not until the healing is stabilized (as for lumbar disk damage).

In upright posture, head, shoulder girdle, pelvis, and feet are precisely vertical to each other. The natural curvature of the spine is maintained, with a slight thoracic kyphosis. Muscles of abdomen and back work together harmoniously. The shoulder blades are not pulled back to support the

extension of the thoracic spine. In this way, the arms can be moved without effort.

7.5.6   Acute Phase

In patients with thoracic disk prolapse, pain is usually not expected to increase in standing and walking, and so relief from weight loading through bed rest is not necessary.

If there is a marked increase in pain compared to the load relief of bed rest, as a result of the strain of standing and walking, the patient should spend a great deal of time lying down during the first 2 or 3 days. If the pain radiates to the ribs, breathing can be impaired. This must be controlled in bedridden patients. If appropriate, the mechanical physical therapy of the spine is supplemented with respiratory therapy.

Useful Guidelines for Conduct During the Acute Phase

Extending the spine is usually the efficacious direction of movement for the centralization and reduction of pain. If there is a pronounced lateral shift, lateral movements like rotation or lateral correction in standing are necessary before extension. The unfavorable direction of movement is usually spinal flexion.

For this reason, any bending of the spine should be temporarily avoided. Since many normal movements in the activities of daily living are associated with stooping, modified forms of these movements, without stooping, are taught. These positions and activities are chiefly lying, lying down and getting up from bed, dressing, undressing, brushing teeth, eating, sitting, and in some cases, coughing and sneezing (for additional critical activities, see Chapter 6.5.6).

Lying

In recumbent position, the bed is positioned flat and at most a small pillow is used for the head. As soon as the patient can lie on their stomach without increased pain, they should spend a great deal of time in this position. The position should be varied occasionally, since movement contributes to pain relief.

Avoiding spinal flexion is best ensured in flat prone and supine position. For this reason, these two positions are preferable to lying on the side.

In lateral position the head should be positioned in line with the extended back, so that flexion is avoided.

Turning

Turning or rolling from the prone to the supine position and vice versa takes place with extended lumbar and thoracic spine flat on the bed. For some patients, the normal sequence is to move from one position to the other via the sitting position.

Note: Turning via sitting should be avoided since this change of position is associated with spinal flexion.

Change of Position

The change of position from *supine* to *sitting* is performed with extended spine via the lateral recumbent position. In learning this unnaturally stiff sequence of movements it helps most patients to imagine that they are moving as though they had swallowed a cane.

Tooth Brushing

In tooth brushing, strain on the thoracic spine can be reduced by leaning the abdomen against the sink, with a slight knee bend and support with the free hand. The spine is extended and only bent forward as far as necessary.

Sitting

Extensive sitting is a well-known risk factor in disk prolapse. Even with successful efforts to maintain an erect posture, the spine is flexed more than in standing. Sitting tends to produce and intensify pain in patients with disk prolapses. This is often only noticed when standing up. For this reason, all patients with thoracic disk damage should be advised to avoid sitting for the time being. If sitting is unavoidable (e.g., at work or while driving to physical therapy) it is best to sit upright with the support of a lumbar roll (see Chapter 9 Rehabilitation and Prevention).

Coughing, Sneezing

Coughing and sneezing often intensify the pain of a disk prolapse. It may be that the spinal flexion associated with coughing and sneezing is the cause for this increased pain. For this reason, it is best for the patient, while coughing or sneezing, to push themselves up from the prone position or extend the spine in standing position, to prevent stooping.

Instructions for the Patient

- *Recumbent:*
  - Lower your bed to be completely flat and do not use more than one small pillow.
  - Alternate between flat prone and supine positions.
  - In lateral position the head should be positioned in line with the extended back, so that flexion is avoided.
  - To alternate positions, roll over the bed with a flat back, so that the lumbar and thoracic spines remain as straight as possible.
- *Standing up and lying down:*
  - Before changing position, extend the spine and keep it extended.
  - To change to sitting from the supine position, first go to the lateral recumbent position and vice versa.
- *Tooth brushing:*
  - Place your feet in a wide stance and lean on the wash basin.
  - Support yourself with one hand on the wash basin.
  - Keep your spine extended with only a slight forward bend.
- *Sitting:*
  - Sit as little as possible.
  - Sit erect and with back support.
  - The best way to support erect sitting posture is to use a lumbar roll.
- *Coughing, Sneezing*
  - When you have an urge to cough or sneeze, extend the thoracic spine as much as possible.
  - Consciously avoid stooping forward with the upper body, which is an automatic movement.

7.5.7   Stabilization

With intermittent pain at reduced intensity that is no longer immediately produced and intensified by movements that were originally unfavorable, the condition can be considered stabilized. In this phase, in addition to the spinal movements, the patient uses both passive and active movements of the extremities, intended to improve nerve-gliding capacity, for testing and self-training see Chapter 7.5.4 Leg, Arm, and Spine Movements Performed by the Patient for Mobilization of the Nervous System.

Rotation of the thoracic spine is practiced first to the affected side and by the next day also to the unaffected side.

7.5.8 Restoration of Original Capacity

Mobility, strength, coordination, balance, and conditioning are prerequisites for the restoration of the patient's capacity and so they must be included in a training program.

In what follows, special exercises for patients with thoracic disk damage are described (see Chapter 9 Rehabilitation and Prevention).

The degree of mobility that can be called *free* is particularly difficult to determine in the thoracic spine, since it is relatively immobile in comparison to the adjacent cervical and lumbar sections of the spine. It is hardly possible to set target values for thoracic spine mobility. Instead, the target values for lumbar and cervical spine are determined (see Chapters 6 and 8: 6.5.8 an 8.5.8 Restoration of Original Capacity) and the mobility of the thoracic spine is simply described.

Marked differences from mobility normally accepted as usual are assessed.

Note: A freely mobile thoracic spine is always free of pain. If end-range movement causes pain, this could be an indication of mechanical impairment of the active and passive motor apparatus.

Free Mobility

Restoration of Extension

Hand Support, Extension While Recumbent (see Fig. 7.5)
- Prone position.
- Place the hands in front of the body or under the shoulders, depending on the region of the thoracic spine where the exercise is intended to have its greatest effect.
- Raise the head as far as possible and extend the spine.
- Slowly extend the elbows and extend the spine at every level to the greatest extent possible.

- Keep back and buttock muscles relaxed.
- Push up as far as possible.
- Lie down again—relax.
- Repeat 10 to 15 times.

Restoration of Rotation

Rotation in Lateral Recumbent Position (see Fig. 7.6)
- Lateral recumbent position.
- Place the hand of the arm lying on top behind your head.
- With the hand of the lower arm hold the legs in position.
- Turn the upper body and head dorsally.
- Move the elbow of the upper arm as far dorsal as possible.
- Return to the middle.
- Repeat 10 to 15 times.
- Change sides.

Note: Because of the physiological thoracic kyphosis, special practice of free mobility of the thoracic spine in flexion may not be necessary.

Restoration of Free Nerve-gliding Ability

The progressive steps of active extremity movements performed by the patient themselves in order to achieve free leg and arm mobility and thus free mobility of the nerve roots and peripheral nerves are the same as the progressive steps of passive movements (see Chapter 6, 6.5.3 Passive Leg Movements for Mobilization of the Nervous System—Progressive Steps of Passive Movements, and the same section under Chapter 8, 8.5.3 Passive Arm Movements for Mobilization of the Nervous System).

In addition to the movement of the extremities, the sequence of movements for the slump test can be practiced again for mobilization of the nervous system.

Strengthening

Note: There are no special exercises to strengthen individual muscles that are paretic as a result of root compression in the thoracic spine.

7.5.9 Rehabilitation, Activities of Daily Living, and Prevention

Reintegration into the activities of daily living is an important goal in the treatment of patients with disk prolapse. The physical therapy program is designed to allow previously working patients to resume their work after the shortest possible period of disability. Detailed instructions for the exercise of free, symmetrical mobility of all joints, coordination, balance, strength, and appropriate cardiovascular capacity are found in Chapter 9 Rehabilitation and Prevention.

The patient receives several instructions for the activities of daily living and a realistic number of individualized prophylactic exercises.

Instructions for the Patient

- Improve your posture and straighten up more frequently than before.
- When sitting, support the forward lumbar curve with a small cushion or roll. This also contributes to the erect posture of the thoracic spine.
- In the morning before getting up and in the evening before falling asleep, lie on your stomach. Relax and read in prone position more often. A thick pillow or a reading wedge under your chest can be helpful.
- Check the mobility in *all* directions of the entire spine. Occasionally run through the entire training program.
- *Regularly extend your entire spine* when you have been sitting for a while or doing something in stooped position. Extend *before* the pain begins. Always compensate for one-sided strains.
- Do not make a habit of sparing yourself, because then the structures of the spine will grow even less capable of dealing with strain. *Use it or lose it!*
- From time to time, treat yourself to a physical therapy session in order to analyze and treat bad posture habits, limitations of movement, asymmetries, and lack of strength.

7.6 After an Operation

Since only case studies of individual patients are available in the literature, no evidence-based recommendations about postoperative course and target treatment can be made. Therefore, if the therapist is planning to use the postoperative treatment concept described here, they should first obtain the agreement of the surgeon.

In cases of thoracic disk prolapse, it seems useful to use postoperative procedures resembling the treatments used for patients operated on for lumbar or cervical disk prolapse.

The *physical therapy examination* of patients operated on for a prolapsed disk is the same as that described in Chapter 5 Therapy. The most complete physical therapy examination possible should be conducted before the operation (see Chapter 4 Diagnosis in Physical Therapy), so that postoperative changes can be documented. Alternatively, this can also be done on the first postoperative day. Postoperative documentation is like documentation of conservative treatment (see Chapter 5).

Postoperatively, to ensure *uncomplicated wound healing* and *prevention of immediate recurrence,* the patient should observe the rules in 7.5.6 Acute Phase—Useful Guidelines for Conduct During the Acute Phase. If possible, the movement transitions should already be practiced with the patient before the operation.

Breathing should be monitored and if pain increases as a result of breathing motions or of limited asymmetrical breathing movements, the patient should receive respiratory therapy.

Patients described in the literature who had undergone surgery for a thoracic disk prolapse usually suffered from paraplegia. If the diagnostic work confirms paraparesis of the legs, all the same measures are applied as in a traumatic paraplegia, such as passive or actively supported leg movement.

If the patient spends a great deal of time lying down after the operation, they should spend at least 1 minute per hour practicing dorsal extension and plantar flexion at the ankle during the first few days for *thrombosis prevention.* In this process, strong muscle tension (especially in the calf muscles) should be built up in order to facilitate venous return and prevent formation of a thrombus.

To *improve venous return*, as vascular training, and to activate trunk muscles, isometric contraction exercises are begun on the first postoperative day.

Simple Isometric Tension Exercises, in Supine Position

Leg Exercises
- Supine position.
- Set feet on flat surface to produce a 30° angle in hip joints.
- Raise toes as high as possible.
- Brace feet against an imaginary resistance diagonally toward the ground and foot end. The legs do not move, the extensor muscles push, and the flexor muscles create the resistance.
- At the same time, push the head toward the head of the bed.
- The muscle tension is transmitted to the trunk muscles and the spine is extended.
- The therapist checks whether abdominal and back muscle tension can be felt.
- Hold the tension for two breaths.
- Release. Relax for two breaths.
- Repeat 5 to 10 times.

Arm Exercise
- Supine position.
- Extend arms on the bed.
- Rotate shoulder joints outward.
- Press extended arms onto the bed.
- Push hands toward the foot of the bed.
- At the same time, push the head toward the head of the bed. The muscle tension is transmitted to the trunk muscles and the spine is extended.
- The therapist checks whether abdominal and back muscle tension can be felt.
- Hold the tension for two breaths.
- Release. Relax for two breaths.
- Repeat 5 to 10 times.

Pushing with Arms and Legs
- Combine the movements described above and perform them simultaneously.

- Hold the tension for two breaths.
- Release. Relax for two breaths.
- Repeat 5 to 10 times.

Note: The patient should repeat the isometric tension exercises 5 to 10 times every hour.

As additional thrombosis and pneumonia prophylaxis and vascular training, the patient should get up and walk as soon as possible. In most cases they will need help at first, since there could be postoperative orthostatic hypotension. If surgery proceeded without complications, the patient can sometimes already get up on the day of the operation or, at the latest, on the first postoperative day.

From the second postoperative day on the isometric tension exercises are supplemented with movement of the thoracic spine. Weight-free mobilization in extension is practiced in lateral recumbent position. The patient is instructed to perform the movements only in a range and with a force such that there is no pain and no pulling at the wound. Usually a patient can assume a prone position without difficulty, which should be done several times a day. The transition from supine to prone position is made with a straight spine (supine–lateral–prone).

From the third postoperative day on physical therapy is conducted according to the same considerations and with the same therapeutic movements as the primary conservative treatment. Emphasis is on the points identified by the diagnosis. The therapy is symptom oriented. If the course of recovery is uncomplicated, one therapeutic movement can be added every day.

8 Cervical Spine

Spinal pain syndromes occur more frequently in the cervical spine than the thoracic spine but less frequently than in the lumbar spine. Accordingly, causes of cervical pain syndromes have been extensively studied.

Cervical disk damage occurs most frequently at intervertebral levels C5–C6 and C6–C7.

> **Definition of Cervicalgia** (Neck pain): Pain centered in the neck.

> **Definition of Brachialgia:** Pain radiating into an arm.

> **Definition of Cervicobrachialgia:** Neck pain combined with shoulder and arm pain.

In this chapter, we will describe the visual findings and diagnostic tests for diseases of the cervical spine, the evaluation criteria for establishing a physical therapy diagnosis, and the course of therapy in a diagnosis of disk damage.

8.1 Diagnostic Assessment Form for the Cervical Spine (Fig. 8.1a–d)

General guidelines for filling out the diagnostic assessment form are given in Chapter 4 Diagnosis in Physical Therapy. This includes personal information and the medical history (**Fig. 8.1a, c**), the body diagram (**Fig 8.1b**), and documentation of pain and sensory disorders (**Fig. 8.1d**). For better understanding, some information from Chapter 4 and Chapter 6 Lumbar Spine will be repeated here.

> The diagnostic assessment form can be downloaded as a PDF file at www.mediacenter.thieme.com.

8.2 Diagnosis by Observation

The visual findings evaluate posture in standing and sitting as well as gait.

Shift

In pathologies of the cervical spine, shift is a lateral displacement of the head with respect to the shoulder girdle. The chin and sternum are used as reference points to determine whether a shift is present. In a right shift, when the face is vertical, the chin is shifted to the right with respect to the sternum.

Protraction

Flexion or a loss of lordosis of the lower and middle cervical spine in the form of a protraction is typical for patients with cervical disk damage. The chin is displaced horizontally ventrally. The lower edge of the lower jaw is almost parallel to the floor while the face is displaced ahead of the body's longitudinal axis.

Guarding Arm Posture

Patients with radicular irritation syndrome in the cervical spine often carry the affected arm bent and close to the body when walking and support its weight with the unaffected arm. When the affected arm hangs down naturally, patients feel increased pain, probably as a nerve tension pain created by the pull of the arm's weight.

8.3 Diagnostic Tests

The diagnostic tests include muscle function and nerve tension tests as well as spinal test movements.

8.3.1 Muscle Function Tests

At the first examination of every patient, muscle function tests are performed for the segment-indicating muscles of nerve roots C6–C8. If compression

Diagnostic assessment—cervical spine   a
Name: _____
Date: _____

Admission data
Therapist: _____

Referral diagnosis on registration: _____

Date of birth: _____

Occupation, hobby: _____

Posture, weight-bearing: _____

On sick leave since: _____

Causative factors: _____

Duration of current episode: _____

Development: better/same/worse:
Prior treatment of current episode: physical therapy/fango/massage/sling table/
chiropractic/injections/medications/other
Medications: benzodiazepines/NSAIDs/steroids since: _____

Prior history: _____

Physical therapy diagnosis: _____

Justification of diagnosis: _____

Diagnostic assessment—cervical spine   b
Name: _____
Date: _____

Body diagram

Markings: ///// Pain ::::: Sensory disorder
Alternatively, pain is marked in red and sensory disorders are marked in blue

Diagnostic assessment—cervical spine   c
Name: _____
Date: _____
Better: Night/morning/daytime/evening/at rest/while moving/
                     stooping/stretching/sitting/lying down/standing/walking
Worse: Night/morning/daytime/evening/at rest/while moving
                     stooping/stretching/sitting/lying down/standing/walking
Coughing/sneezing/straining
Trauma: _____
Operation: _____
Unwanted weight loss   yes/no (_____ kg in _____ weeks)
Reaction to repeated, end-range movements
Starting situation: _____

Movement	NT, CE, EL, PR, PE, NE,↑↓	RI, RW, RNI, RNW
	Change during movement	Change after movement
1 × retraction		
5 × retraction		
1 × extension		
5 × extension		
1 × retraction and extension		
5 × retraction and extension		
1 × rotation right		
5 × rotation right		
1 × rotation left		
5 × rotation left		
1 × lateral flexion right		
5 × lateral flexion right		
1 × lateral flexion left		
5 × lateral flexion left		
1 × flexion		
5 × flexion		
Other:		

Diagnostic assessment—cervical spine: follow-up   d
Name: _____
Date: _____
Medications: benzodiazepines/NSAIDs/steroids   Cervical spine shift: R   L

Vertigo
Pain: document area, activity and intensity

0 1 2 3 4 5 6 7 8 9 10   0 1 2 3 4 5 6 7 8 9 10
Before PT   After PT

0 1 2 3 4 5 6 7 8 9 10   0 1 2 3 4 5 6 7 8 9 10
Maximal   Minimal   in the last 24 hours
Pain radiation in cm before PT _____ after PT _____
Sensory disorder
Area: _____
Characteristics: _____   better/same/worse
Muscle function test

	R	L		R	L
C5 deltoid			Brachioradialis		
C6 biceps brachii			Pronator		
C7 triceps brachii					
C8 interossei					

Signs of nerve extension

ULTT1 right:	ULTT1 left:

Mobility

Retraction	Extension	Flexion	Protraction
Lateral flexion:		Rotation:	
R		R	
L		L	

Fig. 8.1 (a–d) Diagnostic assessment form for the cervical spine.
(NT = not tested; CE = centralized; EL = eliminated; PR = produced; PE = peripheralized; NE = no effect; ↑ = pain increases; ↓ = pain decreases; RI = remains improved; RW = remains worse; RNI = remains not improved; RNW = remains not worse; R = right; L = left; PT = physical therapy; ULTT = upper limb tension test.)

of another root is suspected or a prolapsed disk at a different level is neuroradiologically confirmed, the corresponding segment-indicating muscles are also tested. In comparison of sides, the individual normal range of motion and the individual normal strength are tested.

Testing and Evaluation

Dorsal and Palmar Interossei (C8)

- Seated.
- The patient's palm is turned toward the floor.
- Fingers are extended.
- The patient splays out their fingers (dorsal interossei).
- The therapist exerts resistance at the terminal phalanges around the radial aspect of the second finger and the ulnar aspect of the third finger, and the radial aspect of the third finger and the ulnar aspect of the fourth and fifth fingers.
- The patient adduces (closes) the splayed fingers (palmar interossei).
- The therapist exerts resistance around the ulnar aspect of the second finger and the radial aspect of the fourth and fifth fingers.

Evaluation

- Full strength 5/5: five times full range of motion against strong resistance along the path and at the end.
- 4/5: full range of motion against moderate resistance along the path and at the end.
- 3/5: full range of motion against gravity.
- 2/5: movements are not possible over the whole range of motion.
- 0 to 1/5: it is barely possible to palpate a contraction of the interossei through their position between the metacarpals.

Triceps Brachii (C7)

- Supine recumbent postion.
- 90° elevation (flexion) in the shoulder joint of the arm to be tested, neutral shoulder position with respect to abduction and adduction, inward rotation of shoulder joint.
- The hand on the side to be tested is placed on the contralateral shoulder.
- The patient extends their elbow joint without moving the upper arm.

- The therapist applies resistance at the distal lower arm.

Evaluation

- Full strength 5/5:
  - Five times full range of motion against strong resistance over the path and at the end.
  - Full resistance can only be overcome from 90° elbow flexion.
  - A person of normal strength cannot extend the elbow from complete flexion (hand on the contralateral shoulder) against strong resistance.
  - In case of doubt, comparison of sides indicates whether strength is diminished or not.
- 4/5: full range of motion against moderate resistance along the path and at the end.
- 3/5: full range of motion against gravity.
- 2/5:
  - Examination in supine position with upper arm abducted by 90° and rotated outward.
  - Full range of motion without gravity.
- 1/5: a contraction of the triceps brachii can be detected by palpation of the tendon over the dorsal side of the elbow joint and the muscle fibers on the dorsal aspect of the upper arm.
- 0/5: no palpable contraction.

Note:

- The lower arm flexors are tested together.
- To avoid spinal guarding movements and to compare sides, the testing of the biceps brachii is done bilaterally simultaneously.

Biceps Brachii and Brachioradialis (C6)

- Erect seated position.
- Lower arms in neutral position with respect to supination/pronation.
- The patient bends their elbows without moving the upper arms and upper body.
- The therapist applies resistance at the distal lower arms.

Evaluation

- Full strength 5/5: five times full range of motion against strong resistance along the path and at the end.
- 4/5: full range of motion against moderate resistance along the path and at the end.

- 3/5: full range of motion against gravity.
- 2/5: examination in supine position with upper arm abducted by 90° and rotated outward; full range of motion without gravity.
- 1/5: a contraction of the biceps brachii can be detected by palpation of the tendon in the hollow of the elbow and the muscle fibers on the anterior aspect of the upper arm.
- 0/5: no palpable contraction.

Deltoid Muscle (C5)

Note:

- Usually it is sufficient to test the *middle* and *anterior* portions of the deltoid muscle.
- To avoid spinal guarding movements, the testing is done bilaterally simultaneously.

Middle Portion

- Seated.
- The patient bends their elbow up to 90° and positions the upper arms parallel to the trunk.
- The patient abducts the upper arms up to approximately 90°.
- The therapist applies resistance at the elbow joints.

Evaluation

- Full strength 5/5: five times full range of motion against strong resistance along the path and at the end.
- 4/5: full range of motion against moderate resistance along the path and at the end.
- 3/5: full range of motion against gravity.
- 2/5: examination in supine position: full range of motion without gravity.
- 1/5: a contraction of the middle portion of the muscle can be detected by palpation of the muscle fibers on the lateral side of the upper third of the upper arm.
- 0/5: no palpable contraction.

Anterior Portion

- Seated.
- The patient bends their elbow up to 90° and positions the upper arms parallel to the trunk.
- The patient flexes the upper arms in the shoulder joint up to approximately 90°.
- The therapist applies resistance at the hollow of the elbow.

Evaluation

- Full strength 5/5: five times full range of motion against strong resistance along the path and at the end.
- 4/5: full range of motion against moderate resistance along the path and at the end.
- 3/5: full range of motion against gravity.
- 2/5: examination in lateral recumbent position: full range of motion without gravity.
- 1/5: a contraction of the anterior portion of the deltoid muscle can be detected by palpation of the muscle fibers on the anterior side of the upper third of the upper arm.
- 0/5: no palpable contraction.

8.3.2 Nerve Tension Test of the Upper Extremity

Note:

- Nerve tension tests are always conducted sequentially on both sides.
- Where there is radiating pain, the unaffected arm is tested first.
- Contralateral pain triggered on the affected side by testing of the unaffected side can be a sign of disk prolapse.

Upper Limb Tension Test (ULTT)

This test creates tension on the following nerve roots and peripheral nerves:
- Nerve roots C4–T1.
- Brachial plexus.
- Median nerve.

The pain of nerve tension can be felt in the cervical spine and along the entire course of the brachial plexus and the median nerve. A sensory disorder can be triggered or intensified in the area supplied by the affected nerve root. Most frequently this can be observed in the hand.

Instructions for the Patient

- I am going to move your arm.
- Leave it quite loose.
- I will perform the movement slowly.
- You may feel pulling or pain.
- Please tell me when the movement becomes unpleasant, then I will stop.

- Please tell me if pain arises or is worse on the other side (in one-sided pain and during testing of the unaffected side).
- Please tell me where the pain set in.

Implementation (Fig. 8.2a–d)

- The patient is lying flat on their back.
- The spine is straight, without tilting to the side.
- No cushion under the body.

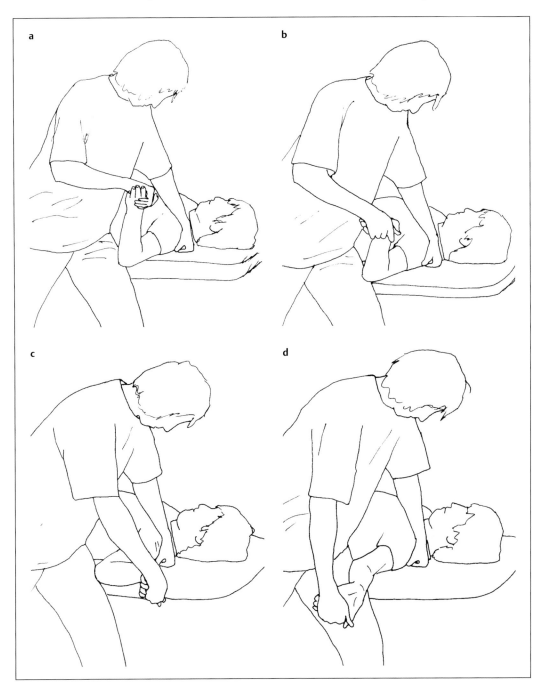

Fig. 8.2 (a–d) Upper limb tension test.

- The patient places the hand that will not be examined next to their body or on their abdomen.
- The therapist moves the shoulder on the side to be tested toward the foot end (depression) until they feel resistance and fixate this position in place.
- The therapist grasps the patient's hand so that the therapist's palm rests in the patient's palm and the therapist can use their own thumb to abduct the patient's thumb.
- Using their own thigh, the therapist guides the patient's upper arm into 90° abduction and fixates it in place there.
- Wrist in dorsal extension.
- Fingers extended.
- Thumb abducted.
- Lower arm in supination.
- The therapist slowly guides the patient's hand toward the patient's head so that outward rotation in the shoulder joint results.
- The therapist slowly extends the elbow joint.

Observations and Criteria for Stopping the Test Movement

- *Avoidance movements:*
  - Movement of the occiput toward the shoulder girdle; neck extension.
  - Inclination of part or all of the spine toward the side being tested.
- *Resistance: elastic end of movement.*
- *Reflex muscle tension:*
  - Suddenly perceptible end of movement.
  - Jerky tension of the finger, wrist, and elbow flexors.

The test is evaluated as *positive* in the following cases:

- The symptoms familiar to the patient are reproduced or intensified.
- A distinct postural response is visible, for example, neck extension.
- A distinct side difference occurs.

To *differentiate* between nerve tension pain and pain due to other causes, the tension is reduced at a point far away from the site of the pain, for instance when the pain is in the lower arm, shoulder elevation or lateral flexion of the cervical spine to the side being tested or when the pain is in the neck, palmar flexion of the hand.

Note:

- In the ULTT, if the pain decreases when nerve tension is reduced, it was probably caused by tension in the nervous system.
- If it remains unchanged, the cause of the pain is more likely to be found in another structure (e.g., muscles or tendons).

8.3.3 Test and Therapeutic Spinal Movements

Certain safety rules must be observed for repeated movements of the cervical spine. End-range extension and rotation of the cervical spine narrows the lumen of the vertebral artery. If there was prior narrowing of the vessel, these movements of the cervical spine can decrease the blood supply to the basilar artery and thus to the brain stem and the cerebellum. This may ultimately result in brain stem symptoms and signs of cerebellar failure such as vertigo, speech disorders, and ataxia, or brain stem symptoms such as diplopia or even loss of consciousness (see Chapter 3 Medical Diagnosis and Treatment).

Note: If new neurological symptoms or signs consistent with brain ischemia arise, the movement tests are immediately stopped and the treating physician is consulted.

In disk prolapse and bony spinal stenoses, there is a danger of myelocompression. This can manifest with sensory disorders and pareses in all four extremities (see Chapter 3). In response to extension of the cervical spine, bony spinal stenosis that narrows the cervical vertebral lumen can compress the spinal cord.

In a disk prolapse, the principal problem is most likely that flexion of the cervical spine displaces disk tissue backward toward the spinal cord.

Note: If symptoms arise in both arms or in the legs, the movement tests are immediately stopped and the treating physician is consulted.

With the help of test movements, the mobility of the spine and the effect of repeated spinal movements on the symptoms, especially pain, are studied.

Evaluation of Mobility

Mobility of the cervical spine in retraction, extension, flexion, lateral flexion, and rotation to both sides is documented in the first therapy session.

Spinal mobility can be evaluated without technically complicated measurement devices (for measures of free mobility see Chapter 8.5.8 Restoration to Original Capacity, Free Mobility).

Observation of whether mobility is limited and whether mobility changes during exercise and in correlation to pain is decisive for diagnosis and treatment in the acute phase.

Repeated Test Movements

Since in disk damage, extension of the affected region of the spine is usually a beneficial movement, retraction and extension are tested first. If the symptoms are asymmetrical, then asymmetrical test movements often lead to centralization and reduction of pain. When symmetrical retraction and extension of the spine do not result in centralization, the next step is to test one-sided rotation or lateral flexion.

The working hypothesis is the idea that movements can exert pressure on the injured region of the anulus fibrosus, thus forcing the displaced gelatinous mass medially or ventrally or both.

Note: In neuroradiologically confirmed diagnosis of disk prolapse, repeated flexion is not tested because of the danger of displacing the disk tissue toward the spinal cord and stretching the spinal cord.

For pain syndromes in the cervical spine, unlike the thoracic and lumbar spine, the weight strain on the spine in a vertical body position does not usually have a significant effect on pain. In addition, less force is required to perform the movements in the seated tests. For this reason, the test movements are first performed while sitting. The weight of the affected arm itself can be relieved by laying the arm in the lap. Testing is only done in reclining position if the patient feels considerably less pain in this position.

Tempo and rhythm of the movements are slow but fluid. The patient should be able to stop the movement at any time. No momentum should be introduced.

The movements are performed with the greatest *range of motion* possible. If the patient stops a movement, the therapist asks why (e.g., because of pain, fear of pain, or limitation of movement).

The *intensity* of the test movements is always increased if a certain movement has a centralizing and reducing effect, but the pain has not disappeared.

The number of *repetitions* is between two and 10. If the pain is intensified or peripheralized by the movement tests and remains changed to this intensity after the movements and there are signs of impaired circulation in the area of the vertebral artery (see Chapter 3, 3.1.1 Medical History), the test is repeated twice at most. If the pain is reduced or centralized, the test is performed 10 times.

The patient is always asked before, during, and after the test movements where and at what intensity on the numerical analog scale (NAS) they are experiencing pain and whether anything changes in these perceptions during the movements. The therapist asks the following questions:

- Is your pain changing?
- Where does it hurt now?
- How intense is your pain now?

Note: Avoid leading questions such as: Is it getting better now? Does the pain go as far into your arm now?

Almost every patient is able to assign a number to the pain intensity between 0 (no pain) and 10 (worst pain imaginable). The therapist should insist that the patient make precise statements about their pain. Statements like "Now it's worse than before" or "It's OK" provide no useful information for planning further treatment.

If, for instance, the neck pain has increased but the radiating arm pain has decreased or stopped, this might be more unpleasant for the patient but must be interpreted as an improvement of symptoms. This should be explained to the patient. Usually the patient can tolerate an increase of central pain if the positive aspect of centralization is explained.

After every test movement, both the pain and the nerve tension sign (upper limb tension test) are measured and documented. The change in mobility of the cervical spine is evaluated and documented. When all test movements have been completed, muscle strength and sensory disorders are reviewed for quality and location and documented.

Instructions for the Patient

- Move your head slowly and without much force.
- Move it as far as possible.
- Tell me how the intensity and location of your pain are changing.
- Stop immediately if you feel dizzy.
- Stop the movement if the pain radiates further.

Protraction is a frequently occurring undesirable posture (**Fig. 8.3**). It is associated with flexion of the lower cervical spine and thoracic spine and thus a potential trigger for disk injuries. Patients with disk damage often remain in this position because it is possible that a displacement of mass to dorsal within the disk blocks extension of the cervical spine. For this reason retraction and extension are important target movements for the treatment of cervical disk damage.

Extension Test

◻ Definition of Retraction:

- The head is moved backward and the lower jaw (in sitting and standing) is positioned parallel to the floor.

- This movement is associated with flexion of the upper and extension of the lower cervical spine.
- The thoracic spine is extended at the same time.

◻ Definition of Protraction:

- The face is moved ventrally.
- This movement is associated with extension of the upper and flexion of the lower cervical spine.
- The thoracic spine is flexed at the same time.

In flexion of the entire cervical spine, there is more flexion in the lower cervical spine than in protraction. In extension of the entire cervical spine there is more extension in the lower cervical spine than in retraction (Ordway et al 1999). For this reason, extension is used for maximal extension of the lower cervical spine.

Rotation and lateral flexion are tested in the most erect position possible. For this reason, retraction is also taught as the first movement direction for rotation and lateral flexion.

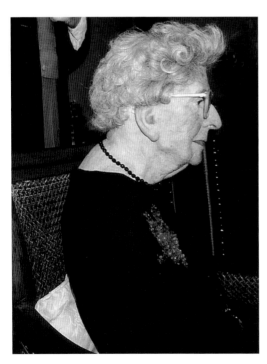

Fig. 8.3 Undesirable posture in protraction.

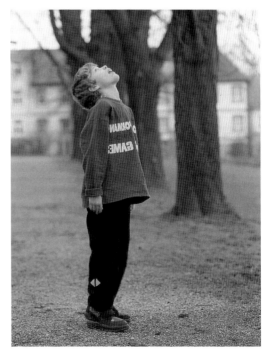

Fig. 8.4 Extension of the entire cervical spine.

Retraction (Fig. 8.5a, b)

- Seated.
- Move the head backward, positioning the lower jaw parallel to the floor.
- This creates a slight pressure at the larynx and a double chin becomes visible.
- Relax.
- Repeat.

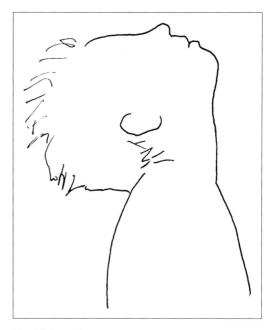

Fig. 8.6 Extension.

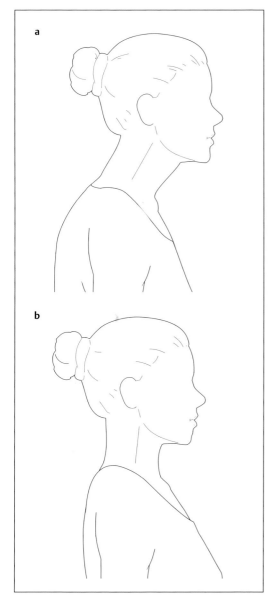

Fig. 8.5 (a, b) Retraction.

Extension (Fig. 8.6)

- Seated.
- Move the head backward, positioning the lower jaw parallel to the floor, upright posture.
- Move the back of the head backward in a large arc until the face is pointing to the ceiling.
- Return to starting position.
- Repeat.

Asymmetrical Tests

Rotation (Fig. 8.7)

Note: Rotating the head to the side affected by disk damage leads to centralization and reduction of pain more often than rotating the head to the unaffected side.

- Seated.
- Move the head backward, positioning the lower jaw parallel to the floor, upright posture.
- Turn the head.
- Return to starting position.
- Repeat.
- Perform the same movement in the other direction.

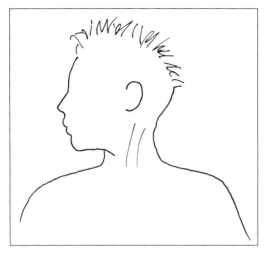

Fig. 8.7 Rotation.

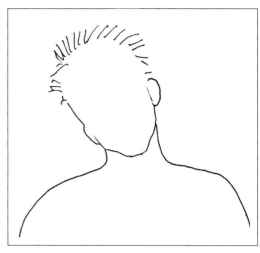

Fig. 8.8 Lateral flexion.

Lateral Flexion (Fig. 8.8)

Note: Lateral flexion to the side affected by disk damage leads to centralization and reduction of pain more often than lateral flexion to the unaffected side.

- Seated.
- Move the head backward, positioning the lower jaw parallel to the floor, upright posture.
- Tip head to the side with the face still oriented ventrally.
- Return to starting position.
- Repeat.
- Perform the same movement in the other direction.

Flexion (Fig. 8.9)

- Seated.
- Move the chin toward the sternum.
- Return to starting position.
- Repeat.

8.4   Establishing the Diagnosis

All findings from the medical history, the physical examination, and the diagnostic tests are taken into account (**Table 8.1**; for fundamental aspects, see Chapter 4 Diagnosis in Physical Therapy).

The diagnosis should be considered a working hypothesis. Discussion with the treating physician may lead to further diagnostic or therapeutic measures.

Summary: Typical Findings in a Diagnosis of Disk Damage

- *Information in the medical history:*
  - Age: 20 to 55 years.
  - Duration: long or short (acute–chronic).

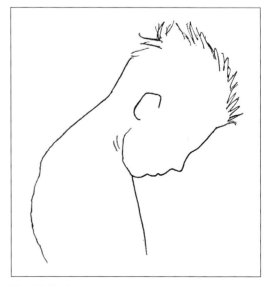

Fig. 8.9 Flexion.

Table 8.1 Simplified guide to interpreting changes in pain caused by test movements

Question	Answer	Conclusions
1. Can the problem be influenced mechanically by movement of the cervical spine?	No	Tumor Inflammatory disease Disease of internal organs Stenosis syndrome of the shoulder, ulnar sulcus, carpal tunnel More examinations **Note:** no mechanical therapy of the cervical spine.
	Yes	**Continue with question 2**
2. Does the same movement always trigger precisely the same pain reaction and does the pain return to its original state after the movement?	Yes	Shortened structures, nerve root adhesions **Note:** mechanical physical therapy Spinal or cervical foraminal stenosis Instability (e.g., after whiplash trauma), facet joint pain More examinations **Note:** In cases of stenosis: posture training, exercise spinal flexion In case of instability: stabilizing strength training
	No	**Continue with question 3**
3. Does the pain centralize or peripheralize within one dermatome?	Yes	Disk damage Check for possible disk prolapse **Note:** mechanical physical therapy
	No	**Continue with question 4**
4. Does the same movement produce different pain reactions with pain that remains the same or increases after the movement?	Yes	Chronified pain syndrome Psychosocial problem More examinations (see Chapter 11 Psychosocial Risk Factors) **Note:** In chronified pain syndrome: different types of activation; unspecific exercise programs, mechanical and strengthening In predominantly psychosocial problems: discuss physical therapy with the treating physician

- Sudden onset.
- Trigger: stooping.
- Changes due to movement.
- Constant or intermittent
- *Character of the complaints:*
  - Pain in the cervical spine.
  - Pain in the cervical spine in combination with dermatome-related radiating pain.
  - Dermatome-related radiating pain without pain in the cervical spine.
  - Dermatome-related sensory disorders.
  - Paresis, chiefly in individual segment-indicating muscles.
- *Findings on inspection:*
  - Protraction/shift deformation.
  - Limited movement.
- *Properties of symptoms upon repeated spinal movement:*
  - Rapid change during the movements.
  - The changes persist after the movements.

- Centralization/peripheralization of the pain.
- Improvement of mobility with decrease in pain and vice versa.
- Nerve tension signs better/worse.
- Sensory perception and strength change from day to day, not within one therapy session.

Differential diagnoses (e.g., stenosis syndromes of tendons that run through the shoulder joint, in the outward rotators, or the biceps brachii), require special differentiating tests. Findings that are typical in a diagnosis of *cervical disk damage* cannot be found in these differential diagnoses. Repeated movements of the cervical spine barely have any effect on symptoms that are caused by irritation of the biceps brachii tendon (for details of differential tests see the literature for manual diagnosis and treatment, for example the Maitland approach; Maitland 2000).

Disorders frequently associated with disk damage such as spinal and foraminal stenosis, spinal instability, facet joint pain, and inflamed or fibrosed nerve roots also cause certain typical pain reactions (see Chapter 10 Diseases Occurring in Association with Prolapsed Disks).

In physical therapy using repeated movements of the cervical spine, the movements that might be beneficial for treatment of disk damage could provoke and intensify symptoms with a different cause (see Chapter 10), reducing the chances of successful conservative therapy in this kind of combined disease. This is particularly true for the cervical spine since the spaces between the nerve roots and the surrounding bony structures, especially in the intervertebral foramina, are particularly narrow.

If the results of diagnostic testing indicate a disk prolapse as the cause of the symptoms, it is determined whether the symptoms are potentially reducible. If the pain centralizes, there is a great likelihood that conservative treatment will be successful. The likelihood of successful mechanical physical therapy is lower for cervical than for lumbar disk prolapse.

In some cases, no movement used in diagnostic testing centralizes or reduces the pain; on the contrary, *every* movement peripheralizes and intensifies the pain. With this kind of pain, the conservative treatment is more difficult. Nevertheless, it is reasonable not to make a decision for or against surgery as an alternative to conservative treatment until after five therapy sessions. The assessment of whether the problem can be reduced often changes in the course of treatment.

Note: If physical therapy diagnosis detects signs and symptoms requiring immediate surgery (e.g., new symptoms or signs of leg, bladder, and bowel disorders, sudden paralysis or a high degree of paresis in one or both arms, unbearable pain), the treating physician should be consulted immediately.

8.5 Therapeutic Procedure with a Diagnosis of Disk Damage

Unlike for patients with lumbar disk prolapse, making the trip to therapy is usually not a problem for patients with cervical disk prolapse. The symptoms do not become worse upon standing and walking, so that the patient can come to the physical therapy practice on foot or by public transport.

Since sitting, especially in a car, is not beneficial for patients with prolapsed disks but rather intensifies symptoms, car trips should be avoided.

In the case of a neuroradiologically confirmed disk prolapse with radicular pain, a short hospitalization for conservative therapy should be considered. In this way, it is possible to ensure that the patient is moving appropriately and relieving pressure. Hourly exercise sessions are not a problem.

Usually the movement tests permit identification of at least *one* specific movement that improves the symptoms. The patient is asked to repeat the movement on their own every hour, usually 10 times in direct succession, with the greatest range of motion possible.

The therapeutically useful movements change in the course of healing. For this reason, to begin with, therapy should be administered for *at least 5 consecutive days.*

Only *one* exercise for independent practice is changed at a time, so that it is clear whether the change has a good or bad effect on the symptoms. Neither medications nor everyday activities, such as returning to work, should be changed at the same time as the exercises.

Practicing unaccustomed movements can cause new complaints that are unrelated to disk injury. For instance, in practicing retraction, the upper cervical spine is flexed. This unaccustomed movement can often cause diffuse pain in the upper cervical spine or headaches. The patient should be informed that these new complaints are to be expected and that they are a normal development and no danger to health.

Summary: Procedure in the Case of a Reducible Disk Problem

- *In the first 5 days:*
  - Acute pain with rapid changes.
  - The pain centralizes when the spine is moved and remains improved after the movements.
  - Well-being and signs such as the upper limb tension test and cervical spine mobility improve.
- *Weeks 2 to 3:*
  - Medications should be first tapered and then discontinued.
  - The improvements in well-being and signs and symptoms stabilize; pain is decreased

to absent and there is no rapid worsening on weight-bearing.

- *Weeks 3 to 6:* restoration of the original capacity for strain and ability to work with normal psychosocial integration are the goal.
- *After 6 weeks:* activities of daily living, which includes some preventive exercises, should be restored with normal capacity and stable psychosocial integration.
- *After 1 year:* complete capacity and complete or extensive reduction of neurological deficits can be expected.

8.5.1 Actively Performed Spinal Movements

The movements of the cervical spine that the patient performs independently correspond to the previously described test movements. The sequence of exercises can deviate from the sequence of tests. For instance, at the beginning of treatment, asymmetrical movements often lead to centralization and reduction of pain while symmetrical retraction and extension of the cervical spine are only introduced after several days for further reduction and elimination of the pain.

In the following, the most frequently useful sequence of *therapeutic* movements for patients with cervical disk prolapse and cervicobrachialgia are introduced.

Asymmetrical Movements

▱ **Note:** Turning the head (rotation) or lateral flexion to the affected side leads to centralization and reduction of pain more often than rotation or lateral flexion to the unaffected side.

Rotation
- Seated.
- Move the head backward, positioning the lower jaw parallel to the floor, upright posture.
- Turn head to affected side.
- Return to starting position.
- Repeat 10 times.

Lateral Flexion
- Seated.
- Move the head backward, positioning the lower jaw parallel to the floor, upright posture.

- Tip head to affected side.
- Return to starting position.
- Repeat 10 times.

Symmetrical Extension

Retraction
- Seated.
- Move the head backward, positioning the lower jaw parallel to the floor, upright posture.
- Return to starting position.
- Repeat 10 times.

Extension
- Seated.
- Move the head backward, positioning the lower jaw parallel to the floor, upright posture.
- Move the back of the head backward in a large arc until the face is pointing to the ceiling.
- Return to starting position.
- Repeat 10 times.

Extension with Rotation at End
- Seated.
- Move the head backward, positioning the lower jaw parallel to the floor, upright posture.
- Move the back of the head backward in a large arc until the face is pointing to the ceiling.
- At the end of the movement, turn the head, with a small range of motion, to the right and the left.
- Return to starting position.
- Repeat 10 times.

8.5.2 Spinal Movements Passively Performed on the Patient by the Therapist

▱ **Note:** Passive movement of the cervical spine may only be performed by therapists who have learned and practiced this technique under an instructor's supervision. Such movements are therefore not presented here. Training in spinal mobilization techniques is offered (e.g., according to the McKenzie and Maitland concepts).

Manipulation of the cervical spine in patients with neck and head pain does not produce better results than mobilization (Hurwitz et al 2002). However, it can result in significant problems (Assendelft et al 1996; Hurwitz et al 1996;

Hufnagel et al 1999; Haldeman et al 2002): the most frequent complication is injury to the vertebral artery, ranging from mild discomfort due to transient ischemia to brain stem and cerebellar infarcts.

Other complications have also been reported, such as spinal cord compression, vertebral fractures, tracheal tearing, diaphragmatic paralysis, hematomas in the carotid artery, and cardiac arrest. The risk of complications is estimated to be 1:40,000 manipulations (Hurwitz et al 1996).

The effect of cervical spine manipulation in patients with cervical disk prolapse has not yet been systematically investigated, but the risk of complication through displacement of the disk toward the spinal cord can be estimated as being higher than in unspecific neck and head pain.

⬦ **Note:** Manipulation of the cervical spine should not be performed.

8.5.3   Passive Arm Movements for Mobilization of the Nervous System

For mobilization of the nervous system, the effect of passive movements is the first to be tested in physical therapy, since passive measures for treating this system are often more effective than active measures. If passive movements of the arms reduce symptoms and if after therapy the nerve tension tests show a greater range of motion than before, the movements are performed again. In addition, the patient is instructed in appropriate self-training methods (see 8.5.4 Arm Movements Performed by the Patient for Mobilization of the Nervous System).

The patient is asked to report immediately any changes in symptoms resulting from the treatment. The treatment method and *intensity* depend on the type and irritability of the symptoms (see Chapter 4 Diagnosis in Physical Therapy). In a very irritable situation, treatment takes place at some distance from the trigger of the symptoms, for instance by dorsal extension of the wrist in the case of cervical disk prolapse.

In principle, the unaffected extremity is moved first, but not sufficiently to trigger additional symptoms. As soon as symptoms only occur as a result of intensive movement and then disappear

rapidly, the movement can also take place in the anatomical area where the symptoms are felt.

The next increase of intensity in the treatment is to increase the number of repetitions. Then the movement is performed with more tension, and the pain or sensory disorder triggered at the end of the movement is tolerated. All symptoms elicited by therapy should disappear immediately after the therapeutic movement is ended.

Progressive Steps of Passive Movements

Improving Mobility in the Upper Limb Tension Test

Step 1
- Supine.
- Dorsal wrist extension.
- Palmar wrist flexion.
- Repeat three to five times.

Step 2
- Supine.
- 90° upper arm abduction.
- Elbow extension and palmar wrist flexion with neutral lower arm position.
- Elbow flexion and dorsal wrist extension with neutral lower arm.
- Repeat 3 to 10 times.

Step 3
- Supine.
- 90° upper arm abduction.
- Lower arm supination.-
- Elbow extension and palmar wrist flexion.
- Elbow flexion and dorsal wrist extension.
- Repeat 3 to 10 times.

Step 4
- Supine.
- Shoulder depression.
- 90° shoulder joint abduction.
- Outward shoulder joint rotation.
- Lower arm supination.
- Elbow extension and palmar wrist flexion.
- Elbow flexion and dorsal wrist extension with finger extension.
- Repeat 3 to 10 times.

Step 5

- Supine.
- Shoulder depression.
- 90° shoulder joint abduction.
- Dorsal wrist extension.
- Extension of fingers.
- Thumb abduction.
- Lower arm supination.
- Outward shoulder joint rotation.
- Elbow extension.
- Elbow flexion.
- Repeat 5 to 15 times.

⏻ **Note:** Improving mobility in the upper limb tension test is similar to the movement pattern for the upper limb tension test (see **Fig. 8.2**).

8.5.4 Arm Movements Performed by the Patient for Mobilization of the Nervous System

If the passive arm movements have reduced symptoms, the patient is given instructions for self-training. The patient is informed that the pain elicited by these exercises sometimes only occurs several hours later or on the next day after the exercise. For this reason, it is advisable to begin carefully. At first, the movements are only practiced three times a day with three repetitions for each arm. The movement is first performed with the unaffected arm and then with the affected arm.

⏻ **Note:** The movements performed by the patient are the same as 8.5.3 Passive Arm Movements for Mobilization of the Nervous System.

- They can be performed seated, standing, or lying down with very little effort.
- In the last step of the treatment plan, movements of the cervical spine are included.
- This sequence of movements is only practiced when lateral flexion of the cervical spine without additional arm movements produces no symptoms.

Performance of Sliders (Fig. 8.10a–c)

- Erect standing.
- Stand approximately one arm's length from the wall.

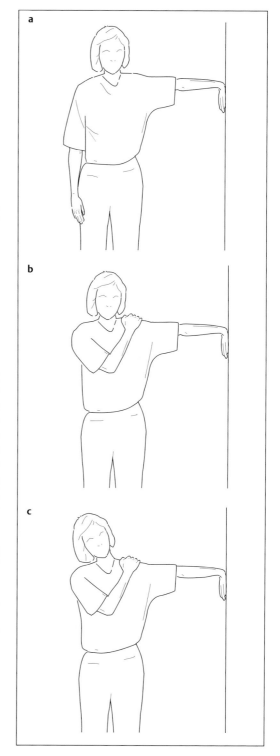

Fig. 8.10 (a–c) Sliders.

- 90° abduction and outward shoulder joint rotation.
- Elbow extension.
- Lower arm supination.
- Place the hand on the wall with extended fingers.
- With the contralateral hand press the shoulder downward.
- Tip head to the opposite side.
- Move back to the starting position.
- Repeat.

8.5.5 Posture Correction

Patients with cervical disk damage are already informed of the advantages of upright posture in the first therapy session. Since the exercises are normally done while sitting or standing and retraction is a movement that contributes to achieving upright position and centralization of pain, reduction of pain can be expected from posture correction. Vertical positioning of the head over the shoulder girdle as well as effortless mobility of the arms with simultaneous straightening of the spine is particularly emphasized for patients with cervical disk damage (see Chapter 9 Rehabilitation and Prevention).

8.5.6 Acute Phase

Note: Weight loading of the spine in the area of the cervical spine usually does not intensify pain, so that bed rest is not part of the therapeutic strategy.

Useful Guidelines for Conduct During the Acute Phase

Retraction and extension of the cervical spine are usually the most beneficial, pain-centralizing and -reducing directions of movement, whereas protraction and flexion lead to intensification of the symptoms. It is therefore a useful preventive measure to temporarily avoid any bending of the spine. Since many normal movements in the activities of daily living are associated with stooping, modified forms of these movements, without stooping, are taught. These activities are chiefly lying, lying down and getting up from bed, brushing teeth, and in some cases, coughing and sneezing. In addition, erect posture in sitting, standing, and walking are practiced (see Chapter 9.1 Posture Training).

Lying

For reclining, the bed is adjusted to flat position. Most of the time, the patient should be lying flat on their back, with at most a small pillow for their head. In lateral reclining position, the head is positioned toward the back, to ensure extension of the cervical spine. A pillow should be placed under the head to fill the space between the neck and the bed such that the cervical spine does not tip to the side.

During the acute phase, the prone position is not possible without an increase of symptoms because of the associated extension and rotation of the cervical spine. The position should be varied occasionally, since movement usually contributes to pain relief.

Turning

Turning or rolling from the lateral reclining to the supine position and vice versa takes place with extended cervical spine flat on the bed. For some patients, the normal sequence is to move from one position to the other via the sitting position. This should be avoided as much as possible since this change of position is associated with spinal flexion.

Change of Position

The change of position from *supine* to *sitting* is performed with extended spine via the lateral recumbent position. In learning this unnaturally stiff sequence of movements it helps most patients to imagine that they are moving as though they had swallowed a cane.

Tooth Brushing

When brushing the teeth, the load on the cervical spine can be reduced by leaning the abdomen against the sink, a slight knee bend, and support with the free hand. The cervical spine is extended and the upper body is only bent forward as far as necessary.

Sitting

Sitting is well known as a causative factor in disk prolapse. Even with successful efforts to maintain an erect posture, the cervical spine, like the lumbar spine, is flexed more than in standing.

Sitting tends to produce and intensify pain in patients with disk prolapses. This is often only noticed when standing up. For this reason, patients with cervical disk damage should sit as little as possible. If sitting is unavoidable, for instance, at work or while riding to physical therapy, it is best to sit upright with the support of a lumbar roll (see Chapter 9 Rehabilitation and Prevention).

Coughing, Sneezing

Coughing and sneezing often intensify the pain associated with disk prolapse. Spinal flexion associated with coughing and sneezing is probably the cause for this increased pain. For coughing and sneezing, the patient should therefore move the back of their head backward, to avoid bending.

Instructions for the Patient

- *Reclining:*
  - Set your bed to be completely flat.
  - Lie flat on your back.
  - When lying on your back, do not use more than a small pillow for your head.
  - In lateral reclining position place your head toward your back.
  - Place a pillow under your head to fill the distance to the bed such that your cervical spine does not tip to the side.
  - To change between these positions, roll over the bed with a flat back, so that the cervical spine remains as straight as possible.
- *Standing up and lying down:*
  - Before changing position, extend the spine and keep it extended.
  - To change to sitting from the supine position, first go to the lateral recumbent position and vice versa.
- *Brushing your teeth:*
  - Lean against the sink.
  - Support yourself with one hand on the wash basin.
  - Keep your cervical spine extended with only a slight forward bend.
- *Sitting:*
  - Sit as little as possible.
  - When you sit, you should hold your head vertically above the shoulder girdle and extend your cervical spine.
- *Coughing, sneezing:*
  - In coughing and sneezing, extend your cervical spine by moving the back of your head toward your back.
  - Consciously avoid bending your cervical spine and upper body forward, which is an automatic movement.

8.5.7   Stabilization

As soon as pain intensity is reduced and the pain is intermittent and no longer constant, and movements that originally peripheralized and intensified the pain no longer have this effect, in addition to spinal movements, passive and active arm movements to improve nerve-gliding capacity are tested and used for self-training (see Chapter 8.5.4 Arm Movements Performed by the Patient for Mobilization of the Nervous System).

Rotation of the cervical spine is practiced first to the affected side and by the next day also to the unaffected side. Then lateral flexion of the cervical spine is practiced to the affected side and by the next day also to the unaffected side.

8.5.8   Restoration of Original Capacity

An exercise program to restore the patient's capacity should take mobility, power, coordination, equilibrium, and conditioning into account.

In what follows, special exercises for patients with cervical disk damage are described; for general points of rehabilitation and prevention of disk damage, see Chapter 9 Rehabilitation and Prevention.

The degree of mobility that can be described as *free* depends on many individual factors, such as the strength of connective tissue structures. There are no standard values for free mobility, but it is useful for therapists and patients to consult the target values given here for target mobility.

> **Note:** A freely mobile cervical spine is always without pain. If end-range movement causes pain, this could be an indication of mechanical impairment of the active and passive motor apparatus.

In rare cases, hypermobility occurs, in which the range of motion extends beyond the generally known range. This can be caused, for instance, by a previous acceleration trauma or related to connective tissue disease.

Free Mobility

Restoration of Extension

- Seated or standing.

- Move the head backward, positioning the lower jaw parallel to the floor, upright posture.
- Move the back of the head backward in a large arc until the face is pointing to the ceiling.
- At the end of the movement, turn the head, with a small range of motion, to the right and the left.
- Return to starting position.
- Repeat 10 to 15 times.

> **Note:** Free mobility in extension has been achieved if in upright, seated position the face is approximately parallel to the floor (see **Fig. 8.6**).

Restoration of Rotation

- Seated or standing.
- Move the head backward, positioning the lower jaw parallel to the floor, upright posture.
- Turn the head.
- Return to starting position.
- Repeat 10 to 15 times.
- Repeat on the other side.

> **Note:** Free mobility is achieved at an 80° angle of rotation. At the end of the movement, an additional lateral flexion to the same side can be seen (see **Fig. 8.7**).

Restoration of Lateral Flexion

- Seated or standing.
- Move the head backward, positioning the lower jaw parallel to the floor, upright posture.
- Tip head to the side.
- Return to starting position.
- Repeat 10 to 15 times.
- Repeat on the other side.

> **Note:** Free mobility is achieved approximately at a 50° angle of lateral flexion (see **Fig. 8.8**).

Restoration of Flexion

Limitation of cervical spine flexion is most likely to be found in the upper cervical spine that is normally extended in the activities of daily living. Even after cervical disk prolapse, limitations of movement in flexion of the lower cervical spine are rare. Mobility in flexion should be tested after the symptoms subside and extension, rotation, and lateral flexion mobility have been restored. If limitation of motion can be observed at that point, this direction of motion is practiced:

- Seated or standing.
- Move the chin toward the sternum.
- Return to starting position.
- Repeat 10 to 15 times.

> **Note:** Free mobility has been achieved if the distance of the chin from the sternum reaches 0 to 5 cm with mouth closed (see **Fig. 8.9**).

Strengthening

In patients with cervical disk prolapse, strengthening of paretic hand and arm muscles is emphasized. The most important measures for this purpose are all the usual activities of daily living like washing, dressing, shopping, and writing.

Individual muscles that have become paretic as a result of root compression are additionally trained with special exercises if their strength is not increased by normal use of the arms.

Strengthening the Muscles that Splay the Fingers (e.g., the Dorsal Interossei)
- Place the hand inside an elastic stocking.
- Extend and splay the fingers—the tissue of the stocking resists the movement.
- Relax.
- Repeat.

Strengthening the Finger Adductor (Closing) Muscles (e.g., the Interossei Palmares)
- Squeeze a sponge or a ball of modeling clay with the whole hand while closing the fingers.
- Relax.
- Repeat.

Strengthening the Elbow Extensors (Triceps Brachii)
- Prone.
- Place hands on the ground at shoulder level.
- Extend elbows; pelvis is not raised.
- Lie down again—stay loose.
- Repeat.

Increasing Intensity (Extension in Prone Position)
- Quadruped position.
- Extend the legs so that the body is supported on hands and feet.

- Extend the spine.
- Contract abdominal muscles so that the lumbar spine does not sag.
- Flex the elbows and extend without changing the position of the trunk.
- Lower the knees until the quadruped stance is achieved.
- Repeat.

Strengthening the Elbow Flexors (Biceps Brachii and Brachioradialis)

- Erect standing.
- Hold weights in your hands.
- Hold arms parallel to trunk.
- Bend elbows.
- Slowly return to extension.
- Repeat.

Increasing Intensity

One way this is done is with different weights, as follows:

- Empty bottle.
- Bottle filled to1 L.
- Bottle filled to 1.5 L.
- Pail containing 5 L liquid.

Strengthening the Arm Abductors (Deltoid)

- Erect standing.
- Hold weights in your hands.
- Hold arms parallel to trunk.
- Keep elbows in extended position.
- Raise arms to side (medial part) or forward (ventral part).
- Slowly return them to the trunk.
- Repeat.

Increasing Intensity

See Strengthening the Elbow Flexors above.

8.5.9   Rehabilitation, Activities of Daily Living, and Prevention

The physical therapy program is designed to allow patients who were employed before the disk prolapse to resume their work after the shortest possible period of disability. Cervical spine exercises have the advantage that they can be performed anywhere, either standing or sitting, over lumbar spine exercises that must be done lying down.

The exercise of free, symmetrical mobility of all joints, coordination, balance, strength, and appropriate cardiovascular capacity are also performed after a cervical spine disk prolapse (see Chapter 9 Rehabilitation and Prevention).

In activities of daily living, the practice effort must be reduced to a realistic level that is individualized for the patient's circumstances. The ideal pattern would be 15-minute exercise units, performed morning, noon, and night, that cover the most important points of the individual training program. In addition, the patient should be given a few important suggestions for the management of everyday living.

Instructions for the Patient

- Improve your posture and straighten up more frequently than before.
- When reading, assume the prone position more often, possibly with a reading wedge.
- *Make a point of maintaining the mobility of the nerve root affected by the disk prolapse.*
- *Regularly extend your cervical spine* when you have been sitting for a while or pursuing an activity in stooped position. Extend *before* the pain begins. Always compensate for one-sided stresses.
- Do not make a habit of sparing yourself, because then the structures of the spine will become even less capable of dealing with strain. *Use it or lose it!*
- From time to time, treat yourself to a physical therapy session in order to analyze and treat bad posture habits, limitations of movement, asymmetries, and lack of strength.

8.6   After an Operation

There are no evidence-based and generally accepted postoperative therapy programs for any surgical treatment of a prolapsed cervical disk. Therefore, if the therapist is planning to use the postoperative treatment concept described here they should first have the agreement of the surgeon.

The *physical therapy examination* of patients operated on for a prolapsed disk is the same as described in Chapter 4 Diagnosis in Physical Therapy. The most complete physical therapy examination possible should be conducted before the operation (see Chapter 4), so that postoperative changes can be documented. Alternatively, this can also be done on the first postoperative day. Postoperative treatment documentation is like documentation of primary conservative treatment (see Chapter 5 Therapy).

To ensure *uncomplicated wound healing* and *prevention of immediate recurrence*, the postoperative patient should observe 8.5.6 Acute Phase—Useful Guidelines for Conduct During the Acute Phase. If possible, the movement transitions should already be practiced with the patient before the operation.

Usually, special measures for the prevention of thrombosis are not necessary after cervical disk operations because the patient can and should get up and walk on the first postoperative day.

To *activate neck and trunk muscles*, isometric tension exercises are begun on the first postoperative day.

Simple Isometric Tension Exercises, in Supine Position

Arm Exercise

- Supine.
- Extend arms on the bed.
- Rotate shoulder joints outward.
- Press extended arms onto the bed.
- Push hands toward the foot of the bed.
- At the same time, push the head toward the head of the bed. The muscle tension is transmitted to the neck and trunk muscles and the spine is extended.
- The therapist checks whether abdominal and back muscle tension can be felt.
- Hold the tension for two breaths.
- Release. Relax for two breaths.
- Repeat 5 to 10 times.

Leg Exercises

- Supine.
- Set feet on flat surface to produce a 30° angle in hip joints.
- Raise toes as high as possible.
- The feet are braced against an imaginary resistance diagonally toward the ground and foot end. The legs do not move, the extensor muscles push, and the flexor muscles create the resistance.
- At the same time, push the head toward the head of the bed.

- The muscle tension is transmitted to the trunk muscles and the spine is extended.
- The therapist checks whether abdominal and back muscle tension can be felt.
- Hold the tension for two breaths.
- Release. Relax for two breaths.
- Repeat 5 to 10 times.

Pushing with Arms and Legs

- Combine the movements described above and perform them simultaneously.
- Hold the tension for two breaths.
- Release. Relax for two breaths.
- Repeat 5 to 10 times.

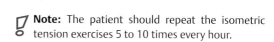 **Note:** The patient should repeat the isometric tension exercises 5 to 10 times every hour.

From the second postoperative day the isometric tension exercises are supplemented with movement of the cervical spine. Mobilization in retraction is practiced in seated position. The patient may only perform the movements in a range and with a force such that there is no pain and no pulling at the wound.

From the third postoperative day physical therapy is conducted according to the same considerations and with the same therapeutic movements as the primary conservative treatment of cervical disk prolapse. Emphasis is on the points identified by the diagnosis. Therapy is symptom oriented. If the course of recovery is uncomplicated, one therapeutic movement can be added every day.

Possible Sequence of Exercises

- *First postoperative day:*
  - Isometric tension exercises.
  - Transition movements from supine to lateral recumbent position to sitting and vice versa.
  - Walking.
- *Second postoperative day:* additional mobilization of the cervical spine in retraction and extension.
- *Third postoperative day:*
  - Continue or discontinue isometric exercises.
  - Increase distance and frequency of walking.
  - Increase mobilization of the cervical spine by rotation to affected side.
- *Fourth postoperative day:*
  - Increase mobilization of the cervical spine by rotation to unaffected side.

– Continue to increase walking.
– If applicable, strengthen weakened muscles and move the corresponding joints to end range.
– **Note:** the shoulder joints should be freely moveable.
- *Fifth postoperative day:* possibly reduce medications but then do not change any exercises.
- *Sixth postoperative day:* increase arm movements for nerve mobilization—three repetitions three times a day.
- *Seventh postoperative day:* increase lateral flexion to affected side.
- *Eighth postoperative day:* practice activities of daily living, such as sitting and lifting; Increase strengthening exercises for the trunk muscles (see Chapter 9 Rehabilitation and Prevention).
- *Ninth postoperative day:*
  – Practice activities of daily living, such as sitting and lifting.
  – Increase strengthening exercises for the trunk muscles (see Chapter 9).
- *Tenth postoperative day:*
  – The wound has healed to the point that the stitches can be removed.
  – Training (see Chapter 9) is conducted step by step.

Rehabilitation sessions at a specialized facility are usually not necessary. An individual training program designed to suit the patient's signs and symptoms, which they can carry out independently, is preferable to group rehabilitation. It is the most efficient way to ensure rapid return to their social environment and the work process.

The duration of disability after surgery for a prolapsed disk, just like the duration of conservative treatment, depends on many factors and is not the same in every case (see Chapter 5 Therapy).

8.7 Case Study

This is the physical therapy treatment of a 39-year-old patient who was hospitalized for 8 days.
- *Diagnosis:* prolapsed disk intervertebral level C6–C7 left with root compression C7 left.
- *MRI diagnosis* (**Fig. 8.11**): disk prolapse in segment C6–C7 left mediolateral, protruding 4 mm intraspinally and partially into foramen, with slight local displacement of the spinal cord and locally reduced cerebrospinal fluid space. Posterior longitudinal ligament detached. The cervical spinal cord is otherwise without contour or signal abnormalities.

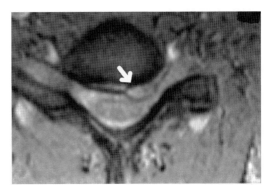

Fig. 8.11 Magnetic resonance imaging shows a mediolateral disk prolapse (arrow).

- *Reason for admission:* investigation of indication for surgery.
- *Medication* during hospitalization: 75 mg diclofenac (NSAID) and 150 mg ranitidine (stomach protection) morning and evening.

Admission Findings

Medical History
- Age: 39 years.
- Occupation: mail delivery person and musician.
- Duration of disability: 13 days.
- Duration of episode and trigger: 14 days ago, during strength training with sit-ups, the patient suffered shooting pains from the neck to the shoulder blade to as far as 5 cm below the elbow in the left arm (corresponding to dermatome C7).
- Previous history: no prior symptoms and no warning signs perceived.
- Treatment to date:
  – Two chiropractic treatments ("several vertebrae were out") without effect.
  – Diclofenac without effect.
- Treatment and course: unchanging symptoms for the past 14 days.

Day 1

Visual Examination
During the examination, the patient sat in a limp, slumped position with protracted head.

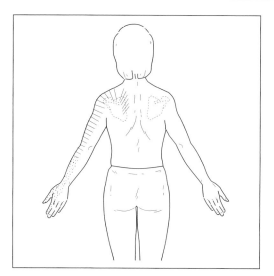

Fig. 8.12 Subjective admission diagnosis: distribution of pain and sensory disorders.

Pain

- Radiating pain (**Fig. 8.12**):
  - From the left medial edge of the shoulder blade over the back of the left upper arm to approximately 5 cm below the elbow.
  - At the medial edge of the shoulder blade the pain intensity was 7/10 and in the arm, 5/10.
- Minimal pain in the last 24 hours; 5/10 in the area indicated above.
- Maximal pain in the last 24 hours; 8/10 in the area indicated above.
- No neck pain.

At night and in the morning the pain was the most pronounced; it improved throughout the day with movement. The patient awakened several times during the night because of the pain. In various positions (sitting, standing, reclining), no preferred or aggravating position could be found.

Sensory Disorder

The patient reported numbness from 5 cm below the elbow to fingers I and II (**Fig. 8.12**). Since a cut injury on the thumb, there has been a distal sensory disorder of the thumb.

Muscle Function Test

Weakness in the left triceps brachii muscle with a score of 3/5 (end-range movement against

gravity possible, no movement against additional resistance).

Nerve Tension Test

The upper limb tension test intensified symptoms, particularly in the shoulder blade at 90° abduction, 0° outward rotation, 90° elbow flexion, dorsal extension in wrist, finger extension, abduction of thumb, and supination of lower arm.

Movement Tests (Fig. 8.13a–f)

- In cervical spine movement tests, response to a single movement was limitation of end-range movement in retraction. This movement produced neck pain and eliminated the lower arm pain.
- Extension was significantly limited and immediately reproduced the lower arm pain.
- Mobility was free for rotation to the left and right and lateral flexion to the left and right. These movements did not change the symptoms.
- Flexion was not limited but it peripheralized and intensified the pain.

Repeated Movements

Retraction (repeated 10 times) eliminated the lower and upper arm pain, reduced shoulder blade pain to 5/10, and produced central neck pain (**Fig. 8.14a, b**). The change persisted after the movements. The range of motion in retraction increased in the course of the repetitions.

Physical Therapy Diagnosis

The symptoms were classified as disk symptoms reducible by mechanical physical therapy.

Comments

The pain changed as a result of repeated retraction of the cervical spine; this is typical for a reducible disk problem. The peripheral pain was eliminated, the shoulder blade pain was reduced, and a new central neck pain was produced. This change persisted after the movements.

The atypical feature was the good cervical spine mobility in flexion, lateral flexion, and rotation.

Reproduction of the lower arm pain in extension was ascribed to the increasing pressure on the irritated nerve root caused by narrowing of the intervertebral foramen.

Physical Therapy

- The patient was asked to assume an erect posture, avoid any flexion of the cervical spine, walk

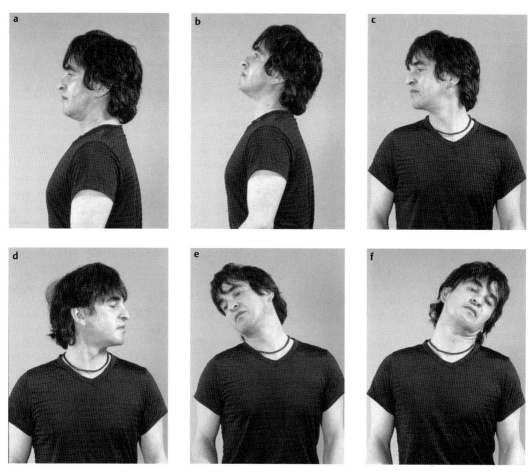

Fig. 8.13 (a–f) Movement tests for the cervical spine.

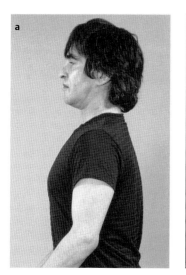

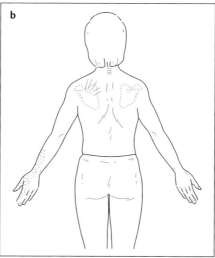

Fig. 8.14 (a, b) Retraction centralizes the pain and is used as the first therapeutic exercise.

a great deal, not to sit, and to lie in bed without a pillow, flat on his back.
- In addition, his homework was to move his head back as far as possible 10 times every hour with his lower jaw remaining parallel to the floor.
- He was to observe his symptoms precisely and only continue exercising if the pain was shifted toward the center or remained the same.
- If the pain radiated further down in the arm, he was to stop the exercise.

Day 2

The patient reported that he was significantly better. He practiced the retraction 10 times an hour, walked a great deal, and did not sit or lie down very much. He had succeeded with the posture correction.

In the last 24 hours, the *maximal pain* was 8/10 from the medial scapula edge to approximately 5 cm below the elbow at night and in the morning before getting up.

The patient reported the *minimal pain* at 3/10 at the medial edge of the scapula to approximately two-thirds of the upper arm. The neck pain did not recur.

At the time of the examination, the patient was feeling pain in the scapula of 3/10 and in the upper arm of 4/10.

The sensory disorder, the decrease in strength, and the nerve tension test of the upper extremity were unchanged.

Repeated Movements
- Retraction repeated five times reduced the upper arm pain to 3/10.
- Retraction and rotation to the left repeated five times had no effect.
- Retraction and rotation to the right repeated five times had no effect.
- Retraction and extension performed once intensified the pain in the whole region with a somewhat greater range of motion than on the day before.
- Retraction and lateral flexion to the left repeated five times reduced the upper arm pain to 2/10 and eliminated the scapula pain (**Fig. 8.15a–c**). This improvement persisted after the movements.

Physical Therapy
In addition to systematic posture monitoring, the patient was asked to practice retraction and lateral flexion to the left every hour, repeated 10 times.

Day 3

Treatment and Course
The patient felt further improvement. He performed the exercises as agreed and obtained pain relief.

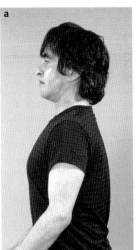
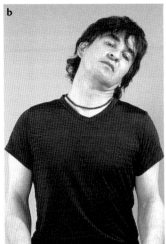
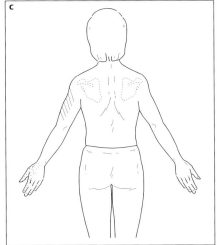

Fig. 8.15 (a–c) Retraction with lateral flexion to the left (the affected side) reduces the upper arm pain and eliminates the pain in the scapula. This movement is used as the second therapeutic exercise.

The *minimal pain* in the last 24 hours was reported in the scapula, at 2/10, in the upper two-thirds of the upper arm at 1/10.

The *maximal pain* in the last 24 hours was reduced to 6/10 in the morning, in the area described above.

The patient slept through the night for the first time.

At the time of the examination, he was feeling pain in the scapula at 2/10 and in the upper arm at 1/10 (**Fig. 8.16**).

The further sensory disorder in the lower arm was not perceived anymore. The patient only reported numbness in the radial dorsum of his hand to fingers I and II (**Fig. 8.16**).

The decreased strength was unchanged.

Nerve Tension Test

Compared to the day before, in the nerve tension test the scapula and upper arm symptoms were only intensified at a large range of motion, at 90° abduction, supination, dorsal extension, extension of the fingers, abduction of the thumb, 90° outward rotation in the shoulder joint, and 130° elbow extension (50° elbow flexion).

Repeated Movements

- Retraction and lateral flexion to the left repeated five times eliminated the scapula pain but had no effect on the slight (1/10) upper arm pain.

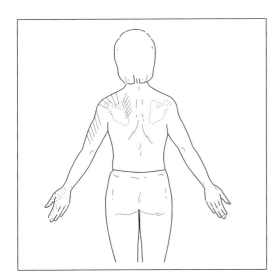

Fig. 8.16 Control findings for the subjective parameters pain and sensory disorder on Day 3.

- After this, the pain in supine position decreased.
- For the first time in 16 days, the patient had no pain (0/10).
- A slight pulling pain (0.5/10) in the upper arm returned in seated position.

Physical Therapy

Because of the good results, no additional test movements were performed and the self-training was not changed.

Comments

Before the start of the physical therapy described, the patient suffered constant, intense pain for 14 days. During and after each therapy session and independent exercises, he experienced distinct improvement of his symptoms. Since the administration of pain medication was not changed, the improvement that occurred was probably due to the movements he practiced.

Day 6

Treatment and Course

The patient felt well and on the previous day he had gone for a 30-minute car ride, in order to work at the sound studio. During and after the drive, the upper arm pain became more intense but did not radiate below the elbow.

He did the exercises as agreed and obtained pain relief through them. The most intense pain in the last 24 hours was once more at 6/10 in the upper arm; the minimal pain was 0/10.

At the time of the examination, the patient was feeling upper arm pain at an intensity of 3/10 and of 0/10 in the scapula.

Mobility of the cervical spine was unchanged and free in retraction, rotation to the left and right, and lateral flexion to the left and right.

Flexion was not tested. Limitation of extension was not as pronounced as on Day 3 (**Fig. 8.17a, b**).

The upper arm pain only became more intense when the range of motion increased.

The sensory disorder was unchanged in the radial dorsum of the hand and fingers I and II.

Muscle Function Test

Here there was a pronounced improvement of the strength of the triceps brachii to 4/5.

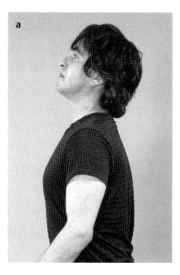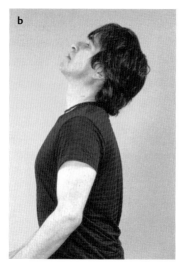

Fig. 8.17 (a, b) Comparison of extension mobility on Day 1 and Day 6.

Nerve Tension Test

The upper arm pain was intensified and the pain in the scapula was reproduced. However, the range of motion was greater than on Day 3: 90° abduction, supination, dorsal extension, 90° outward rotation in the shoulder joint, and 150° elbow extension (30° elbow flexion).

Repeated Movements

- Retraction repeated five times had no effect.
- Retraction and lateral flexion to the left repeated five times reduced the upper arm pain to 2/10 but did not change the location of the pain (no centralization).

Physical Therapy

Nerve-gliding techniques (sliders, **Fig. 8.18a, b**) for the left arm eliminated the upper arm pain.

The patient became free of pain (**Fig. 8.19a, b**).

After the movements this improvement also persisted in seated position.

In addition to systematic posture monitoring, the patient was asked to perform retraction and lateral bending to the left 10 times every hour and three repetitions of the slide movement three times a day with the right and left arms (see **Fig. 8.10a–c**).

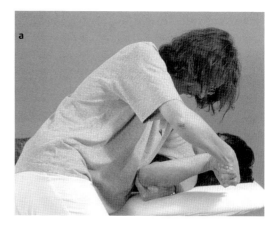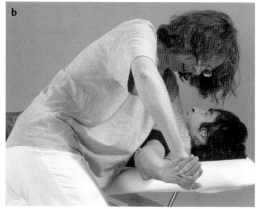

Fig. 8.18 (a, b) Passive arm movements (sliders) to improve nerve-gliding capacity.

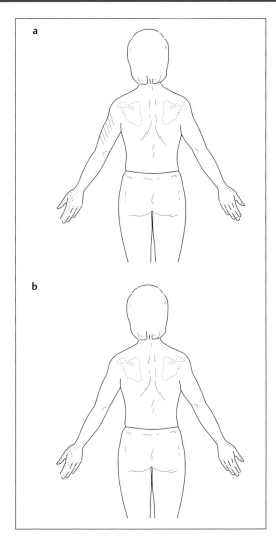

Fig. 8.19 The arm movements eliminate the upper arm pain. **(a)** Pain before the movements. **(b)** Pain after the movements.

Comments

Only in the first therapy session was the pain centralized such that the peripheral pain disappeared and a new, central pain in the area of the spine developed. In the course of treatment, centralization developed such that the peripheral pain (below the elbow) no longer occurred and the maximal pain radiation extended to the upper two-thirds of the upper arm. After this, the pain was eliminated without any further central shift.

Movements of the affected arm eliminated the upper arm pain. This effect was possibly caused by mobilization of the affected nerve root.

Day 7

Treatment and Course
The patient reported that he had been completely without pain on the day before. He had performed the movements as agreed. In the evening, he forgot to take his pain medicine and in the morning of the examination day, he noticed slightly increased pain.

He rated the *maximal upper arm pain* in the last 24 hours at 5/10.

At the time of the examination, he felt no pain (0/10).

The range of motion of the cervical spine was unchanged. On extension of the cervical spine, the upper arm pain continued to be reproduced.

Flexion of the cervical spine was not tested.

The sensory disorder was unchanged.

Muscle Function Test
There was a further improvement of triceps brachii strength.

Nerve Tension Test
At approximately the same range of motion as on the day before, the pain was reproduced, but exclusively in the upper arm and no longer in the scapula.

Physical Therapy
The passive arm movements for nerve mobilization were performed with repetitions. Because of the good results of the previous exercises, no additional test movements were performed and the self-training was not changed.

Because of the satisfactory improvement of pain, strength, and sensory function, it was decided in a consultation among the patient, the treating physician, and the physical therapist not to consider an operation.

Discharge from the hospital was planned for the following day and further conservative therapy was planned.

Day 8

The patient reported that he was largely free of pain. He had performed the movements as agreed.

He rated the *maximal pain* in the last 24 hours at 2/10 as a slight pull in the upper arm.

At the time of the examination, the patient had no pain.

Rotation of the cervical spine to left and right, lateral flexion to left and right, and retraction were free and caused neither pain nor sensory disorders.

On this day, extension was free for the first time and caused no symptoms in the arm, only a slight pulling centrally, in the region of the cervical spine.

Flexion of the cervical spine was not tested.

The sensory disorder was unchanged in the radial dorsum of the hand and fingers I and II (**Fig. 8.20a, b**).

Strength had improved more and was now only minimally reduced.

The nerve tension test showed the same result as on the day before.

Repeated Movements

- With repeated retraction and extension, the central pulling sensation around the cervical spine was felt less and less, and after 10 repetitions it no longer occurred.
- After the movements, the patient was free of symptoms, as before.
- Resting on the reading wedge was tested; the patient found it comfortable.

Comments

The fact that movement in extension was free and reproduced no symptoms in the arm was interpreted as follows: the swelling in the nerve root had subsided and the root was no longer compressed by the disk material, so that the narrowing of the intervertebral foramen upon extension no longer exerted pressure on the nerve root.

Planning Further Treatment

- The therapeutic asymmetric movements of retraction and lateral flexion were replaced with the symmetrical movement of retraction and extension.
- Recommended self-training for the next 2 weeks was 10 repetitions of retraction and extension per hour as well as arm movements for nerve mobilization in intensified form (five repetitions, five times a day) with the right and left arms.
- The patient was told to lie on the reading wedge for reading and writing.
- He was asked to report immediately if his condition worsened.
- A follow-up examination and treatment appointment was scheduled for 2 weeks later.

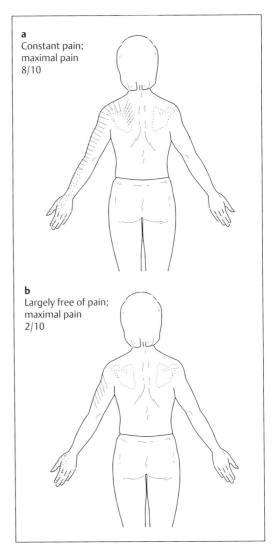

a
Constant pain;
maximal pain
8/10

b
Largely free of pain;
maximal pain
2/10

Fig. 8.20 (a, b) Comparison of the subjective parameters pain and sensory disorders at Day 1 and Day 8. The pain recorded is always the region of maximal pain.

- The morning dose of pain medication was to be discontinued from the following day, and with constant improvement, after 2 days the medication was to be discontinued entirely.

Follow-up Examination 14 Days after Discharge

The patient performed the exercises systematically, with a positive effect. He only experienced pain in car trips that lasted more than 2 hours. The resulting pain was in the upper arm and neck.

The patient continued to take the pain medication for 1 week after discharge and then stopped.

Mobility of the cervical spine was free in all directions.

In the muscle function test of the triceps brachii, the strength of the triceps brachii was normal.

Sensory disorders in the hand had improved so that there was a sensory disorder only in the thumb, but this had already existed before the disk prolapse after a cut injury.

The patient was able to work, experienced no limitation in playing guitar, and was satisfied with his treatment and progress.

For further stabilization of the successful healing process, he was given a training program designed to promote strengthening and better conditioning (see Chapter 9, 9.6 Strength).

It was assumed that hand coordination was sufficiently trained through regular guitar playing.

No additional physical therapy was necessary. The patient was asked to get in touch immediately if the symptoms returned.

9 Rehabilitation and Prevention

Restoration of normal capacity and reintegration into work and social life (rehabilitation) are the long-term goals when treating patients with intervertebral disk disease. Therapy in which reduction of symptoms by means of mechanical maneuvers is emphasized is followed by a period of increasing the capacity.

Once the symptoms have disappeared to a large extent or completely, or if there is no further therapeutic option for the reduction of symptoms, efforts are focused on the ability to work and a normal capacity. In other words, the patient goes into training.

In this phase of therapy, pain is a less important topic. Rather, the measurement and documentation of mobility, strength, the distance that can be walked, and the time that can be spent seated without pain play the dominant role. Physical activity in daily living improves the stability of the vertebrae and intervertebral disks (Porter et al 1989).

> **Note:** Stability (from the Latin *stabilitas*, meaning endurance, sturdiness, resistance) of the spine and well-being are being developed. The spine is stable when it resists pressure and tension stresses and limits the mobility of the supporting structures in such a way that neuronal structures are not damaged or irritated and the supporting structures themselves remain intact.

Often, earlier habits of posture and movement patterns must be changed. An individualized exercise program should be integrated into activities of daily living. This requires complicated integrative and psychological learning processes.

> **Note:** The rehabilitation and prevention phase is not intended to protect or unburden the individuals, but to impose stresses that are appropriate to their abilities.

> **Definition of Prevention:** This concept covers measures of avoidance (here, avoidance of disease).

The prevention of back pain should begin in childhood and youth. In Denmark, for instance, approximately 50% of 18- to 20-year-olds have already experienced episodes of back pain (Leboeuf-Yde and Kyvik 1998). Here, after disk damage has become symptomatic, prevention has the goal of avoiding recurrence of symptoms (relapse) or, worse, the development of disk prolapse.

Back School

Back school also pursues the goal of prevention and rehabilitation of back pain. In these programs, group therapy offers patients information about the structure and function of the spine, and postures and movements that protect the back. Other activities are group games, exercises for body consciousness, and strength and fitness training.

Not all back school programs are the same. There is no consensus about the best lifting techniques and the optimal seated position. The information and exercises used in the programs are based on individual opinions of trainers and often not on scientific studies.

Data from systematic literature searches that include only controlled studies do not substantiate the efficacy of back school programs (Van Tulder et al 2000; Maier-Riehle and Harter 2001; Heymans et al 2005).

Individual treatment that takes the patient's specific problems into account achieves the goal of rehabilitation more rapidly than group therapy, which always includes exercises that are not appropriate for one patient or another. Further, peer group pressure should not be underestimated. As long as complete restoration of load-bearing capacity has not been achieved, there is a possible danger of excessive stress and the accompanying symptoms.

Groups may possibly be of use in prevention, but here too, the participants should be as homogeneous as possible. For instance, exercises that are beneficial for participants with disk prolapse can be contraindicated for patients with vertebral instability. If the makeup of the group is not homogeneous, conflicts can arise because certain exercises will produce symptoms in some participants, who will then have to be asked to sit out during the exercises that are contraindicated for them.

Normal Movement

A person is able to perform complex movements that are more or less necessary in daily living. Normal movement requires coordination, balance, mobility, strength, and endurance.

Definition of Normal Movement: This concept covers movements that are a matter of course, self-evident, appropriate, and familiar. They are efficient and selective.

The judgment as to whether a movement is natural or normal requires observation and familiarity with numerous variations of movement types. A functional feedback system (deep and superficial sensitivity), pain-free mobility to the age-appropriate limit, and strength and endurance appropriate to the demands are the most important requirements.

In a case of disk damage, all the basic requirements for normal movement sequences may be disrupted. A small sensory deficit can lead to coordination disorders (sensory ataxia). Paresis and painful limitations of movement can make certain movements impossible and depending on the duration and manifestation of the disease, the patient's condition can be significantly diminished.

Exercise Programs

In designing an exercise program intended to restore normal capacity or to avoid disk damage, the many demands made on the spine must be taken into account. Reliable statics (standing still) and dynamics (movement) must be ensured. Posture and movement behavior must be modified. Even the individuals' attitude toward their own health must be modified. Every day some time should be set aside for exercise and often-repeated movements and postures, such as those that are typical at work, should regularly be briefly interrupted to perform compensatory movements and increase postural tone. These are the aspects to be strengthened by the exercise program:

- Daily living–relevant, symmetrical mobility of all joints.
- Coordination.
- Balance.
- Strength, endurance, and speed of the entire musculature.
- Appropriate cardiovascular capacity.

A deficiency in one of these areas leads to compensatory movement patterns that can bring about painful functional limitations and degenerative changes. Activities such as standing, walking, and lifting are part of everyone's daily life. Performing them in such a way that the load is equally distributed over all structures of the motor apparatus is a matter of training. In addition to these common activities, every affected person should also practice special movements that are the opposite of the daily, individual, one-sided movements.

The exercises designed to work up to free mobility of individual sections of the spine affected by disk damage and strengthen muscles affected by a root compression have already been presented in Chapters 6 to 8. In the following, we present tips and instructions for exercises that concentrate on optimizing the capacity of the whole body without focusing on isolated sections of the spine.

9.1   Posture Training

Definition of Good Posture: Good posture is erect, and head, shoulders, pelvis, and feet are plumb in relation to each other. The spine describes an S curve with lumbar lordosis, thoracic kyphosis, and cervical lordosis.

When lumbar lordosis is eliminated, the entire spine goes into flexion except for the upper cervical spine, which is forced into compensatory extension. The structures of both the active and passive supporting structures contribute equally to ensuring upright posture. Muscles of the abdomen and back work together harmoniously to make the trunk the stable center from which arms and legs can be moved in coordination and without effort. The muscles are oriented in their optimal direction of pull and can perform their function with the least effort possible. Muscle activity holds or leads the joints so as to distribute loads over a number of different joints and the leverage effects are as small as possible.

In addition to maintaining body position, posture is also an expression of an individual's overall manner. If a newly learned posture leads to an artificial and inadequate outward appearance, the person gives the impression of being nonauthentic. This means that patients must change their posture gradually and in a way that corresponds to their character. This is supported by the conviction and the feeling that erect posture relieves pain and contributes to the avoidance of new pain.

9.2   Stability

After a disk prolapse, the passive supporting structures are weakened and the result can be segmental instability with back pain. Special tonic muscle groups lying deep and close to joints are responsible for the control of posture and movement. These must be specifically activated and their tone must be increased, in order to provide for stability. The local stabilizing muscles work in co-contraction and thus control movement from front and back simultaneously, in contrast to the muscles needed to produce movement. These function antagonistically. In the lumbar spine and the lower thoracic spine, the most important stabilizing muscle groups are the multifidi muscles, the short back muscles, and the transversely running abdominal muscles (see **Fig. 9.1**). In ad-

dition, the muscles of the pelvic floor hold the lower trunk. In the cervical spine and the upper thoracic spine, the multifidi, the anterior neck muscles, and the pectoral muscles are the chief stabilizers.

In a healthy person, the tension in the stabilizing muscles already increases when an arm movement is planned, before the movement begins. In individuals with back pain, no matter what the cause, the arm movement usually begins before the stabilizing muscles have adapted their tone to an additional stress. This causes an uncontrolled application of force on the spine that can lead to pain and, in the long term, to damage of the passive supporting structures (Richardson et al 2004). Activation of the local stabilizing muscles must be practiced (**Fig. 9.2a, b**); it does not begin functioning again spontaneously (Hides et al 1996; Richardson et al 2004). Patients who are training their segmental stabilization have less pain and exhibit better function than patients who are carrying out general strengthening of the abdominal and back muscles, muscle tension, and joint mobility (Kladny et al 2003).

Activation of the local spine-stabilizing muscles:
• Stand erect.
• Contract the transverse abdominal muscles such that the navel moves toward the spine and the waist becomes small.
• The spine remains unmoving.

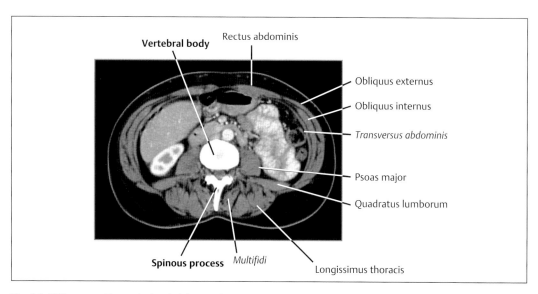

Fig. 9.1 MRI cross-section at the level of the navel.

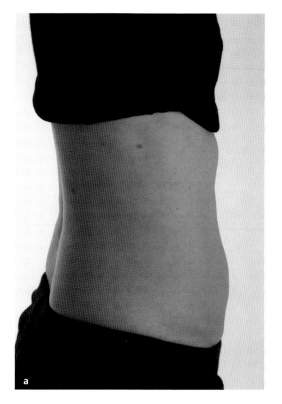 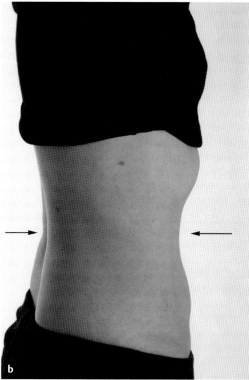

Fig. 9.2 Activation of the local spine-stabilizing muscles. **(a)** Without activation. **(b)** With activation.

- The muscles of the pelvic floor and the short back muscles automatically also contract.
- Continue quiet abdominal breathing.
- Release. In the course of time, the muscle tone should decrease less and less on relaxation.
- This activity should be regularly repeated throughout the day.

Increasing intensity of the exercise, strengthening the trunk and neck muscles:
- Stand erect.
- Be conscious of the trunk muscle contraction.
- Pull the navel toward the spine.
- Raise the arms forward.
- An increase in tension will be felt in the trunk muscles, especially in the abdominal muscles and the neck muscles.
- The thorax remains plumb over the pelvis and the head is positioned vertically over the shoulder girdle.

- Rapidly move the extended arms up and down, with a small range of motion.
- Another increase in tension is felt.
- Release.
- Repeat 5 to 10 times.

Activities that challenge balance and coordination also encourage activation of the stabilizing muscles and the tone simultaneously. This is presumably because the cerebellum is controlling balance, coordination, and muscle tone at the same time. The best activities for achieving erect posture and increasing tone are: mini knee bends with the body erect until the heels leave the ground, standing on one leg, standing on tiptoe alternating with mini knee bends, jumping in place with a soft landing. One of these activities should be used for 20 seconds at a time to interrupt repeated typical postures.

9.2.1   Juggling

Juggling also involves the challenges listed above. It is true that balance is not intensely challenged, but concentration and motor learning are trained all the more (Draganski et al 2004).

Everyone is familiar with the fact that concentration is accompanied by increased muscle tension. This mechanism should be controlled in juggling in such a way that the positive effect of increased stability sets in without causing a sensation of tension. Additional beneficial effects of juggling are, among other things, that the patient is having fun, concentrating on a single, nonjudgmental process and thus being distracted from any unpleasant thoughts while improving general coordination. If the ball falls, one should not react with a hectic flexion of the spine but go into a controlled knee bend to pick it up. This provides the added benefit of countless knee bends.

Complicated movement sequences are best learned by practicing partial sequences and then combining them (Huys et al 2004). Throw and catch exercises are done first with the dominant hand, usually the right hand, then repeated with the other hand. After this, a ball is tossed from one

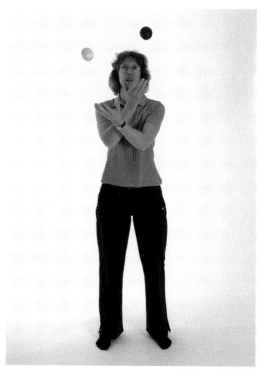

Fig. 9.3 Juggling with two balls.

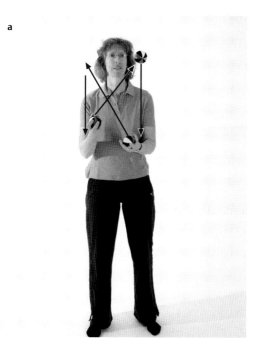

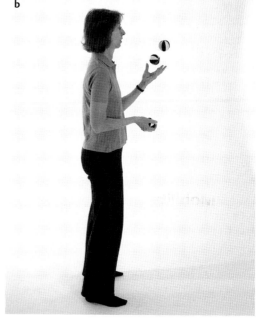

Fig. 9.4 Juggling with three balls. **(a)** Seen from the front. **(b)** Seen from the side.

hand to the other, two balls are thrown with both hands, straight up or crossed, and finally, three balls are used for juggling. Books and DVD courses provide precise instruction for juggling exercises (Ehlers 2008). Here we present only two exercises to begin with and to stimulate interest in doing more.

Basic Position
- Stand erect, feet a hip-width apart, knees slightly bent.
- Hold upper arms loosely next to the trunk.
- Bend elbows approximately 90°.
- The hands are always returned to the basic position, at waist level.
- The balls are thrown to somewhere above eye level and caught at waist level.

Juggling with Two Balls
- Hold a ball in each hand.
- Throw both balls straight up at the same time.
- Cross hands.
- Catch both balls at the same time with crossed hands.
- Throw the balls straight up from this position.
- Move the hands back to the starting position.
- Catch the balls.

Sequence when Juggling with Three Balls
- In juggling with three balls, the balls are thrown and caught in a pattern that resembles a horizontal "8" in a rhythmic, harmonious motion sequence.
- Throw the ball with the right hand at waist height to the left at shoulder level.
- When this ball begins to fall, the ball in the left hand is thrown to the right at shoulder level and shortly thereafter the first ball is caught in the left hand.
- Repeat the sequence.

9.3 Mobility

Daily living–relevant mobility of all joints is necessary for equal distribution of loads over various structures of the supporting structures. It provides freedom from pain and allows the optimal balance reactions that make for good coordination. This means, for instance, that to avoid back pain, not only spinal mobility but also mobility of the hip and knee joints are essential.

Examples
- A flexion contracture of the hip joint can result in flexion of the entire spine.
- A lack of flexion in hip and knee joints makes it impossible to squat when lifting loads, so that the load on the spine increases.
- If mobility is lacking in a section of the spine, the corresponding movement is compensated by another section.

Note: Free mobility of all joints is practiced. Exercises for free mobility of the entire spine in rotation should be practiced as shown in Chapter 6.5.8 Restoration of Original Capacity, Free Mobility (lumbar spine). If at the same time the arms are extended in abduction, the shoulder joints are also mobilized. The spine and the hip joints are extended by extension in the prone position (see **Fig. 6.18**). This also provides additional extension of the cervical spine. The mobility of the shoulder, ankle, hip, and knee joints should be tested, and exercised if necessary.

9.4 Sitting

Recommendations for back-protective sitting positions and furniture are widely discussed. In one subject, pressure measurements in the disk during relaxed sitting in flexion showed a lower pressure than in erect standing (Wilke et al 1999). This finding led to a wide-ranging discussion of the erect seated posture favored by physical therapists and back school programs and of the claim that standing is preferable to sitting.

However, in the test, the measuring probe was placed in the middle of the nucleus pulposus (ibid.) so that the usefulness of the measurement is questionable since it does not permit a nuanced statement about pressure distribution and direction. The measurement only showed that in relaxed sitting in flexion, there is a decrease in pressure in the middle of the disk, compared to the standing position. The dorsal displacement of the nucleus pulposus that can be expected in sitting (Adams and Hutton 1985; Fennell et al 1996) would lead, rather, to the expectation of a pressure increase in the dorsal and dorsolateral part of the disk.

Moreover, pressure stress in this area is of special significance for the development of disk damage. In addition, relaxed sitting in flexion occurs naturally, since actively maintaining an erect posture for the whole day is unlikely.

Note: Relaxed sitting in flexion should not be explicitly recommended for prevention of back pain.

The hip joint flexion associated with sitting eliminates physiological lumbar lordosis because of the resulting position of the pelvis. A gradual extension of the lumbar spine is only possible through the force of the back extensors. The continual maximal activity of the back extensors is not desirable because of the associated pressure increase in the disks and facet joints. In addition it is unrealistic because in sitting, one works at other tasks besides maintaining one's posture. Therefore, in sitting, the back should be supported.

Requirements for Controlled Sitting

- In sitting, the back should be supported by a back rest that reaches as far as the shoulder blades.
- The lumbar lordosis is passively supported by a foam roll. The best dimensions for the foam roll are a density of 30 (the measure of hardness), with a diameter of 8 cm and a length of 30 cm. In many chairs, the so-called lumbar support of the back rest starts directly on the sitting surface (i.e., in the pelvic area) and ends at the lumbar spine, but this does not support the lumbar lordosis.
- The back rest must be slanted backward or be adjustable to lean backward.
- The sitting surface should be deep enough for almost the whole thigh to lie on it when the buttocks are situated as far back as the back rest. Small individuals with short thighs need a sitting surface that is not so deep that it is impossible to slide the buttocks back as far as the back rest because leaning back to the back rest would produce a bent sitting posture.
- The sitting surface should be horizontal or with a slant adjustable toward the front. If the sitting surface slants backward or if there is a hollow for the buttocks, the lumbar spine will be flexed. This should be avoided.
- Adjustable seat height prevents a person from sitting too low, which would result in increased flexion of the lumbar spine.
- When sitting without a back rest, it is best to sit on the front part of the seating surface. The feet are placed flat on the floor, under the knees. In this way, part of the body weight can be carried

by the legs. The pelvis is tipped forward, so that the lumbar spine is moved toward extension. In some circumstances, weight can be taken off the spine by supporting the elbows on a table and the chin on the hands.

Note: In acute disk problems, sitting should be broadly discouraged, since sitting and standing up from a seated position are frequent pain triggers. Basically it is best to interrupt sitting regularly with standing, walking around, or lying prone.

9.5   Lifting

Every independent person can encounter the need to lift weights of up to 15 kg (e.g., a crate of beverage bottles) in daily living. For this reason, lifting, carrying, and putting down of heavy weights should be practiced with every patient who has suffered disk damage. All the passive (ligaments, joints, disks) and active (muscles) support structures must be prepared for this load by training. Moreover, good mobility, especially in hip and knee joints, and trained balance are essential for controlled lifting, carrying, and setting down.

Consequently, individuals who do not shift heavy objects in their daily lives have less capacity for doing so. A person who works sitting down for 12 hours every day who wants to help in a household move should not carry any heavy weights (over 15 kg), because neither vertebral end plates nor disks nor the small vertebral joints and their associated muscles are able to do so without being damaged.

Lifting Technique

Before lifting a weight, the local stabilizing muscles are consciously activated: the spine is straightened, the navel is pulled in toward the spine, and the pelvic floor muscles are contracted. When practicing the lifting technique that imposes the least stress on the spine, the patient is also practicing carrying and, most importantly, setting down the weight. These three phases of shifting a weight are very different from each other:
- *Lifting:* the muscles that extend the body against gravity function dynamically and concentrically.
- *Carrying:* the anti-gravity muscles function largely statically and concentrically.

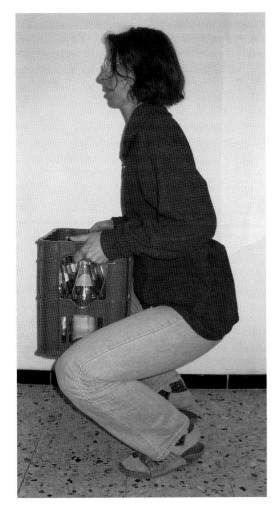

Fig. 9.5 In lifting weights, the spine should be kept vertical with the knees bent.

- *Setting down:* the muscles function dynamically and eccentrically.

In setting down a load, if fatigue has already set in, the muscles have the most difficult task to perform. Moreover, the individuals carrying the load often concentrate on optimal posture only while lifting it and not while setting it down. In this way, they risk disk damage.

Correct Carrying
- In lifting and setting down loads, the knee and hip joints are flexed in such a way that the load is lifted and lowered with an extended, vertical spine.

- The weight is brought close to the body as quickly as possible, kept there while carrying, and moved outward from the body as late as possible when setting it down (**Fig. 9.5**). This movement sequence requires not only mobility and strength but also sufficient balance to rise from squatting in a controlled manner.
- If pivoting is necessary to transport the weight (e.g., lifting a case of bottles out of the shopping cart and into the luggage compartment), one lifts the weight and steps away with body erect, so as to turn the body without rotating the spine.

Note: The weight of the load that a person can lift without problems depends on the individual's constitution, strength, and coordination.

In contrast to lifting, nonweight-bearing activities require a flexed spine in order to maintain mobility (**Fig. 9.6**).

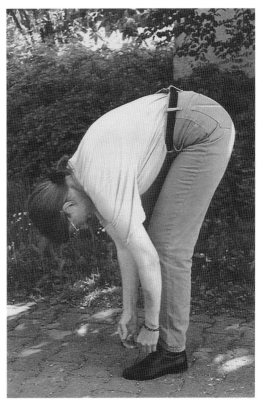

Fig. 9.6 It is fine to bend over to tie shoe laces.

9.6 Strength

In many back school programs and in prescriptions for patients with back pain, the emphasis is on strengthening the back and abdominal muscles.

Helewa et al (1999) studied the question of whether strengthening the trunk muscles contributes to avoiding back pain. They found that back school with a strengthening program was not superior to training without such a program.

In the therapy design described here, deficient maximal strength and power are not considered as important as insufficiently targeted movement for generating disk damage. Improvement of strength endurance, reactive strength, and tone of the stabilizing tonic muscles is described above under 9.2 Stability. After receiving instruction, the patient should work independently at home on strengthening. The same exercises also serve to improve coordination. The exercises to strengthen the abdominal muscles are performed without flexing the spine.

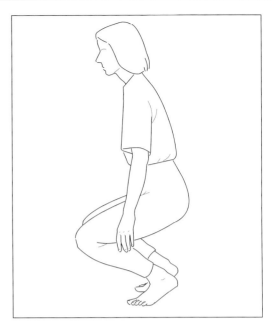

Fig. 9.7 Knee bends to strengthen the leg and trunk muscles and train balance.

Strength Exercises

Knee Bends to Strengthen the Leg and Trunk Muscles and Train Balance (Fig. 9.7)
- Erect standing position.
- Extend the arms forward.
- Bend the knees, keeping the body vertical (shoulder girdle over the pelvis).
- The tone of the stabilizing muscles in abdomen, back, and neck rises automatically and in some cases can be increased by additional, conscious contraction.
- Return to erect position.
- Repeat.

Increasing Intensity
In the same exercise, let the arms hang next to the body. This makes it significantly more difficult to maintain balance.

Strengthening the Spine and Hip Extensors in Prone Position (Fig. 9.8)
- Prone.
- Place outward-rotated arms next to the body.
- Bend elbows, hands pointing toward head.
- Extend neck and back.
- Raise head.
- Thorax remains in place.

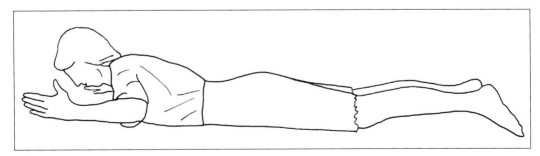

Fig. 9.8 Strengthening the spine and hip extensors in prone position.

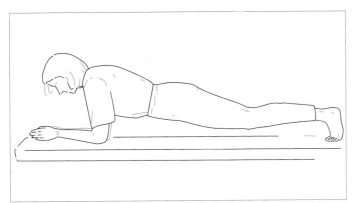

Fig. 9.9 Strengthening the abdominal muscles while supported on lower arms.

- Raise arms.
- Return to original position—relax.
- Repeat.

Increasing Intensity

Extend arms alternately toward the head and move them back next to the body.

Strengthening the Abdominal Muscles While Supported on Lower Arms (Fig. 9.9)

- Quadruped position.
- Lower arm support.
- Move the shoulders away from the ears toward the foot end.
- Contract the abdominal muscles.
- Extend legs and support feet on toes so that only the lower arms and the toes are in contact with the table.
- Slowly return to quadruped position.
- Repeat.

Strengthening the Abdominal Muscles while Supine (Fig. 9.10)

- Supine.
- Pull the navel toward the spine and keep it there.
- Set feet on the ground one after the other.
- Raise the knees toward the abdomen, one after the other.
- Extend one leg and slowly lower it while the contraction of the abdominal muscles maintains the lumbar spine in position and avoids additional extension.
- Flex the leg toward the abdomen again.
- Change legs.
- Repeat.

Push-ups to Strengthen the Trunk, Leg, and Arm Muscles (Fig. 9.11)

- Support yourself on hands and feet.
- Extend the spine.

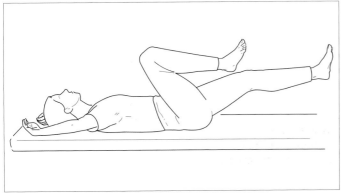

Fig. 9.10 Strengthening the abdominal muscles while supine.

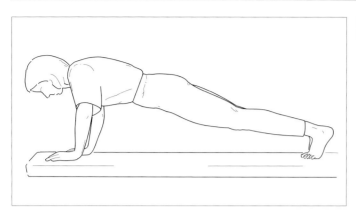

Fig. 9.11 Push-ups to strengthen the trunk, leg, and arm muscles.

- Move the shoulders away from the ears toward the foot end.
- Contract the abdominal muscles such that the lumbar spine does not sag.
- Pull the navel toward the spine and keep it there.
- Flex the elbows and extend without changing the position of the trunk.

Note: With push-ups, the abdominal muscles must generate a bridging tension that prevents the spine from sagging.

9.7   Coordination and Balance

After a disk prolapse, coordination and balance can be disrupted, especially in case of associated pain, sensory disorders, and paresis in one or both legs. Often patients report a feeling of strangeness in the affected leg. This can lead to insecurity and asymmetrical movement patterns. Patients support themselves with their hands when rising from a chair, hold tight to the railing when climbing stairs, and lose their balance when getting up from a squatting position.

Note: Rising from a chair, holding tight to the railing when climbing stairs, and getting up from squatting and so on are practiced in such a way that supporting and holding tight are not necessary. Additional training in balance and coordination is provided by juggling (see 9.2.1), knee bends (see under 9.6 Strength), and practicing running (see under 9.8 Conditioning below).

9.8   Cardiovascular Fitness

After a disk prolapse that involves more than 2 weeks of illness, the patient's cardiovascular fitness is markedly reduced. The first step of fitness training consists of walking. If patients have been prevented from walking for several weeks because of pain they already feel very tired after a 30-minute walk and on the next day, their leg muscles are sore. This discomfort is normal and recedes after 1 or 2 days.

Note:
- The distance walked during fitness training is constantly increased.
- Climbing stairs is a useful form of fitness training.

Running

When symptoms have largely disappeared, running can be started as a form of training. Running has an aerial phase in which both feet are in the air, whereas in walking one foot is always touching the ground. Walking and running are the natural means of human locomotion and thus they are not detrimental, but necessary for health.

Even after a conservatively or surgically treated disk prolapse, running is a beneficial sports activity. The muscle tone of the arms, trunk, and legs is optimized. The spine straightens and abdominal and back muscles stabilize the trunk.

The slight rotation of the spine, rhythmically alternating from right to left, can contribute to the reduction of residual symptoms. In addition, running

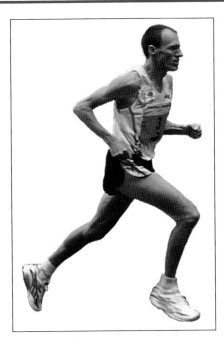

Fig. 9.12 Running.

improves the circulation and supports regulation of blood pressure and body weight. This sport is economical and can be independently and safely practiced by every patient after one or two lessons.

Training by Running (Fig. 9.12)

- Start with very slow running or running in place.
- Land gently with the feet and cushion every step. Running should only make a very soft noise.
- Alternate 1 minute of running with 1 minute of walking.
- Run according to the landscape. This means first walk on uphill and downhill slopes. Run on level terrain. Joints and muscles need time to adapt.
- Breathe naturally and do not count steps per breath.
- You should be able to chat at any time; this means that breathing and heart rate are appropriate.

Note: *No false pride! Start running slowly—running speed will increase on its own as your condition improves.*

- Gradually increase effort, depending on the condition.
- First increase the distance run, and then the tempo.

- Goal: aim for 20 to 45 minutes of running three times a week.

9.9 Individual Compensatory Movements

Patients with disk damage are asked about the posture, movements, and load-bearing stress associated with their work and hobbies. This information determines the instruction they receive about practicing individual compensatory movements.

Examples

- A cashier who must mostly turn to the left at work regularly practices the same movement to the right to compensate for this one-sided stress.
- A violinist who holds the violin by tipping the cervical spine to the right regularly practices tipping the cervical spine to the left.
- Individuals who stoop, lift, and sit a great deal in daily living (**Fig. 9 13a, b**) regularly practice extension of the spine.
- Young people who must sit for hours at school should do their homework in a prone position (**Fig. 9.14**). Many pupils do this instinctively. They should not be stopped from doing this for the sake of better-looking handwriting.
- A veterinarian has learned to squat while treating a horse's leg (**Fig. 9.15a**). In this way, she can treat the horse with an almost extended spine. For her own safety, she has practiced jumping up rapidly from this position. Between treatments, she takes a break in her car and creates additional extension of her spine by bending both knees in prone position (**Fig. 9.15b**).
- While operating, a right-handed surgeon must bend forward and turn to the left frequently and for long periods of time (**Fig. 9.16a**). This often leads to disk displacement to the right and posterior in the cervical and lumbar spine. He should take advantage of a short pause in his work to straighten up and turn to the right (**Fig. 9.16b**). In addition, after every operation, he should repeat this movement approximately 10 times, with a wide range of motion.

- Individuals who write and have to think, and who usually sit while they work, should change their position at least once an hour. It is easily possible to work at an adjustable-height desk (**Fig. 9.17**). Prone position, using a reading wedge (shown on the left of the figure against the wall), is a useful and feasible alternative to constant sitting.

Pope et al (1998) showed with electromyograms that vibrations of the whole body under an unexpected weight strain lead to slower contraction of the back muscles. For instance, because of this, truck drivers who carry heavy loads after they have been sitting with long periods of exposure to vibration have a particular risk of developing disk damage.

Moreover, it was also shown that even 5 minutes of walking before carrying the loads eliminates this effect (ibid.).

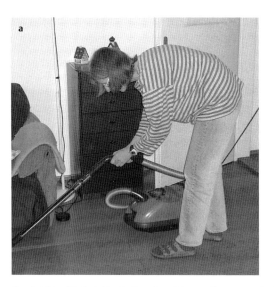
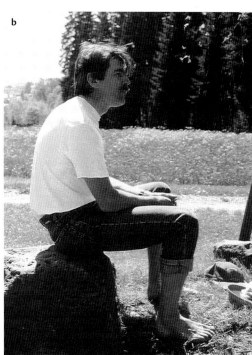

Fig. 9.13 (a, b) Activities in flexed position and long periods of sitting.

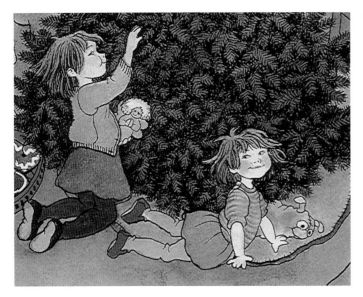

Fig. 9.14 Children in prone position.

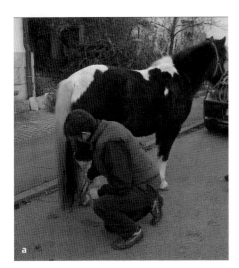
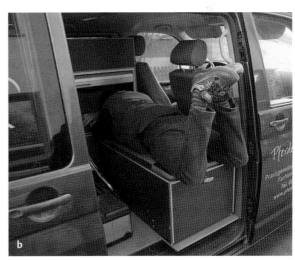

Fig. 9.15 (a) Veterinary treatment of a horse. **(b)** Compensatory extension movement of the spine after providing veterinary treatment.

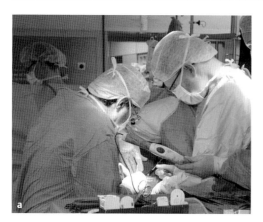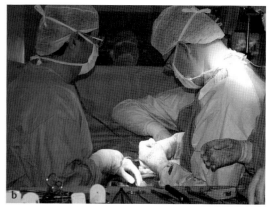

Fig. 9.16 (a) The surgeon turns and bends to the left while operating. **(b)** The surgeon straightens up during a short waiting period.

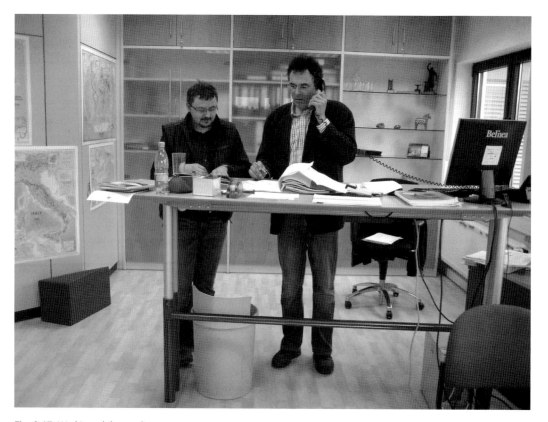

Fig. 9.17 Working while standing.

10   Diseases Occurring in Association With Prolapsed Disks

Mechanical disorders often associated with prolapsed disks such as spinal and foraminal stenosis, spinal instability, facet joint pain as well as impaired nerve mobility cause stereotypical pain reactions when repeated spinal movements are performed.

When the physical therapy methods described here are used, the movements that were beneficial for treatment of disk damage can trigger and intensify symptoms resulting from other causes. Conservative therapy in this type of co-morbidity is accordingly more difficult than therapy for disk damage without additional mechanical impairment.

Beside additional mechanical diseases, other diseases, such as neurological diseases, can make the treatment of patients with disk damage more difficult.

10.1   Additional Diseases With Mechanical Effects on the Spine

Among the co-morbidities most frequently associated with disk damage are:
- Bony spinal and foraminal stenosis.
- Facet joint pain.
- Inflamed or fibrosed nerve roots.

The typical pain behavior in certain co-morbidities and the resulting incompatibility with movements that are therapeutically beneficial in disk damage are summarized below.

Spinal or Foraminal Stenosis

Since the lumen of the spinal canal and the intervertebral foramina are narrowed when the spine is extended, symptoms are triggered by extension of a stenosed section of the spine, as well as by standing and walking for some time. This causes spinal pain and sensory disorders or pain that radiates into the arms and legs. A cervical spinal stenosis can lead to centrally triggered symptoms in the legs.

If stenosis syndrome and a disk prolapse occur concomitantly, repeated spinal movements can have the consequence that moderate extension of the spine centralizes and reduces the pain, whereas pain is intensified and peripheralized as a result of end-range extension. Both areas, the one in which the symptoms are felt and the one related to the disk prolapse, are distant from each other if the spinal or foraminal stenosis is located at a different level than the disk prolapse.

After the movement tests, the symptoms that were first triggered by end-range movement rapidly resolve. In sitting and moderate spinal flexion, the pain caused by long standing and walking is reduced. End-range flexion of the spine intensifies and peripheralizes the pain caused by the disk prolapse.

In physical therapy, the spinal movements are practiced in such a way that radiating pain and sensory disorders are not triggered.

Spinal Instability and Facet Joint Pain

One or more segments of the spine can be unstable or exhibit unnatural movement as a result of displacement of the vertebrae in relation to each other. This displacement may not be very pronounced and may not be visualized by imaging procedures but is clearly visible in MRI or X-ray images in spondylolysthesis (**Fig. 10.1**). This type of sliding in a direction transverse to natural movement exerts excessive pressure and tension on the facet joints, which can cause inflammation, feelings of blockage, and pain. Over the course of years, the body compensates for the unnatural

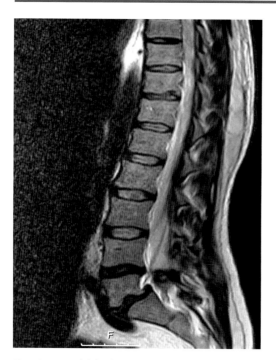

Fig. 10.1 Spondylolysthesis at L5–S1.

mobility by generating bone in these joints, in the form of osteochondroses. This can result in foraminal and spinal stenosis syndromes (Kalichman and Hunter 2008).

The dull facet pain can extend along the spine and up to 10 cm lateral to it. Some affected individuals describe it as a feeling that the spine will snap. Typical triggers are static stress of long duration, especially standing and walking slowly. In movement tests, extension intensifies the pain. Sitting for a short time or spinal flexion relieve the pain (ibid.).

Clinically, the visible mobility of the spine can be normal, hypermobile, or hypomobile. Instability can be segmental (i.e., in a single section of the spine) or global (i.e., present in several or all sections of the spine). In the latter case, the individuals are usually hypermobile overall, for instance, with hyperextensible elbow and knee joints.

There are reliable tests for clinical diagnosis of an instability (Luomajoki et al 2008; Algarni et al 2011). The results of palpation are only informative when evaluated in connection with symptom provocation (Schneider et al 2008). Since the goal of physical therapy is to reduce symptoms,

establishing a hypothesis and a treatment plan is based largely on symptoms. Often patients report that their spines click when they move; some frequently trigger this during the day with jerking movements of head or trunk. This gives affected individuals a feeling of liberated movement after a "blockage." Such unblocking is also the objective of chiropractic maneuvers. But it must be assumed that repeated, jerky movements weaken the passive support system and irritate the facet joints. For this reason, exercises that activate and strengthen the active support system should be preferred to such passive movements.

Three points must be borne in mind in connection with a disk prolapse:

- If a patient has a combination of a disk displacement and facet joint pain, this mechanical conflict will make treatment more difficult. The disk displacement is most likely to be reduced by extension of the spine, but at the same time, this exerts more pressure on the facet joints. Facet pain is reduced by decreased stress in flexion, but this intensifies the displacement of the disk. In this case, twisting movements and moderate spinal extension are helpful.
- After the acute phase of a disk displacement, the initially intensive practice of extension, with 10 repetitions per hour, must be reduced at the right time so as not to trigger facet pain. After centralization and reduction of the pain, the frequency of the exercises is reduced after about 5 days to every 2 hours and then, rapidly, to three times a day.
- A disk prolapse weakens the passive support system, thus reducing spinal stability. For this reason, after a prolapsed disk has been healed, stability must be practiced and trained as a preventive measure (see Chapter 9 Rehabilitation and Prevention).

Inflamed or Fibrosed Nerve Roots

An inflamed or fibrosed nerve root can occupy space in the intervertebral foramen; in spinal extension and rotation it can be compressed intervertebrally because the lumen of the intervertebral foramen has become smaller. In flexion and rotation away from the affected side, tension is applied to the affected nerve root, which also triggers symptoms. This can cause pain and sensory disorders in the affected section of the spine and along the course of the peripheral nerves that branch from this affected nerve root.

If an inflamed or fibrosed nerve root is associated with a disk prolapse, repeated spinal movements can cause the following pain behavior: the pain centralizes and is reduced by moderate spinal movement while end-range movement elicits radiating radicular pains and possibly sensory disorders. Depending on the irritability of the symptoms, they persist after the movement tests or resolve.

In physical therapy, the spinal movements are practiced in such a way that radiating pain and sensory disorders are not triggered. Often the symptoms can be improved by movements of the extremities that can possibly reduce swelling of the nerve roots, thus making it possible to practice end-range spinal movements.

10.2 Nonmechanical Additional Diseases

In addition to mechanical spinal disorders, other associated diseases can influence the course and success of physical therapy for disk damage:
- Neurological diseases that prevent patients from controlling their posture and movements.
- Diseases that force patients to sit more.

A disease that seems to be more frequently associated with disk damage is *idiopathic Parkinson's disease.* This neurodegenerative disease, principally affecting the motor system, is associated with stooping posture. Patients are unable, or only barely able, to control their movements and posture. The consequences are often sciatica and disk prolapse, especially in the lumbar spine.

The conservative therapy described here can often not be systematically carried out because patients are not able to do the exercises regularly. Therefore, physical therapy for affected patients emphasizes prevention. Patients should be instructed to lie prone often, to exercise extension in prone position every morning, and to read either while supported with the forearms or while resting on a reading wedge.

This also applies to patients who are forced by their disease to sit a great deal, as, for instance, in the case of neurological diseases such as paraplegia or multiple sclerosis, or after injuries, for instance, fractures of the lower extremities.

Note: The diagnostic methods and therapy described for pain syndrome associated with disk damage should also be the goal for patients with non-mechanical secondary diseases, even though in these cases paralysis, sensory disorders, and impaired ability to communicate can make successful conservative treatment difficult.

11 Psychosocial Risk Factors

In popular speech, the spine has many psychological associations. Sayings like "He's got a broad back" or "She has plenty of backbone" are used to express strength and perseverance. Weakness and failure, on the other hand, are expressed by sayings like "She is bowed down with grief," or "What a spineless coward."

Spinal pain syndrome is also frequently associated with psychological factors (Waddell et al 1980; Waddell 1987, 1998; Boos et al 1995; Hildebrandt et al 1996; Hasenbring et al 1999). Especially when the usual diagnostic strategies do not yield an answer, the somatic cause of the symptoms is not clear, and various treatment strategies are not successful, psychological mechanisms are singled out as the cause of back and neck pain.

When there is a suspicion that psychosocial factors are present, patients and therapists are usually not sure whether psychological, social, or somatic causes are responsible for the symptoms and what forms of therapy could decrease the symptoms. This uncertainty can place considerable stress on the healthcare system through consultation of a number of different physicians and submission to numerous treatment possibilities, not to mention the resulting disability.

Although it is difficult to identify psychological factors, physical therapists and physicians can recognize some psychological mechanisms and plan therapy accordingly. Especially in chronic pain syndrome, which due to a long period of pain and helplessness can lead to psychological changes such as depression, it is often not clear whether the somatic problem has led to psychological problems or vice versa. For this reason it is important to try to determine whether the problem is a physical disease, a psychological disorder, or a combination of the two. If the problem is a combination, it is necessary to clarify whether the psychological or the physical problem is currently more intense so that treatment can emphasize therapy of the dominant problem.

Therapists should also be aware of risk factors for psychological disorders that can result from pain syndromes so that they can plan their therapy, especially information and instruction for patients, in such a way as to prevent development of anxiety, depression, and avoidance behavior. In planning a disk operation, psychosocial risk factors should be taken into account in order to prevent a predictable poor outcome of surgery. Patients with psychosocial problems should undergo a psychotherapeutic examination, either instead of or in addition to an operation, and if necessary, they should receive supportive treatment before and after surgery (Waddell et al 1980; Junge et al 1996).

In this chapter, we will describe evaluation criteria and tests that allow the examiner to diagnose psychosocial influences. The specialized psychological and psychotherapeutic literature and programs for the treatment of chronic back pain should be used to plan a targeted therapy for problems dominated by psychosocial factors (Hildebrandt et al 1996; Hasenbring et al 1999; Grawe 2000).

Nonorganic Physical Signs According to Waddell

Waddell et al (1980) have developed a reliable standardized examination to differentiate between organic and nonorganic signs in patients with back pain (**Fig. 11.1**). These simple examinations are helpful for physical therapists and physicians who are not trained in psychology when they attempt to identify patients whose symptoms are chiefly characterized by psychosocial factors.

The examination tests five parameters: *sensitivity, simulated stress, discrepancy between straight leg raise test and sitting with legs extended, association of disorders with anatomical structural relationships*, and *behavior when pain is triggered*. Every positive test result counts.

Sensitivity	Negative	Positive
Superficial	☐	☐
Not anatomical	☐	☐
Simulation test	☐	☐
Axial weight-bearing	☐	☐
Rotation	☐	☐
Discrepancy between straight leg raise test and sitting with legs extended	☐	☐
Regional disorders	☐	☐
Deviations from neuroanatomical situation	☐	☐
Sensory disorders	☐	☐
Muscle weakness	☐	☐
Overreaction	☐	☐

Fig. 11.1 Diagnostic examination form for documentation of the tests.

Note:

- If the test results for three of the five parameters are positive, the test is considered positive overall. This means that the patient's symptoms are chiefly influenced by psychosocial factors and that psychotherapy seems advisable.
- A single positive test result is ignored. These tests are less reliable in patients who are older than 60 years, or suffering from severe neurological diseases.

Examination

Superficial *sensitivity* is tested by moving the skin of the back. This test is normally not painful. In addition, the area of pain radiation is assessed. If the patient reports many different, large, painful areas, the test is considered positive.

Simulation tests mimic loading of the lumbar spine. An axial load is applied in the form of light pressure on the head of a patient standing erect. Axial rotation is simulated by applying passive rotation to arms passively held close to the pelvis, in such a way that there is no rotation in the spine, but only in the hips and ankles. If the patient reports that spinal pain is intensified in one of these tests, the test is considered positive.

A *discrepancy* between the report of pain in the straight leg raise test and when sitting with legs outstretched or with knees extended while sitting on the edge of the bed is considered positive if the angular difference is 40° or more.

Regional disorders (e.g., sensory disorders and muscle weakness) are evaluated as to whether they are compatible with the neuroanatomical configuration. If a leg suddenly gives way, this is considered a positive test result just as much as sensory disorder in the whole leg.

Examples of *overreaction* are excessive verbalization of the pain, intense grimacing, general muscle tension, tremor, collapse, and sweating. Especially in the assessment of these overreactions, it must be noted that patients with organic disorders can also develop these behaviors to express the pressure of pain. Therefore, overreaction alone seems unsuitable as a means of ruling out an organic disease.

The patient's answers to the interview and medical history can also point to psychosocial risk factors (**Fig. 11.2**). Typical responses of patients with psychosocial risk factors and pathological symptoms, in addition to the above-mentioned deviations from known anatomical configurations, are constant pain lasting for months to years, therapy resistance, and emergency hospitalization (Waddell 1998). Patients report that for years they have not been pain free for a minute. The pain is rated very high on the numerical analog scale (NAS; 5 to 10/10).

	Positive	Negative
Does your tailbone hurt?	☐ Yes	☐ No
Do you have pain in your whole leg?	☐ Yes	☐ No
Does your whole leg get numb?	☐ Yes	☐ No
Does the whole leg give way in walking and standing?	☐ Yes	☐ No
In the past year, have you had any time without pain?	☐ No	☐ Yes
Has any treatment been helpful?	☐ No	☐ Yes
Have you had an emergency hospitalization?	☐ Yes	☐ No

Fig. 11.2 Diagnostic examination form for documenting the interview.

In these patients, treatment regularly leads to adverse effects and increase of pain. Medications trigger vertigo or stomach aches and physical therapy is associated with pain, even if it is only felt many hours after treatment.

Other Psychosocial Factors

Constantly changing reports of symptoms, constant high rating of pain (8–10 on the NAS), variable behavior when patients are observed (e.g., limping) and when they think they are not being observed are additional indications of a nonorganic disorder. If desire for a pension or a so-called morbid gain through increased attention exists, for instance by a spouse when pain is reported, the psychosocial factors contribute to maintenance of the illness event.

In psychology, the secondary morbid gain is also interpreted in the light of *operant conditioning*, learning through success, which is characterized by retention of certain behaviors on the grounds of reward (Hasenbring et al 2001).

Fear of pain and the resulting avoidance behavior can also be the cause of back pain and its chronification or at least support it (Waddell et al 1993; McCracken et al 1996; Crombez et al 1999; Pfingsten et al 2000). Some authors suspect that the fear of pain that might be triggered by stress

causes more impairment than the pain itself (Crombez et al 1999).

Persistent *excessive stress* during the work day or in the social sphere, dissatisfaction at work, depression, and misdirected coping behavior in a state of pain are relevant predictors for the onset of acute back pain and chronification (Hasenbring et al 2001).

Depression can express itself on the following four levels:
- Emotional: depressed mood.
- Motivational: loss of drive.
- Cognitive: thoughts of helplessness and hopelessness.
- Behavior related: withdrawal behavior.

There is a useful self-testing scale for the diagnosis of depression (Zung and Wonnacott 1970; Zung 1983). It uses factors such as liability to cry, sleep and appetite disorders, decreased libido, agitation, indecision, and irritability as indications of depression.

Note: In patients with spinal cord disorders, psychosocial factors can play an important part, especially in chronification. The task of both physical therapists and physicians consists in recognizing in time the patients who need professional psychological or psychotherapeutic support.

Scientific interest in spinal disorders and their treatment is very high, and in the last 20 years, this has led to a great increase in knowledge. Yet, many publications on the topic of back pain begin with the statement that back pain is highly prevalent and represents a huge drain on the healthcare system and on society and end by calling for more well-designed studies.

Randomization is commonly considered an important feature of a good, informative study. This requires at least two groups of patients to be randomly assigned to one of the several therapeutic methods to be compared. Often, the conservative methods are insufficiently described and in inexact terms such as exercises, physical therapy, manipulation, manual therapy, or educational brochures. The nature and intensity of exercises a patient has performed for treatment of precisely which symptoms and in which phase of their illness is seldom specified. Yet, such information is essential to derive treatment recommendations.

Sometimes a battery of exercises with previously defined movements is called physical therapy and practiced with the patient for a standardized period of time. This strategy is not helpful since the acute phase of a spinal disorder calls for different exercises than the advanced healing phase. For instance, extension in prone position at a rate of 10 repetitions an hour is often advisable in the first week of a disk prolapse, leading to centralization and elimination of pain. If the patient exercises at this intensity over a period of 6 weeks, the small vertebral joints will be overloaded and new pains will develop. Exercises that are helpful in a specific situation may become ineffective or even harmful in the further course of disease.

Hosseinifar et al (2013) compared the usefulness of McKenzie's exercises with regard to pain, disability, and thickness of the stabilizing muscles with the usefulness of stabilizing exercises. It is not surprising that repetitive spinal movements performed with the arms did not strengthen the trunk since this is not their purpose. Moreover, it can be shown that repeated end-range spinal movements over a period of 6 weeks do not increase the capac-

ity for the stress of everyday living. And yet, it is inadmissible to conclude that stabilizing exercises are more efficacious than McKenzie's exercises in improving pain and function and in increasing the mass of the transverse muscles.

Another important weakness that leads to the unsatisfactory quality of many therapy studies is the lack of a standardized clinical-diagnostic approach, especially in the area of nonspecific and chronic back pain, but also in disk prolapse. Review articles often assemble the results of several randomized studies and thereby try to derive conclusions from them.

Funding is challenging, and blinding of either therapists or patients is impossible for most therapeutic approaches. Therefore, some insight must also be derived from small, single-arm studies in addressing the question of how to examine a patient in order to develop an optimal treatment for them. Some valuable insights were already obtained years ago and some old ideas about back pain are still valid to date, and are therefore presented here together with more recent studies.

A PubMed search for studies published between 1966 and 2015 yielded about 26,746 studies on the topic of low back pain. There are only about 20,607 studies on neck pain. If the topic is narrowed down to disk prolapse (*disk herniation*), the number of studies falls to about 17,400. Disk prolapse and exercise (*disk herniation exercises*) yields 300 hits. It is difficult to find the studies that have practical application to physical therapy work in this flood of information. The studies listed below may serve as examples for an overview of the clinical and scientific knowledge obtained through studies of back and neck pain and disk prolapse.

The selected studies provide a basis for the diagnostic and treatment approaches described herein, support the usefulness of this treatment, or provide a starting point for discussion of topics such as the advantages and disadvantages of an operation. Our own magnetic resonance imaging (MRI) study in flexed, extended, and neutral position of the spine with previously unpublished data is presented in detail, as well as our own study of the usefulness of muscle relaxants.

The contents of the articles are briefly presented, the authors' interpretation is given in the Conclusions sections, and the studies are evaluated from our point of view in the Comments sections.

12.1 Breig A, Troup JDG. Biomechanical considerations in the straight-leg-raising test. Cadaveric and clinical studies of the effects of medial hip rotation. Spine. 1979;4:242–250

Publication Type

Experimental anatomical and clinical prospective single-arm study.

Issue

Do clinical and anatomical investigations of tension changes in the sacral plexus when testing the Lasègue sign (straight leg raise test) have concurrent results?

Background

In 1864, Lasègue described the painful effect of knee extension and hip flexion in patients with ischialgia. Since then, the straight leg raise (SLR) test has become a recognized method for investigating lumbar nerve root irritation syndromes. In 1901, Fajersztajn described the increased pain in dorsal extension of the ankle and flexion of the neck and in raising the unaffected leg. Woodhall and Hayes (1950) ascribed the pain response on raising the unaffected leg in disk prolapse to the lateral tension that is exerted on the affected nerve root by this maneuver.

In anatomical studies, the cause of the clinically observed pain reaction was investigated in more depth. Breig (1960, 1978), Breig and Marions (1963), and Breig and Troup (1979) investigated the effect of extremity and head movement on the dura mater and the sacral nerves of recently deceased individuals. When hips and knees were flexed, the sacral plexus remained relaxed. In contrast, when knees were extended, the sacral plexus, the lower lumbar, and sacral nerve roots came under tension, and the fasciae surrounding the nerve roots were pulled caudally. When a disk prolapse was simulated, the nerve root and its surrounding fascia were pulled upward through the intervertebral foramen. Through mechanical damage, transforaminal fasciae or the root sheath can become triggers for painful irritation, for instance through a disk prolapse, with a possible consequence of fibrosis and contraction of the root pouch.

Method

Biomechanical studies were performed on six cadavers to confirm the increased tension on the sacral plexus when the hip is rotated inward. First the sacral plexus was dissected and markers were sutured to the nerve for photographic documentation of the change when the hip was rotated inward. Then a standardized SLR test was performed: neutral hip rotation, supine position, body and extremities in the same plane. Three more tests were performed: dorsal extension of the ankle, inward hip rotation, and neck flexion.

Results

The tension in the sacral plexus resulting from inward rotation of the hip increased palpably in all six cadavers. In four cases, the changes were photographically documented. The sacral plexus was placed under tension, and the displacement of the markers varied from 2 to 10 mm.

Clinical Study Method

Four hundred and forty-two patients who returned to work after an episode of back pain were examined. The SLR test was administered with neutral hip rotation in supine position, with body and extremities in straight extension. The degree of pain-free mobility was measured with a goniometer. All patients with a pain reaction below an angle of 60°, with a side difference in pain or mobility, were subjected to three further tests. The leg was raised to 5° below the pain threshold. Then the foot was passively moved to dorsal extension, the hip rotated inward, and, finally, the neck was passively flexed. Every pain was recorded. In addition, the neck of the patient, seated in a maximally flexed position, was bent.

Results

One hundred and twenty (27%) of the 442 patients exhibited a side difference of more than 10° in the SLR. Seventy patients exhibited positive results in the additional tests. Fifty patients exhibited negative results in the additional tests. In 22 of the 442 patients, the side difference consisted only of a difference in pain reproduction. However, without exception, these patients exhibited positive results in the additional tests. Of 78 patients with neurological deficits of an unspecified nature, 31 exhibited positive results in the additional tests. When the neck was bent with the patient in a flexed, seated position, 92 (20%) of 442 patients reported back pain. Only 25 of them had positive results in the SLR test and positive results in the additional tests, and 67 patients had pain on rotation only when their necks were flexed.

Conclusions

The cadaver studies indicate that in most individuals, the tension in the sacral plexus increases with inward rotation of the hip. If neck flexion in seated position and the SLR with all additional tests, as well as the SLR test on the unaffected side, cause or intensify pain in the affected leg, there is no doubt that increased tension in the nerve root is the cause. Back pain in the tension tests might be caused by adhesion of the dura mater or the root sheath to the anulus fibrosus, the ligamentum flavum, or the capsule of the apophyseal joints.

Comments

The potential significance of the standardized administration of nerve tension tests was presented anatomically and clinically. If the leg deviates in adduction and inward rotation, the tension on the sacral plexus and the nerve roots that constitute it is increased and pain is triggered sooner than when the leg is in neutral position. If the leg deviates in abduction and outward rotation, the opposite effect is produced. Measurement values of the SLR can thus only be compared if the test is performed in exactly the same way every time.

The fact that 47% of the individuals examined after an episode of back pain exhibited positive signs of nerve tension can be seen as an indication that limited nerve mobility is often associated with back pain. Thus, nerve mobility should be included in diagnosis and therapy in cases of back and neck pain, as described in the design presented here.

12.2 Maigne JY, Deligne L. Computed tomographic follow-up study of 21 cases of nonoperatively treated cervical intervertebral soft disk herniation. Spine. 1994;19:189–191

Publication Type

Retrospective case study.

Issue

Computed tomography (CT) examination of patients with cervical disk prolapse successfully treated with conservative therapy: comparison of the initial findings with findings 1 to 30 months after reduction of symptoms.

Background

Although disk prolapses are a frequent cause of radicular pain, the connection between the magnitude of the disk prolapse and the clinical symptoms and signs is unclear. In addition, the mechanism leading to clinical changes during therapy is unknown. It is known that lumbar disk prolapses can become smaller over the course of several months (Maigne et al 1992).

Patients and Method

In a period of 3 years, 45 patients with cervical root compression syndrome were included in the study. In 37 patients, a disk prolapse with root compression was diagnosed using CT. Two of these patients underwent surgery. The remaining 35 patients were treated conservatively with steroidal or nonsteroidal anti-inflammatory medications, neck brace, and traction. Twenty-one patients who felt well after 1 to 30 months were subjected to a second CT examination. The criterion for healing was complete disappearance of the radiating symptoms, even if local neck pain was still experienced.

The disk prolapses were classified according to their anteroposterior extension. Prolapses that filled more than half the spinal canal were defined as *large*, prolapses that filled less than a quarter of the spinal canal were defined as *small*, and prolapses between these two were defined as *medium*. In the control CT, the size decrease of the prolapse compared to the first examination was given in percent.

Results

The initial CT examination showed nine small, seven medium, and five large prolapses. In comparison to the first examination, there was a diminution of prolapses from 0 to 35% in five cases, of 35 to 75% in six cases, and from 75 to 100% in 10 cases. All large prolapses shrank by at least 75%.

Conclusions

The shrinking of the cervical disk prolapses showed the same development as that observed earlier in lumbar disk prolapses (Maigne et al 1992). The fact that large prolapses shrank by at least 75% could be because these were disk sequestrations that had slid away or because large prolapses lose their connection to the hydrostatic mechanism of the spinal disk and consequently lose water more rapidly and in larger amounts. This study shows the tendency of most cervical disk prolapses to resolve. Since the second examination involved only patients whose conservative treatment had been successful, the morphological change in the prolapsed disk cannot be correlated with the clinical course.

Comments

The time to the follow-up examination varied considerably. There is no clear statement of the extent to which the interval to follow-up examination was determined by disappearance of the symptoms. The authors do not explain why only patients without radiating pain were examined and patients with continuing peripheral pain were not.

Treatment with steroids is not described in detail, so it remains unclear whether increased shrinking of large prolapses is associated with administration of steroids.

The article provides no conclusions as to whether the shrinkage of prolapsed disks is associated with improvement of symptoms. In order to make such a judgment, a follow-up examination of all patients, including those who continued to suffer radiating pain, would have been necessary.

12.3 Donelson R, Aprill C, Medcalf R, Grant W. A prospective study of centralization of lumbar and referred pain. Spine. 1997;22:1115–1122

Publication Type

Prospective study.

Issue

Is it possible to make reliable statements about the condition of the anulus fibrosus of the spinal disk using repeated end-range spinal movements and with evaluation of centralization and peripheralization of pain, as described by McKenzie?

Background

The clinical sign of "centralization" that McKenzie was the first to describe occurs frequently during mechanical examination using repeated end-range spinal movements in patients with radicular pain. Radiating or radicular pain disappears rapidly from distal to proximal during movement, that is, toward or up to the midline of the back. McKenzie also postulated that pain in the midline of the back, under the same test conditions, can disappear as a result of repeated end-range movements in a single direction. The opposite development is called peripheralization. This change persists after the spinal movements. McKenzie proposed that a statement about the condition of the anulus can be made on the basis of the centralization and the preferred direction of movement. The following are the components of McKenzie's hypothesis:

- Centralizing pain emanates from the spinal disk and only occurs when the anulus is intact.
- Pain that is only peripheralizing also emanates from the spinal disk but the anulus is no longer functionally intact.
- Radiating pain whose location cannot be rapidly changed by repeated end-range movements does not emanate from the disk.
- Diskography with provocation of the pain described by the patient is the only reliable method of arriving at a statement about the condition of the anulus and about whether the reported pain is emanating from the disk.

Patients and Method

Sixty-three patients who had been suffering from back pain and back and leg pain for longer than 3 months were examined mechanically by two McKenzie therapists and then diskographically by radiologists. All patients were examined by MRI. All examiners documented their results independently and were not informed of the evaluations made by the other examiners (blinded). Subsequently the findings were reviewed to check for agreement.

The McKenzie therapists classified the pain during mechanical examination as follows:

- Centralizing pain.
- Peripheralizing pain.
- Radiating pain whose location cannot be rapidly changed by repeated end-range movements.

In the diskographic examination, contrast medium was injected into the disk, the pain reaction was documented, and the integrity of the painful disk was visualized with CT.

A diskogram was evaluated as positive under the following conditions: the pain reported by the patient could be reproduced exactly and imaging showed tears in the outer third of the anulus with the outer edge still intact or tears running entirely through the anulus.

Results

A high correlation was found for both centralization and peripheralization with positive diskograms (tears in the anulus fibrosus) and a high correlation of "unchanged pain" with negative diskograms ($p < 0.001$). Patients with centralizing pain more frequently had a stable outer anulus than patients whose pain peripheralized ($p < 0.042$) (**Table 12.1**). The results of MRI examinations are not described in detail but only summarized as "no disk prolapses"

Conclusions

Noninvasive imaging procedures such as native X-rays, CT, or MRI do not permit visualizing which structures the pain is emanating from. An advantage of the McKenzie Method® is the fact that it leads to a diagnosis regarding disk integrity and to an appropriate treatment without the disadvantages of invasive diskography, which entails a pain response. Although pain is a subjective sensation, stereotypical pain patterns can have a diagnostic and prognostic value.

Comments

A focused therapy plan is an important goal in treating patients with back pain or radiating pain (Waddell 1996; Cherkin et al 1998). The first step toward achieving this goal is a diagnosis. It is well known that disk damage is associated with back pain and that expansion of the damage can lead to radicular pain. The observation that this pain behavior can be reversed by means of repeated end-range spinal movements was first described by McKenzie (1981). We have made use of this phenomenon in several clinical studies and found it helpful for patients, over years of clinical work.

The concept of centralization is not clearly defined in the present study. The authors do not specify whether by centralization they mean only a retreat of the pain to the midline of the spine or whether they include simple disappearance of peripheral pain. The graphic (Fig. 1 in the article) that explains peripheralization and centralization still shows back pain at the broadest extension of pain to the foot. It remains unclear how centralization proceeds or is defined when no back pain but only leg pain is experienced.

Terms for the condition of the anulus are occasionally used in a contradictory way. McKenzie assumed that centralization only takes place when

Table 12.1 Results of the mechanical and diskographic examinations

Results of the mechanical examination (McKenzie)	Number of patients	Positive diskograms (neuroradiological examination)	Stable outer anulus (neuroradiological examination)
Centralization	31 (49.2%)	23/31 (74%) $p < 0.007$	21/23 (91%) $p < 0.001$
Peripheralization	16 (25.4%)	11/16 (69%) $p < 0.004$	6/11 (54%) $p < 0.093$
No change	16 (25.4%)	2/16 (12.5%) $p < 0.001$	2/2 (100%)
Total	63 (100%)	36/63 (57%)	29/63 (46%)

Note: The p values represent the correlation between the results of mechanical and diskographic examinations.

the nucleus pulposus is contained in an intact anular shell. The present study worked with the hypothesis that centralizing pain originates in the disk and that in patients with centralizing pain the anulus is intact. A positive diskogram with *intact outer* anulus was offered as confirmation of the correctness of this hypothesis. A diskogram was evaluated as positive if the outer third of the anulus showed tears or the anulus was torn through to the outside. Presumably in patients with centralizing pain, the entire anulus was not intact—only the exterior shell.

Meanwhile, the concept of centralization was extensively discussed. The following definition seems useful to us: "The distal pain is eliminated during movements of the spine and remains absent after the movements." May et al (2008) offer the following definition in a review paper: "Centralization is the abolition of distal pain in response to repeated movements or sustained postures." Whether the tear in the anulus fibrosus is partial or complete is not decisive for the prognosis or the selection of exercises. This can be concluded from our studies on patients with radiologically and clinically confirmed disk prolapses as well as sequesters (Brötz et al 2003, 2008; Brötz, Burkard, et al 2010; Brötz, Maschke, et al 2010).

12.4   Brötz D, Küker W, Maschke E, Wick W, Dichgans J, Weller M. A prospective trial of mechanical physiotherapy for lumbar disk prolapse. J Neurol. 2003;250:746–749

Publication Type
Prospective single-arm study.

Issue
Is physical therapy with repeated spinal movements (McKenzie Method®) and nerve-gliding movements in patients with neuroradiologically confirmed lumbar disk prolapse efficacious and can the probability of efficacy be prospectively determined?

Background
In most publications about conservative therapy of back pain, neither the patients' clinical signs and symptoms nor the therapy applied are described with satisfactory precision. A broad range of therapeutic measures, administered in various combinations, is available to patients with disk prolapses. At present, there are no generally recognized guidelines for the selection of conservative therapies.

Patients and Method
In a single-arm prospective study, 50 consecutive patients with neuroradiologically confirmed lumbar disk prolapse were treated according to the McKenzie Method® (1981). After the acute phase, therapeutic leg movements (Maitland 1994) were increased. The objective of the leg movements was improvement of nerve-gliding capacity.

The patients included had a neuroradiologically confirmed (CT or MRI) disk prolapse, sciatica, with and without neurological deficit. An additional inclusion criterion was centralization of radiating pain within the first five physical therapy sessions taking place on 5 consecutive days. Patients with bladder and colon disorders with suddenly occurring high-grade (strength degree 1 or less) paresis or paralysis were excluded. These patients underwent surgery immediately. Another exclusion criterion was the absence of centralization of the radiating pain within the first five therapy sessions. All patients attended daily physical therapy sessions lasting 45 minutes. These sessions were conducted according to the guidelines described here, by two physiotherapists. In addition, all patients independently practiced the spinal and leg movements assigned during therapy. Most of the patients also received pain medications and muscle relaxants. All findings were documented on admission, discharge, 6 weeks after discharge, and 1 year after discharge.

Results
Of 150 patients with the suspected diagnosis of disk prolapse, 64 patients were excluded because the neuroradiological examination did not definitively show a disk prolapse, no radiating pain was experienced, or another pathology was identified as the cause of

Table 12.2 Results of the admission examination and the second follow-up examination[a]

Patient status	On admission	At the second follow-up examination
Paresis (grade 4)[b]	16/50 (32%)	5/43 (11%)
Paresis (grade 3 and worse)[b]	14/50 (28%)	0/43 (0%)
Pain 5–10[c]	27/49 (55%)	1/43 (2%)
Pain 1–4[c]	22/49 (44%)	4/43 (9%)
Sensory disorder	38/50 (76%)	17/43 (39%)
SLR (median ± SEM in cm)[d]	44 ± 22 (10–92)	88 ± 11 (30–103)
Use of muscle relaxants	44/50 (88%)	0/43 (0%)
Use of pain medication	48/50 (96%)	5/43 (11%)
Employed	36/50 (72%)	30/43 (69%)
In physical therapeutic treatment	50/50 (100%)	9/43 (20%)
Self-training physical therapy	N/A[e]	38/43 (88%)
Surgery	N/A	5/48 (10%)
Satisfaction with regard to back problem, nonoperated patients	N/A	40/43 (93%)
Satisfaction with regard to back problem, operated patients	N/A	3/4 (75%)

Notes:

[a] Only the nonoperated patients are listed in the third column.

[b] Paresis grade 4: complete range of motion against resistance but without complete strength; paresis grade 3: complete range of motion against gravity but inability to move against resistance.

[c] Pain was measured on a numerical analog scale (0 means no pain, 10 means the strongest possible pain). SEM: Standard Error of the Mean, a statistical measure.

[d] The nerve tension sign straight leg raise (SLR) was measured as the distance in centimeters between the outer malleolus and the pad.

[e] N/A, not applicable.

the pain. Thirty-six patients were treated surgically for disk prolapse. Fifty patients satisfied the inclusion criteria and were taken into the study.

The size of the disk prolapses was measured according to their anteroposterior extension in the spinal canal. This was < 25% in 39 patients, 25 to 50% in six patients, 50 to 75% in two patients and > 75% in three patients. Two patients had foraminal disk prolapses. Nineteen patients had a sequester. The median time spent as an in-patient was 10 days; the average period of disability and limitation of activities of daily living was 35 days after discharge.

The results of the admission examination and the second follow-up examination approximately 1 year after discharge are given in **Table 12.2**.

Conclusions

Contrary to the assumptions of McKenzie (1981) and Donelson et al (1997) the phenomenon of centralization was seen even in patients with a pronounced disk prolapse, sometimes greater than 50% of the spinal canal diameter, or with sequestered disk prolapse. This examination shows that these patients too are candidates for the conservative therapy described here and that the outlook for success can be easily judged prospectively.

Comments

We assume that this symptom-oriented therapy, which requires the patient's active participation, has a high potential to avoid operations for disk prolapse and prevent chronification of back pain. In the meantime the condition of the patients in this study was also described at a 5-year follow-up; they had continued independent exercise, remained satisfied, and had a low operation rate (Brötz, Burkard, et al 2010).

It would be desirable to have randomized studies in which homogeneous patient groups comparable to this study receive either no therapy, a different, customary conservative therapy, surgical treatment, or the therapy applied here. In the past, this kind of therapy has failed because when the therapy fails, patients do not remain in the arm of the study to which they were assigned (see above).

12.5   Weinstein JN, Tosteson TD, Lurie JD, Tosteson ANA, Hanscom B, Skinner JS et al. Surgical versus nonoperative treatment for lumbar disk herniation. The Spine Patient Outcomes Research Trial (SPORT): a randomized trial. JAMA. 2006b;296:2441–2450

Publication Type
Prospective, randomized, two-arm study.

Issue
Investigation of the efficacy of surgical therapy compared to nonoperative therapy in patients with lumbar disk prolapses.

Background
In the United States, diskectomy is the most frequent surgical treatment for patients with back and leg pain. The operation rate varies from one state to another, by factors of up to 15. The question arises whether some operations were contraindicated. In this article, the results over an observation period of 2 years are presented. The Spine Patient Outcomes Research Trial (SPORT) was begun in 2000 in order to compare the results of surgical versus conservative treatment of lumbar disk prolapse, spinal canal stenosis, and degenerative spondylolisthesis.

Patients and Method
The study was conducted at 13 multidisciplinary centers in 11 US states. Patients included were older than 18 years with radiologically confirmed lumbar disk prolapse and symptoms that had persisted for at least 6 weeks in spite of conservative treatment. The conservative treatment before inclusion in the study was not specified. Seventy-six percent of patients had received physical therapy. The inclusion criteria defined were radicular pain radiating into one leg, noticeable nerve tension signs, or neurological deficits. Exclusion criteria were prior spine operations, cauda equina symptoms, scoliosis over 15°, segmental instability, vertebral fractures, infections and tumors, inflammatory spondylarthropathy, pregnancy, concomitant illness making surgery impossible, and refusal to undergo surgery.

The treatment method was either a standard open diskectomy or customary nonoperative therapy and was intended to be randomized. This customary therapy included active physical therapy, information with instructions for exercising at home, and nonsteroidal anti-inflammatory medications, if tolerated.

The primary target parameter was the 36-point questionnaire (SF-36) and a modified Oswestry Disability Index (see Chapter 2, **Fig. 2.15**). The end points evaluated were changes, compared to the baseline, after 6 weeks, 3 months, 6 months, 1 year, and 2 years. Secondary outcome parameters were self-evaluated improvement, ability to work, and satisfaction with the symptoms and treatment. The intensity of the symptoms was measured with the Sciatica Bothersomeness Index.

Potential candidates were given a choice of participating in the randomized study or in a nonrandomized observational group.

Results
Of 1991 eligible patients, 501 (25%) consented to be randomized. Of these, 472 (94%) took part in at least one follow-up examination. At each examination date, 73 to 86% of patients were available. Their average age was 42 years; most of them were male, Caucasian, and employed. Sixty-one percent of the disk prolapses were at the level of L5–S1.

The nonoperative treatment strategies were information (93%), anti-inflammatory medication (61%), and injections (56%). Only 44% received active physical therapy although 67% had received this treatment before inclusion in the study.

The average operation time was 75 minutes. Complications were injury to the dura mater with loss of spinal fluid in 4% of patients. Within 1 year, 4% of patients were re-operated on.

A significant fraction of the patients in both groups changed the assigned treatment strategy. In the group that was to be surgically treated, 32% had been operated on by the 6-week check-up, after 3 months, 50%, after 6 months, 57%, after a year, 59%, and after 2 years, 60% of patients. In the group that was to be conservatively treated, 18% had been operated on by the 6-week check-up, after 3 months, 30%, after 6 months, 39%, after 1 year, 43%, and after 2 years, 45% of patients. The patients who switched from the conservative to the surgical arm tended to have a lower income, more pain, and more limitations at the start of and during the study and poorer function than the patients who did not transfer. Conversely, the patients who transferred to conservative treatment had higher incomes, less pain, and fewer limitations at the start and during the study.

The data were analyzed statistically both according to intention to treat and according to the treatment actually received. For all target parameters, there were no statistically significant differences, with a tendency to better results in the operated group. At all the measurement dates and in all measurement parameters, both groups improved significantly. Satisfaction with symptoms and treatment was somewhat higher among operated patients, whereas the ability to work developed better in the nonoperated patients.

After 3 months, 43% of nonoperated patients compared to 54% of operated patients were satisfied with the symptoms; after a year 59% of the nonoperated versus 65% of the operated; and after 2 years 64% of the nonoperated versus 68% of the operated patients were satisfied. After 1 year, 87% of the nonoperated versus 90% of the operated patients were satisfied with their treatment.

Conclusions

The results of this study are comparable to earlier studies of the same issue (Weber 1983; Carragee et al 1996; Atlas et al 2001 [the Maine Lumbar Spine Study]). Placebo effects cannot be ruled out since blinding regarding therapy by such means as a mock operation is impossible for ethical reasons. The large number of conservative methods and the variety of ways in which they are used can be considered individualized therapy and may have

great advantages. Recommendations for operative or conservative therapy cannot be made on the basis of these data.

Comments

The first randomized, controlled, prospective study comparing the course of healing in an operated group with healing in a conservatively treated group of patients with confirmed disk prolapse was conducted by Weber (1983). Here, in spite of the inferiority of the conservative therapy, after 1 year 60% of the conservatively treated patients exhibited satisfactory results. After 10 years almost all pareses had resolved and no significant differences between the groups could be measured.

In the SPORT study, satisfaction with symptoms was relatively low in both groups (59% and 65% respectively), while satisfaction with treatment was relatively high (87% versus 90%). It is of interest to know how patients explained satisfaction with treatment. As the authors remarked, it is possible that the more intense surgical treatment automatically produces greater satisfaction as placebo effect.

It was not possible to determine whether a nonspecific conservative treatment is superior or inferior to a specific surgical therapy, either in this study, earlier studies, or the later study by Peul et al (2007). Moreover, a global question like this one is not of interest to the individual patient. Even if one treatment arm had statistically better results, there would be too many open variables. For instance, the postoperative therapy was not described. Surely it affects the outcome of the operation? Possibly a defined surgical method with reasonable aftercare might produce a better outcome.

The lack of clarity concerning the conservative therapy is even more important. Most of the treatments were passive. Only 44% of the patients received physical therapy. This treatment was also not described in detail, so that possibly both beneficial and counterproductive physical therapy methods came into play. It remains to be determined how good the results of conservative treatment could have been if exclusively beneficial strategies had been applied and the patients had learned the mechanical causes of a disk prolapse and how they themselves could contribute to healing with exercises and by the way they perform their daily activities.

12.6 Functional Investigation of the Lumbar Spine and the Spinal Canal in Flexion, Extension, and Neutral Position in Patients with Lumbar Disk Prolapse, Using Magnetic Resonance Tomography: Capture of Morphological Changes

(Report at the 2008 annual conference of the Radiological Society of North America and previously unpublished data. Concept and patient recruiting: D. Brötz, S. Burkard; radiology: S. Miller, J. Döring, C. Bretschneider, B. Klumpp, C.D. Claussen; data evaluation: M. Stark.)

Study Type
Prospective exploratory study.

Issue
Does spinal flexion or extension influence the prolapsed tissue in a lumbar disk prolapse? And is there a correlation with changes in symptoms?

Background
There have been several studies using MRI to visualize position-determined changes of the nucleus pulposus within the disk or the diagnosis of disk shift (Fennell et al 1996; Jinkins et al 2005). In our own study (Brötz et al 2008), morphological changes in the disk prolapse were monitored over the course of 5 days of mechanical physical therapy, using MRI. Other studies investigated the long-term course of disk prolapse by means of imaging (Bush et al 1992; Maigne et al 1992; Maigne and Deligne 1994; Slavin et al 2001; Reyentovich et al 2002; Henmi et al 2002). Before we began our study in 2007, no study had examined changes in bulging disk substance during and after end-range spinal positions in flexion and extension. In the meantime there have been two small single-arm studies of this issue (Fasey et al 2010; Takasaki et al 2010).

Most patients with radiologically confirmed lumbar disk prolapse associated with sciatica and neurological deficits can achieve sustained improvement of their symptoms, even to the point of being symptom free, by means of physical therapy that is oriented to symptoms and posture (Brötz et al 2001, 2003; Brötz, Burkard, et al 2010; Brötz, Maschke, et al 2010). In each therapy session, the physical therapist and the patient evaluated the spinal movements that centralized or reduced the pain. These movements were rotation and extension of the spine. Patients were instructed to repeat these spinal movements, first at a rate of 10 times an hour and later less often. In addition, the patients were advised to adjust their daily behavior to avoid the disadvantageous movements of flexion and sitting. With time, stabilizing muscle activity and leg movements to mobilize neural pathways were added to the exercise program.

Patients and Method
Patients with MRI-confirmed lumbar disk prolapse and the appropriate symptoms, who were eligible for conservative therapy on the basis of their symptoms and were treated according to the principles described here, were candidates for this study. The treating physical therapists, DB or SB, informed the eligible patients, who were then informed about the course of the investigation by the radiologists SM or JD.

Inclusion Criteria
- 18 to 80 years.
- Sciatica.
- With or without neurological deficit.
- Lumbar disk prolapse corresponding to the symptoms, visualized with MRI.
- Centralization, reduction, or elimination of pain by means of spinal movements.
- Toleration of positions in flexion and extension of the spine.
- Agreement to be studied.

Exclusion Criteria
- Contraindication for MRI.
- Pregnant or lactating women.
- Prior operations for disk prolapse.
- Prior traumatic spinal injuries.
- Use of corticosteroids.
- Bladder or large intestine paralysis.
- High-grade paresis (strength level 1) or paralysis appearing in the past 24 hours.
- Pacemaker, intracranial metal implants.
- Claustrophobia.

- Ferromagnetic implants, depending on the build (e.g., hip or knee prostheses older than 20 years) except tooth implants.
- Lacking written informed consent.

Radiology

All patients were informed about the MRI examination in the customary way. The examinations were performed with a 1.5 Tesla scanner (MAGNETOM Espree, Siemens AG, Erlangen) with a gradient strength of 40 mT/m. The study participants were examined in supine position; a body coil was used for signal acquisition. Disk morphology was investigated by visualizing sections of the spinal column at the level of the affected intervertebral disk space in sagittal and axial planes, using T2w SE technology. Examination was performed in immediate sequence, in flat supine position, flexion, extension, and once more in flat supine position (see **Fig. 12.1a–d**). During and after the individual examinations, the patient was asked about symptoms and the answers were documented. The examination was terminated if the patient exhibited claustrophobia or intensified symptoms.

Evaluation

The angles between the vertebrae at the level of the disk prolapse were measured in the different positions. The size of the disk prolapse was determined by measuring the prolapsed disk tissue. The LEONARDO Workstation (Siemens, Erlangen) was used. First the maximal measurable distance between the prolapsed portion of the disk and the vertebral body in the various positions in the sagittal section was measured. The same measurement was repeated in the transverse section. In the sagittal images, the surface area of the disk projecting into the spinal canal was measured. In the transverse images, the surface area of the spinal canal was determined. In the next step, the volume of the prolapsed disk was measured in the sagittal images. In the transverse section, the volume of

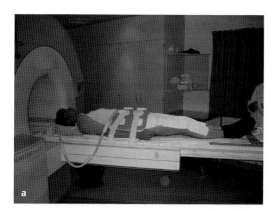
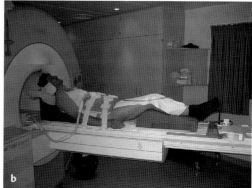
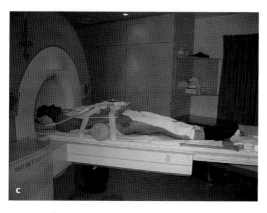
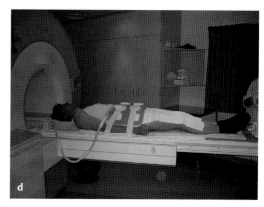

Fig. 12.1 **(a)** Flat supine position. **(b)** Flexion position. **(c)** Extension position. **(d)** Flat supine position.

the missing surface area of the spinal canal was measured in the four positions.

A change in clinical symptoms, pain intensity (numerical analog scale), location of pain, and sensitivity with position change were documented.

Results

All patients assigned to be examined were able to be examined according to the protocol. Twenty patients (mean age 41/25–65 years, 15 male) with symptoms of acute disk prolapse were examined. In physical therapy sessions and during the examination, 70% of patients exhibited centralization of the radiating pain in extension. All these patients also achieved improvement and elimination of symptoms. Six patients failed to achieve sustainable pain relief. Four of these patients underwent surgery. Three of the operated patients failed to show pain centralization.

Distance of Disk Prolapse Sagittal Section

The maximal distance of the prolapsed disk tissue from the vertebra decreased by −4.44% (SD ± 10.90%) in 80% of patients between the flat supine position before the examination and the flat supine position after positioning in extension. The difference was even greater between positioning in flexion and in extension. In 90% of patients, the

distance of the prolapsed disk tissue decreased by 10.59% (SD ± 10.29%) (**Fig. 12.2**).

Distance of Disk Prolapse Transversal Section

The maximal distance of the prolapsed disk tissue from the vertebra decreased by −13.55% (SD ± 18.57%) in 80% of patients between the flat supine position before the examination and the flat supine position after positioning in extension. In 85% of patients, between the position in flexion and the position in extension the maximal distance decreased on average by −9.04% (SD ± 27.05%). On average, the maximal distance of the prolapsed disk tissue decreased from 0.61 cm to 0.59 cm (sagittal section) and from 0.38 cm to 0.33 cm (transverse section).

Surface Area of the Prolapsed Disk Tissue

The surface area of the prolapsed disk tissue in flat supine position is greater before and less after positioning in extension (sagittal section) in 45% of patients with an average difference of −0.22% (SD ± 10.06%) and in 85% of patients (transverse section) with an average difference of −13.55% (SD ± 18.57%). Between the position in flexion and the position in extension the surface area (sagittal section) decreased in 90% of patients with an average difference of −12.72% (SD ± 11.50%) and

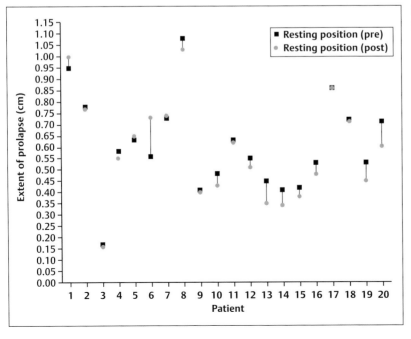

Fig. 12.2 Distance of disk prolapse sagittal section.

(transverse section) in 85% of patients with an average difference of –9.04% (SD ± 27.05%).

Volume of the Prolapsed Disk Tissue

The calculated volume of the prolapsed disk tissue decreased between flat supine position before and after positioning in extension in 50% of patients in the section by an average difference of +1.83% (SD ± 21.86%). In 70% of patients, between the position in flexion and the position in extension, the volume decreased by an average difference of –8.46% (SD ± 19.57%)

Discussion and Conclusions

Using dynamic MRI, changes in the prolapsed disk tissue were shown to correlate with the symptom changes of centralization and reduction of radiating pain. The hypothesis that the disk prolapse changes position as a result of spinal flexion and extension was confirmed. Since with extension the maximal distance and the surface area of the prolapsed tissue decrease, thus decreasing the potential damage to nerve pathways, this movement should be a goal for patients with lumbar disk prolapse.

13 Significance, Types, and Objectives of Clinical Studies

In light of the high significance for health economics of back pain in general and of disk prolapse in particular, it is remarkable that only a few therapies commonly used today are supported by adequate clinical studies demonstrating their efficacy. Considering the increasing cost pressure in healthcare, efficacy is an increasingly important criterion for health insurance companies in determining whether to accept or decline to cover the cost of treatment. This emphasis is also reflected in the increasing importance of therapeutic guidelines established by the relevant specialist societies that will be advising funding organizations in the distribution of healthcare resources. The following procedures exist for evaluation of treatment efficacy:

Evaluation of Efficacy

↑↑ Declaration of efficacy is supported by several adequate, valid (e.g., randomized) clinical trials or by one or more valid meta-analyses or systematic reviews. Positive judgment is well documented.

↑ Declaration of efficacy is supported by at least one adequate, valid (e.g., randomized) clinical trial. Positive judgment is documented.

↓↓ Negative declaration of efficacy is supported by several adequate, valid (e.g., randomized) clinical trials or by one or more valid meta-analyses or systematic reviews. Negative judgment is well documented.

↔ There are no adequate trial results to confirm efficacy or inefficacy. This can be caused by the lack of adequate trials or by the existence of several contradictory trial results.

Hierarchy of Evidence Levels

(I = highest evidence level, V = lowest evidence level)
I. At least one systematic review article based on high-quality randomized clinical trials.
II. At least one sufficiently large or high quality randomized clinical study of high quality.
III. Studies without randomization (cohorts, case and control studies) of high methodological quality.
IV. More than one nonexperimental study of high methodological quality.
V. Opinions of respected authorities (through clinical experience), expert commissions, descriptive studies.

Jadad Scale for Evaluation of Controlled Studies

(5 points = high quality, 0 points = poor quality)

Randomization	1
Adequate description of the randomization	1
Double blinding	1
Adequate description of the blinding	1
Description of individuals who withdraw from a study	1

Prospective Studies

Clinical studies in the narrow sense deal with the treatment of patients in accordance with a previously defined *study protocol*. This means that establishing a protocol is a prerequisite for implementing the study. Such studies, called prospective, are generally more conclusive than retrospective studies.

Retrospective Studies

In this type of study, patient files are evaluated retrospectively with regard to a specific question in order to confirm or rule out a suspected connection. The results often serve to generate hypotheses that can later be investigated in prospective studies.

Study Arm

A clinical study can investigate one or more types of treatment. A group of patients treated according to the same principle is called a study arm.

First-time investigation of a new treatment usually involves a *single-arm* study, whereas comparison of several forms of treatment involves a *multi-arm* (usually two-arm) study. The established treatment is considered the *standard arm* and the new treatment represents the *experimental arm.*

Randomization
In multi-arm studies, patients are assigned to the study arm at random. This is called randomization and usually takes place on the basis of previously established randomization lists.

Reliability
In diagnostic and therapeutic strategies for clinical studies, particularly in the area of physical therapy, the intertester and intratester reliability should be ensured. This means that a number of different investigators examining the same patient and the same investigator performing repeated examinations should all obtain the same result.

Placebo Effect
This concept covers all effects of therapeutic measures that are interpreted not as a specific result of the measure itself but as an unspecific reaction of the patient to the therapeutic measure. Specific factors that produce a placebo effect are the patient's expectation, the personality of the therapist, and the external circumstances surrounding delivery of the treatment.

Thus academic rank, name recognition, and social status favor confidence in the therapist's competence. Moreover, there is a greater expectation of improvement if the therapeutic measure involves a high level of instrumentation and personnel than if it simply involves administration of a pill by clinical study personnel.

Blinding
To minimize the placebo effect, patients should ideally not know to which therapy arm they have been assigned. Naturally, this blinding is only possible when the two therapies being compared are outwardly similar, such as two analgesics for the treatment of back pain. On the other hand, patient blinding is not possible if conservative and surgical treatments or various forms of physical therapy are being compared.

The ideal experimental design uses *double blinding*, in which neither patient nor therapist knows to which treatment arm the patient has been assigned. This procedure can be strictly followed in drug studies or where different therapists perform and evaluate the treatment.

Phases of Clinical Studies
Depending on the issues being investigated, clinical studies are often categorized in four different phases. **Table 13.1** summarizes the most important characteristics of these phases and gives examples of the corresponding issues.

Table 13.1 Characteristics of the phases of clinical studies

	Objective	Example
Phase I	Use in humans Toxicity Determination of maximum tolerated or optimal dose (pharmaceuticals)	New analgesics
Phase II	Signal of efficacy	New physical therapy technique
Phase III	Randomization (comparison with a standard) Expanding indication	Comparison between conservative and surgical treatment Comparing the combination of physical therapy and pharmaceutical compound with a single therapy mode
Phase IV	Optimization of therapy (dose and application form of drug) Detection of rare side-effects Cost–benefit analysis Interaction studies Special patient groups (children, the elderly, patients unable to give consent)	Expanding indication for a physical therapy technique

Criteria for Inclusion/Exclusion

The planning of a clinical study should include careful consideration of which patients are most suitable for investigation of the underlying issue. This is formally confirmed by the definition of inclusion/exclusion criteria in the study protocol. The criteria are related to such things as the differentiation of related diseases, upper and lower age limits, prior illnesses, co-morbidities, and concurrent medications.

Target Parameters

Additional requirements for the successful conduct of a clinical study are the clear statement of the issue to be investigated as well as target parameters (end points) on which the study results are determined. Examples of this type of end point are parameters such as survival time in cancer, the time to next flare-up of the illness in multiple sclerosis, consumption of analgesics, or the duration of disability in the case of back pain.

Prior consultation with experts in biometrics is necessary for planning the end point and evaluating the results. On the basis of the results expected by the sponsors, biometricians can calculate in advance how many patients must be included in a study in order to prove or disprove the hypothesis.

Significance

The sequence of treatment and follow-up examinations must be precisely specified in a protocol. In the evaluation of clinical studies, biometric methods are used to determine whether an observed difference in the values of a target parameter between the study arms was significant.

A difference observed in the study is significant if it reflects an actually existing difference with a previously defined (small) probability of error (p value). The smaller the p value, the greater is the difference and the smaller is the probability of an erroneous assumption of a difference that in fact does not exist.

If the investigator assumes that they have detected a difference even though there is none, this is called a false positive. Conversely, a false negative exists if the investigator concludes that the study hypothesis is false, even though it is in fact correct.

The primary sources of false-negative study results are an insufficient number of patients because of unrealistic expectations in planning the number of cases as well as the establishment of inappropriate target parameters.

Declaration of Informed Consent

The patient information document and the patient's declaration of consent are important components of the study protocol. Both documents must be submitted to the responsible *Ethics Committee* for review. The study can only begin when this committee has granted its agreement in writing. The *Guidelines for Good Clinical Practice* (GCP) were developed by the World Health Organization in 1995 for the planning and implementation of clinical studies.

Glossary

Active physical therapy: hands-on therapy where the patients themselves must physically move their joints and muscles as part of the treatment process.

Allodynia: pain triggered by stimuli that normally do not cause pain.

Analgesia: lack of pain sensation in response to physiologically painful stimuli.

Arm (of a study): group of patients treated uniformly according to a protocol (e.g., single-arm study, two-arm study).

Back school: various programs for the prevention of back pain, using information about the origin of the pain, training in lifting, sitting, and posture, strength and relaxation training.

Blinding: in *simple* blinding, patients do not know to which treatment arm of a multi-arm study they have been assigned. The ideal experimental design uses *double blinding*, in which neither patient nor therapist knows to which treatment arm the patient has been assigned.

Brachialgia: arm pain.

Brown-Séquard syndrome: spinal hemiplegia with ipsilateral disturbance of proprioceptive sensibility and paresis and contralateral disturbance of pain and temperature sensation.

Centralization: shift of the distal extent of radiating or radicular pain further to proximal. In this process, central pain, more toward or in the center of the affected spinal segment, can arise or increase. This change is triggered by spinal movements and persists after the movements (antonym: peripheralization).

Cervicobrachialgia: neck pain combined with radiating arm pain.

Cohort: patient group with common characteristics and symptoms.

Compliance: assent, obedience, especially the willingness of patients to follow instructions regarding treatment.

Computed tomography (CT): imaging procedure that records the attenuation of X-rays emanating from different directions and passing through body tissue; used for diagnosis of various neurological diseases.

Contracture: Limitation in the movement of joints caused by shortening and shrinking of muscles, ligaments, and joints, or by ossification. A contracture is labeled according to the direction of movement that is shortened. For instance, in a flexion contracture, end-range extension is not possible, whereas free flexion is possible.

Coping: conscious effort to master or tolerate disease, especially chronic disease, disability, and illnesses with doubtful prognosis.

Depression: psychological condition with dejected mood, loss of drive, thoughts of helplessness and hopelessness, and withdrawal.

Derangement: according to McKenzie (1986), designation for damage to an intervertebral disc.

Diagnosis: identification of an illness on the basis of symptoms.

Diagnostics: procedures used to determine the cause or classification of an illness. These include the medical history and physical examination as well as instrumental diagnostics and laboratory studies.

Diskogram/Diskography: radiological procedure to determine the integrity of the spinal disk, in which contrast medium is introduced into the intervertebral disk. The intervertebral space is then observed for possible leakage of contrast medium. At this point, it can be determined whether the patient's familiar pain is reproduced.

Distal: a position designation indicating a point distant from the body center, lying toward the extremities (antonym: proximal).

Dysesthesia: unpleasant, abnormal sensation, spontaneous or triggered by external stimuli.

Dysfunction: incorrect function; according to McKenzie (1986), especially a term for contracted structures such as joint capsules, muscles, tendons, ligaments.

Electromyography (EMG): an electrodiagnostic medicine technique for evaluating and recording the electrical activity produced by skeletal muscles to produce a record called an electromyogram.

Electroneurography (ENG): is a non-invasive test used to examine the integrity and conductivity of a peripheral nerve.

Evidence: verified facts relating to a situation.

Fango pack: clay or mud pack, especially using a clay obtained from certain hot springs in Battaglio, Italy, used as a hot application.

Fibromyalgia: pain in muscles (usually generalized), connective tissue and bones; diagnostically uncertain concept of illness.

GCP: Good Clinical Practice; standards for the planning and implementation of clinical studies.

Hyperalgesia: intensified pain sensation in response to physiologically painful stimuli.

Hyperpathia: intensified reaction to external painful or nonpainful stimuli such as repeated stimuli.

Inclinometer: a device for measuring the angle of inclination of something, especially from the horizontal.

Intertester reliability: the extent to which different testers arrive at the same result; see also *reliability.*

Intratester reliability: the extent to which one and the same tester arrives at the same result in repeated testing; see also *reliability.*

Irritability: especially in Butler (1998) and Maitland (2000): the extent to which symptoms can be affected by mechanical maneuvers.

kPa: kilopascals, the SI derived unit of pressure, internal pressure, stress.

Locked-in syndrome: the inability to move or speak, but with consciousness preserved. The cause is usually a stroke in the territory supplied by the basilar artery.

Low back pain: back or sacral pain.

Lumbago: back or sacral pain.

Magnetic resonance imaging (MRI): imaging procedure that records electromagnetic waves emanating from the body after the application of a magnetic field, used to diagnose various neurological diseases (also known as *magnetic resonance tomography* or *nuclear spin tomography*).

Magnetic resonance tomography: see *magnetic resonance imaging.*

Manipulation: in this context, pulsed passive movement of a joint performed at high speed within or beyond the limit of passive mobility.

Medical history: history of a disease.

Meta-analysis: Secondary analysis of clinical studies with critical evaluation. A meta-analysis is usually conducted with a large number of studies of a specific issue.

mm HG: millimeters of mercury, a unit of pressure.

Mobilization: active or passive movement of a joint.

Neuralgia: pain in the area supplied by a peripheral nerve.

Noninvasive: designation for examination and treatment procedures in which the patient's body is not injured.

Nonspecific pain: ambiguous pain that cannot be classified as a symptom of a named disease.

Nonsteroidal anti-inflammatory drugs (NSAIDs): pain relievers that are not based on steroids such as cortisone and also have an anti-inflammatory effect.

Nuclear spin tomography: see *magnetic resonance imaging.*

Numeric analog scale (NAS): scale for the classification of pain intensity in which the pain is matched with specific numerical values.

Operant conditioning: learning by success, retention of certain behaviors for which one is rewarded.

Passive physical therapy: so-called because the modalities are done to the patient by the therapist.

Peripheralization: shift of the distal extent of radiating or radicular pain further distally. In this process, central pain, more toward or in the center of the affected spinal segment, can disappear. This change is caused by spinal movements and persists after the movements (antonym: centralization).

Placebo effect: all effects of therapeutic measures that are not a specific result of the measure itself but are interpreted as a nonspecific reaction of the patient to the therapeutic measure.

Polytopic pain syndrome: report of pain at many points on the body that cannot be diagnostically classified.

Positron emission tomography (PET): a nuclear medicine, functional imaging technique that produces a three-dimensional image.

Prevention: avoidance measures.

Prone knee bend (PKB): bending the knee in prone position; nerve tension test for the nerve roots of the upper lumbar and thoracic spinal segments and the femoral nerve.

Prospective studies: one form of prospective study follows ongoing outcomes in patients who are treated according to a predefined study protocol.

Protective muscle spasm: reflex muscle activity that can be considered a protective mechanism.

Proximal: indicates positional relationship to the center of the body (antonym: distal).

Randomization: assignment of patients to study arms on the basis of chance. This usually takes place by previously established randomization lists.

Randomized controlled trial (RCT): a type of medical experiment where the people being studied are randomly allocated to one or other of the different treatments under study.

Rehabilitation: restoration; more broadly, restoration of patients to their condition before an illness by means of therapeutic measures.

Relapse: recurrence of an illness after a cure.

Reliability: trustworthiness; quality criterion for a test or measurement procedure, determined by monitoring its ability to arrive at the identical result on repetition; see also *test–retest reliability, intertester reliability*, and *intratester reliability*.

Retrospective study: backward-looking evaluation of patient files related to the same specific issue to confirm or rule out a suspected connection.

Review: 1. An overview article, in contrast to publications that present new (original) data. 2. Process of evaluating a scientific manuscript submitted for publication.

Sciatica: low back pain radiating to the buttocks, hips, and/or outer side of the legs, along the course of the sciatic nerve.

Sensitivity: among other things, a measure of the probability that an existing illness can be detected by a diagnostic procedure.

Sensory evoked potential (SEP): examination technique in which the response to peripheral nerve stimulation delivered by an electrode attached to the skin is recorded at various levels further proximal (e.g., at the spine or at the brain via the scalp).

Signs: objective and objectifiable accompanying phenomena of a disease (measurable, visible to an observer).

Specificity: among other things, a measure of the probability that if a diagnostic test is positive, the suspected illness is present.

Specific pain: a pain that can be unambiguously classified within a named disease, for instance, pain caused by a disk prolapse.

Spondylolisthesis: forward displacement (sliding) of a vertebra, especially the fifth lumbar vertebra, often occurring after trauma.

Straight leg raise (SLR): raising the extended leg; nerve tension test for the nerve roots of the lower lumbar spine (L5 and S1), the sacral plexus, the sciatic nerve, the peroneal nerve, the tibial nerve; the test for the Lasègue sign.

Symptoms: subjective phenomena associated with an illness, experienced by the patient but not visible or measurable by an observer, in contrast to signs of illness, which are objectively verifiable.

Target parameters: end points defined in a study protocol that are monitored at specified times.

Test–retest reliability: reliability that when the test is repeated, the result will be the same; see also *reliability*.

Upper limb tension test (ULTT): nerve tension test of the upper extremity, for the nerve roots of the middle and lower cervical spine, the brachial plexus, and the median nerve.

Validity: quality criterion for a test or measurement procedure, assessing its ability to verify the extent to which a measurement or conclusion corresponds accurately to the real world.

Visual analog scale (VAS): a visible scale used to classify the intensity of pain.

Bibliography/References

Adams MA, Dolan P. Could sudden increase in physical activity cause degeneration of intervertebral discs? Lancet. 1997;350:734–735

Adams MA, Hutton WC. Prolapsed intervertebral disc: a hyperflexion injury. Spine. 1982;7:184–191

Adams MA, Hutton WC. Gradual disc prolapse. Spine. 1985;10:524–542

Adams MA, Dolan P, Hutton WC. The lumbar spine in backward bending. Spine. 1988;13:1019–1026

Adams MA, Freeman BJC, Morrison HP, Nelson IW, Dolan P. Mechanical initiation of intervertebral disc degeneration. Spine. 2000;25:1625–1636

Adams MA, Green TP, Dolan P. The strength in anterior bending of lumbar intervertebral discs. Spine. 1994;19:2197–2203

Adams MA, McMillan DW, Green TP, Dolan P. Sustained loading generates stress concentrations in lumbar intervertebral discs. Spine. 1996;21:434–438

Adams MA, May S, Freeman BJC, Morrison HP, Dolan P. Effects of backward bending on lumbar intervertebral discs. Relevance to physical therapy treatments for low back pain. Spine. 2000;25:431–437

Alexander H, Jones AM, Rosenbaum DH. Nonoperative management of herniated nucleus pulposus: patient selection by the extension sign. Orthop Rev. 1992;21:181–188

Algarni AM, Schneiders AG, Hendrick PA. Clinical tests to diagnose lumbar segmental instability: a systematic review. J Orthop Sports Phys Ther. 2011;41:130–140

Amanzio M, Benedetti F. Neuropharmacological dissection of placebo analgesia: expectation-activated opioid systems versus conditioning-activated specific subsystems. The J Neurosci. 1999;19:484–494

Andersson GB, Schulz AB, Nachemson AL. Intervertebral disc pressures during traction. Scand J Rehab Med. 1983;(Suppl.)9:88–91

Aota Y, Onari K, An HS, Yoshikawa K. Dorsal root ganglia morphologic features in patients with herniation of the nucleus pulposus: assessment using magnetic resonance myelography and clinical correlation. Spine. 2001;26:2125–2132

Arbeitsgemeinschaft der Wissenschaftlichen Medizinischen Fachgesellschaften (AWMF). Website. Available at http://www.awmf.org/leitlinien_leitlinien-suche.html_AWMF 2012. Accessed September 3, 2015

Assendelft WJ, Bouter LM, Knipschild PG. Complications of spinal manipulation: a comprehensive review of the literature. J Fam Pract. 1996;42:475–480

Atlas SJ, Keller RB, Chang YC, Deyo RA, Singer DE. Surgical and nonsurgical management of sciatica secondary to a lumbar disc herniation: five-year outcomes from the Maine Lumbar Spine Study. Spine. 2001;26:1179–1187

Barlocher CB, Krauss JK, Seiler RW. Central lumbar disc herniation. Acta Neurochir (Vienna). 2000;142:1369–1374

Basler HD, Jakle C, Kroner-Herwig B. Incorporation of cognitive-behavioral treatment into the medical care of chronic low back patients: a controlled randomized study in German pain treatment centers. Patient Educ Couns. 1997;31:113–124

Bell MA, Weddell AGM. A morphologic study of intrafascicular vessels of mammalian sciatic nerve. Muscle Nerve. 1984;7:524–534

BenDebba M, Van Alphen HA, Long DM. Association between peridural scar and activity-related pain after lumbar discectomy. Neurol Res. 1999;21(Suppl.)1:37–42

Bischoff HP. Manuelle Therapie für Physiotherapeuten. Balingen: Medizinische Verlagsgesellschaft; 1994

Boden SD, Davis DO, Dina TS, Patronas NJ, Wiesel SW. Abnormal magnetic-resonance scans of the lumbar spine in asymptomatic subjects. J Bone Joint Surg Am. 1990;72-A:403–408

Bogduk N. The innervation of the lumbar spine. Spine. 1983;8:286–293

Bogduk N. Klinische Anatomie von Lendenwirbelsäule und Sakrum. Berlin: Springer; 2000

Bogduk N, Tynan W, Wison AIS. The nerve supply to the lumbar intervertebral discs. J Anat. 1981;132:39–56

Bogduk N, Windsor M, Inglis A. The innervation of the cervical intervertebral discs. Spine. 1988;13:2–8

Boos N, Rieder R, Schade V, Spratt KF, Semmer N, Aebi M. The diagnostic accuracy of magnetic resonance imaging, work perception, and psychosocial factors in identifying symptomatic disc herniations. Spine. 1995;20:2613–2625

Borenstein DG. Epidemiology, etiology, diagnostic evaluation, and treatment of low back pain. Curr Opin Rheumatol. 1999;11:151–157

Brandt T, Dichgans J, Diener HC. Therapie und Verlauf neurologischer Erkrankungen. Stuttgart: Kohlhammer; 2003

Breig A. Biomechanics of the Central Nervous System: Some Basic Normal and Pathologic Phenomena. Stockholm: Almquist & Wiksell; 1960

Breig A. Adverse Mechanical Tension in the Central Nervous System. Stockholm: Almqvist & Wiksell; 1978

Breig A, Marions O. Biomechanics of the lumbosacral nerve roots. Acta Radiol Diagn (Stockh). 1963;1:1141–1160

Breig A, Troup JDG. Biomechanical considerations in the straight-leg-raising test. Cadaveric and clinical studies of the effects of medial hip rotation. Spine. 1979;4:242–250

Brisby H, Olmarker K, Larsson K, Nutu M, Rydevik B. Proinflammatory cytokines in cerebrospinal fluid and serum in patients with disc herniation and sciatica. Eur Spine J. 2002;11:62–66

Brotchi J, Pirotte B, De Witte O, Levivier M. Prevention of epidural fibrosis in a prospective series of 100 primary lumbosacral discectomy patients: follow-up and assessment at reoperation. Neurol Res. 1999;21(Suppl.)1:47–50

Brötz D, Burkard S, Weller M. A prospective study of mechanical physiotherapy for lumbar disk prolapse: five year follow-up and final report. NeuroRehabilitation. 2010;26:155–158

Brötz D, Hahn U, Maschke E, Wick W, Küker W, Weller M. Lumbar disk prolapse: response to mechanical physiotherapy in the absence of changes in magnetic resonance imaging. Report of 11 cases. NeuroRehabilitation. 2008;23:289–294

Brötz D, Küker W, Maschke E, Wick W, Dichgans J, Weller M. A prospective trial of mechanical physiotherapy for lumbar disk prolapse. J Neurol. 2003;250:746–749

Brötz D, Maschke E, Burkard S, Engel C, Mänz C, Ernemann U et al. Is there a role for benzodiazepines in the management of lumbar disc prolapse with acute sciatica? Pain. 2010; 149:470–475

Brötz D, Weller M, Küker W, Dichgans J, Götz A. Mechanische physiotherapeutische Diagnostik und Therapie bei Patienten mit lumbalen Bandscheibenvorfällen. Aktuel Neurol. 2001; 28:74–81

Brügger A. Die Funktionskrankheiten des Bewegungsapparates: eine Standortbestimmung. In: Die Funktionskrankheiten des Bewegungsapparates. Vol. 8. Jena: G. Fischer; 1997

Burton AK, Waddell G, Tillotson M, Summerton N. Information and advice to patients with back pain can have a positive effect. A randomized controlled trial of a novel educational booklet in primary care. Spine. 1999; 24:2484–2491

Bush K, Cowan N, Katz DE, Gishen P. The natural history of sciatica associated with disc pathology. A prospective study with clinical and independent radiologic follow-up. Spine. 1992;17:1205–1212

Butler D. Mobilisation des Nervensystems. Berlin: Springer; 1998

Byröd G, Rydevic B, Nordborg C, Olmarker K. Early effects of nucleus pulposus application on spinal nerve root morphology and function. Eur Spine J. 1998;7:445–449

Carragee EJ, Helms E, O'Sullivan GS. Are postoperative activity restrictions necessary after posterior lumbar discectomy? A prospective study of outcomes in 50 consecutive cases. Spine. 1996;21:1893–1897

Cavafy J. A case of sciatic nerve-stretching in locomotor ataxy: with remarks on the operation. BMJ. 1881;17:973–974

Cherkin DC. Primary care research on low back pain. The state of the science. Spine. 1998;23:1997–2002

Cherkin DC, Deyo RA, Battié M, Street J, Barlow W. A comparison of physical therapy, chiropractic manipulation, and provision of an educational booklet for the treatment of patients with low back pain. N Engl J Med. 1998;8:1021–1029

Cherkin DC, Deyo RA, Street JH, Hunt M, Barlow W. Pitfalls of patient education: limited success of a program for back pain in primary care. Spine. 1996;21:354–355

Cherkin DC, Deyo RA, Wheeler K, Ciol MA. Physician variation in diagnostic testing for low back pain. Who you see is what you get. Arthritis Rheum. 1994;37:15–22

Chrubasik S, Junck H, Zappe HA, Stutzke O. A survey on pain complaints and health care utilization in a German population sample. Eur J Anaestesiol. 1998;15:397–408

Crombez G, Vlaeyen JWS, Heuts PHTG, Lysens R. Pain-related fear is more disabling than pain itself: evidence on the role of pain-related fear in chronic pain disability. Pain. 1999;80: 329–339

De Pascalis V, Chiaradia C, Carotenuto E. The contribution of suggestibility and expectation to placebo analgesia phenomenon in an experimental setting. Pain. 2002;96:393–402

Devulder J. Transforaminal nerve root sleeve injection with corticosteroids, hyaluronidase, and local anesthetic in the failed back surgery syndrome. J Spinal Disord. 1998;11:151–154

Deyo RA, Diehl AK, Rosenthal M. How many days of bed rest for acute low back pain? A randomized clinical trial. N Engl J Med. 1986;315:1064–1070

Deyo RA, Phillips WP. Low back pain: a primary care challenge. Spine. 1996;21:2826–2832

Diener HC, Leonhardt H. Schmerztherapie. In: Brandt T, Dichgans J, Diener HC. Therapie und Verlauf neurologischer Erkrankungen. Stuttgart: Kohlhammer; 1998

Dommisse GF. The blood supply of the spinal cord. In: Grieve GP, ed. Modern Manual Therapy of the Vertebral Column. Edinburgh: Churchill Livingstone; 1986

Donelson R, Aprill C, Medcalf R, Grant W. A prospective study of centralization of lumbar and referred pain. Spine. 1997;22:1115–1122

Donelson R, Grant W, Kamps C, Medcalf R. Pain response to sagittal end-range spinal motion. A prospective, randomized, multicentered trial. Spine. 1990;16:206–211

Donelson R, Silva G, Murphy K. Centralization phenomenon: its usefulness in evaluating and treating referred pain. Spine. 1990;15:211–213

Draganski B, Gaser C, Busch V, Schuierer G, Bogdahn U, May A. Changes in grey matter induced by training. Nature. 2004;427:311–312

Dreyfuss P, Michaelson M, Pauza K, McLarty J, Bogduk N. The value of medical history and physical examination in diagnosing sacroiliac joint pain. Spine. 1996;21:2594–2602

Dubourg G, Rozenberg S, Fautel B et al. A pilot study on the recovery from paresis after lumbar disc herniation. Spine. 2002;27:1426–1432

Ehlers S. Learn to Juggle: Success Guaranteed. Norderstedt: BoD; 2008

Elfering A, Semmer N, Birkhofer D, Zanetti M, Hodler J, Boos N. Risk factors for lumbar disc degeneration. A 5-year prospective MRI study in asymptomatic individuals. Spine. 2002;27:125–134

Elvey RL. Physical evaluation of the peripheral nervous system in disorders of pain and dysfunction. J Hand Ther. 1997;10:122–129

Faas A. Exercises: which ones are worth trying, for which patients, and when? Spine. 1996;21:2874–2879

Faas A, Van Eijk JTM, Chavannes AW, Gubbels JW. A randomized trial of exercise therapy in patients with acute low back pain. Efficacy on sickness absence. Spine. 1995;20:941–947

Fairbank JCT, Pynsent PB. The Oswestry Disability Index. Spine. 2000;25:2940–2952

Fairbank JCT, Davies JB, Couper J, O'Brien JP. The Oswestry Low Back Pain Disability Questionnaire. Physiother. 1980;66:271–273

Fajersztajn J. Über das gekreuzte Ischiasphänomen. Wien Klin Wochenschr. 1901;14:41–47

Fazey PJ, Takasaki H, Singer KP. Nucleus pulposus deformation in response to lumbar spine lateral flexion: an in vivo MRI investigation. Eur Spine J 2010;19:1115–1120.

Fennell AJ, Jones AP, Hukins DW. Migration of the nucleus pulposus within the intervertebral disc during flexion and extension of the spine. Spine. 1996;21:2753–2757

Friberg O, Nurminen M, Kurhonen K, Soininen E, Mänttäri T. Accuracy and precision of clinical estimation of leg length discrepancy and lumbar scoliosis: comparison of clinical and radiological measurements. Int Disabil Stud. 1988;10:49–53

Fritz JM, Delitto A, Vignovic M, Busse RG. Intertester reliability of judgements of the centralization phenomenon and status change during movement testing in patients with low back pain. Arch Phys Med Rehabil. 2000;81:57–61

Furlan AD, Brosseau L, Imamura M, Irvin E. Massage for low back pain: a systematic review within the framework of the Cochrane Collaboration Back Review Group. Spine. 2002;27:1896–1910

Furusawa N, Baba H, Miyoshi N, Maezawa Y, Uchida K, Kokubo Y et al. Herniation of cervical intervertebral disc: immunohistochemical examination and measurement of nitric oxide production. Spine. 2001;26:1110–1116

Gerber B, Wilken H, Barten G, Zacharias K. Positive effect of balneotherapy on post-PID symptoms. Int J Fertil Menopausal Stud. 1993; 38:296–300

Gertzbein SD, Tait JH, Devlin SR. The stimulation of lymphocytes by nucleus pulposus in patients with degenerative disk disease of the lumbar spine. Clin Orthop Relat Res. 1977;123:149–154

Grawe K. Psychologische Therapie. Göttingen: Hogrefe; 2000

Gronblad M, Virre J, Seitsalo S, Habtemariam A, Karaharju E. Inflammatory cells, motor weakness, and straight leg raising in transligamentous disc herniations. Spine. 2000;25:2803–2807

Grundy PF, Roberts CJ. Does unequal leg length cause back pain? Lancet. 1984;4:256–258

Hadjipavlou AG, Simmons JW, Pope MH, Necessary JT, Goel VK. Pathomechanics and clinical relevance of disc degeneration and annular tear: a-point-of-view review. Am J Orthop. 1999;28:561–571

Hagen KB, Thune O. Work incapacity from low back pain in the general population. Spine. 1998;23:2091–2095

Haldeman S, Kohlbeck FJ, McGregor M. Unpredictability of cerebrovascular ischemia associated with cervical spine manipulation therapy: a review of sixty-four cases after cervical spine manipulation. Spine. 2002;27:49–55

Hall TM, Elvey RL. Nerve trunk pain: physical diagnosis and treatment. Man Ther. 1999;4:63–73

Hampton D, Laros G, McCarron R, Franks D. Healing potential of the anulus fibrosus. Spine. 1989;14:398–401

Hasenbring M, Haller D, Klasen B. Psychologische Mechanismen in Prozessen der Schmerzchronifizierung—Unter- oder überbewertet? Schmerz. 2001;15:442–447

Hasenbring M, Ulrich HW, Hartmann M, Soyka D. The efficacy of a risk factor-based cognitive behavioral intervention and electromyographic biofeedback in patients with acute sciatic pain. An attempt to prevent chronicity. Spine. 1999;24:2525–2535

Hee HT, Ill-Whitecloud TS, Myers L, Roesch W, Ricciardi JE. Do worker's compensation patients with neck pain have lower SF-36 scores? Eur Spine J. 2002;11:375–381

Helewa A, Goldsmith CH, Lee P, Smythe HA, Forwell L. Does strengthening the abdominal muscles prevent low back pain—a randomized controlled trial. J Rheumatol. 1999; 26:1808–1815

Henmi T, Sairo K, Nakano S, Kanematsu Y, Kajikawa T, Katoh S et al. Natural history of extruded lumbar intervertebral disc herniation. J Med Invest. 2002;49:40–43

Heymans MW, Van Tulder M, Esmail R, Bombardier C, Koes B. Back schools for nonspecific low back pain: a systematic review within the Cochrane Collaboration Back Review Group. Spine. 2005;30:2153–2163

Hides JA, Richardson CA, Gwendolen CJ. Multifidus muscle recovery is not automatic after resolution of acute, first-episode low back pain. Spine. 1996;21:2763–2769

Holm S, Nachemson A. Variations in the nutrition of the canine intervertebral disc induced by motions. Spine. 1983;8:866–874

Holm S, Nachemson A. Nutrition of the intervertebral disc: acute effects of cigarette smoking. An experimental animal study. Ups J Med Sci. 1988;93:91–99

Hildebrandt J, Pfingsten M, Franz C, Saur P, Seeger D. Das Göttinger Rücken-Intensiv-Programm (GRIP)—ein multimodales Behandlungsprogramm für Patienten mit chronischen Rückenschmerzen. Part 1. Der Schmerz. 1996; 10:190–203

Holm S, Maroudas A, Urban JP, Selstam G, Nachemson A. Nutrition of the intervertebral disc: solute transport and metabolism. Connect Tissue Res. 1981;8:101–119

Hossseinifar M, Akbari M, Behtash H, Amiri M, Sarrafzadeh J. The Effects of Stabilization and Mckenzie Exercises on Transverse Abdominis and Multifidus Muscle Thickness, Pain, and Disability: A Randomized Controlled Trial in Non Specific Chronic Low Back Pain. J. Phys. Ther. Sci. 2013;25:1541–1545.

Hrobjartsson A. What are the main methodological problems in the estimation of placebo effects? J Clin Epidemiol. 2002;55:430–435

Hufnagel A, Hammers A, Schonle PW, Bohm KD, Leonhardt G. Stroke following chiropractic manipulation of the cervical spine. J Neurol. 1999;246:683–688

Hurwitz EL, Aker PD, Adams AH, Meeker WC, Shekelle PG. Manipulation and mobilization of the cervical spine. Spine. 1996;21:1746–1760

Hurwitz EL, Morgenstern H, Harder P, Kominski GF, Yu F, Adams AH. A randomized trial of chiropractic manipulation and mobilization for patients with neck pain: clinical outcomes from the UCLA neck-pain study. Am J Public Health. 2002;92:1634–1641

Huys R, Daffertshofer A, Beek P. Multiple time scales and subsystem embedding in the learning of juggling. Hum Mov Sci. 2004;23:315–336

Ikeda T, Nakamura T, Kikuchi T, Umeda S, Senda H, Takagi K. Pathomechanism of spontaneous regression of the herniated lumbar disc: histologic and immunohistochemical study. J Spinal Disord. 1996;9:136–140

Indahl A, Kaigle AM, Reikeras O, Holm SH. Interaction between the porcine lumbar intervertebral disc, zygapophysial joints, and paraspinal muscles. Spine. 1997;22:2834–2840

Indahl A, Velund L, Reikeraas O. Good prognosis for low back pain when left untampered. A randomized clinical trial. Spine. 1995;20:473–477

Jinkins JR, Dworkin JS, Damadian RV. Upright, weight-bearing, dynamic-kinetic MRI of the spine: initial results. Eur Radiol 2005;15:1815–1825.

Johannsen F, Remvig L, Kryger P, Beck P, Lybeck K, Larsen LH et al. Supervised endurance exercise training compared to home training after first lumbar discectomy: a clinical trial. Clin Exp Rheumatol. 1994;12:609–614

Jonsson B, Stromqvist B. Repeat decompression of lumbar nerve roots: a prospective two-year evaluation. J Bone Joint Surg (Br). 1993;75:894–897

Jonsson B, Stromqvist B. Clinical characteristics of recurrent sciatica after lumbar discectomy. Spine. 1996;15:500–505

Junge A, Fröhlich M, Ahrens S, Hasenbring M, Sandler AJ, Grab D et al. Predictors of bad and good outcome of lumbar spine surgery. A prospective clinical study with 2 years' follow-up. Spine. 1996;21:1056–1065

Kalichman L, Hunter DJ. Diagnosis and conservative management of degenerative lumbar spondylolisthesis. Eur Spine J. 2008;17:327–335

Kaptchuk TJ. The placebo effect in alternative medicine: can the performance of a healing ritual have clinical significance? Ann Intern Med. 2002;136:817–825

Kayama S, Konno S, Olmarker K, Yabuki S, Kikuchi S. Incision of the anulus fibrosus induces nerve root morphologic, vascular, and functional changes. An experimental study. Spine. 1996;21:2539–2543

Kilpikoski S, Airaksinen O, Kankaanpaa M, Leminen P, Videman T, Alen M. Interexaminer reliability of low back pain assessment using the McKenzie method. Spine. 2002;27:E207– E214

Kjellby-Wendt G, Styf J. Early active training after lumbar discectomy. A prospective, randomized, and controlled study. Spine. 1998;23:2345–2351

Kjellman G, Oberg B. A randomized clinical trial comparing general exercise, McKenzie treatment and a control group in patients with neck pain. J Rehabil Med. 2002;34:183–190

Kladny B, Fischer FC, Haase I. Wertigkeit der muskulären segmentalen Stabilisierung zur Behandlung von Rückenschmerz und Bandscheibenerkrankungen im Rahmen der ambulanten Rehabilitation. Z Orthop 2003;141:401–405.

Kleinrensink GJ, Stoeckart R, Mulder PG, Hoek G, Broek T, Vleeming A et al. Upper limb tension tests as tools in the diagnosis of nerve and plexus lesions. Anatomical and biomechanical aspects. Clin Biomech (Bristol, Avon). 2000;15:9–14

Koes BW, Assendelft JJ, Van der Heijden GJMG, Bouter LM. Spinal manipulation for low back pain: an updated systematic review of randomized clinical trials. Spine. 1996;21:2860–2873

Koes BW, Van Tulder MW, Ostelo R, Kim-Burton A, Waddell G. Clinical guidelines for the management of low back pain in primary care: an international comparison. Spine. 2001;26:2504–2513

Komori H, Okawa A, Haro H, Shimomiya-Ki K. Factors predicting the prognosis of lumbar radiculopathy due to disc herniation. J Orthop Sci. 2002;7:56–61

Kopp JR, Alexander H, Turocy H, Levrini MG, Lichtman DM. The use of lumbar extension in the evaluation and treatment of patients with acute herniated nucleus pulposus. Clin Orthop Relat Res. 1986;202:211–218

Kotilainen E, Alanen A, Erkintalo M, Valtonen S, Kormono M. Association between decreased disc signal intensity in preoperative T2-weighted MRI and a 5-year outcome after lumbar minimally invasive discectomy. Minim Invasive Neurosurg. 2001;44:31–36

Krismer M, Van Tulder M. Low back pain (non-specific). Best Pract Res Clin Rheumatol. 2007;21:77–91

Lasègue C. Considerations sur la sciatique. Arch Gen de Med Paris. 1864;2:558–580

Laslett M, Öberg B, Aprill CN, McDonald B. Centralization as a predictor of provocation discography results in chronic low back pain, and the influence of disability and distress on diagnostic power. Spine J. 2005;5:370–380

Leboeuf-Yde C. Body weight and low back pain. A systematic literature review of 56 journal articles reporting on 65 epidemiologic studies. Spine. 2000;25:226–237

Leboeuf-Yde C, Kyvik KO. At what age does low back pain become a common problem? A study of 29,424 individuals aged 12–41 years. Spine. 1998;23:228–234

Leboeuf-Yde C, Lauritsen JM. The prevalence of low back pain in the literature. Spine. 1995; 20:2112–2118

Leino PL. Is back pain increasing? Results from national surveys in Finland. Scand J Rheumatol. 1994;23:269–276

Levi N, Gjerris F, Dons K. Thoracic disc herniation. Unilateral transpedicular approach in 35 consecutive patients. J Neurosurg Sci. 1999;43: 37–42

Loeser JD. Pain due to nerve injury. Spine. 1985;10:232–235

Loeser JD. What is chronic pain? Theor Med. 1991;12:213–225

Loeser JD. Pain: an overview. Lancet. 1999;353:1607–1609

Loeser JD. Pain and suffering. Clin J Pain. 2000;(Suppl.)16:S2–S6

Loeser JD, Volinn E. Epidemiology of low back pain. Neurosurg Clin N Am. 1991;2:713–718

Long AL. The centralization phenomenon. Its usefulness as a predictor of outcome in conservative treatment of chronic low back pain. A pilot study. Spine. 1995;20:2513–2520

Long A, Donelson R, Fung T. Does it matter which exercise? A randomized control trial of exercise for low back pain. Spine. 2004;29:2593–2602

Lundborg G. Structure and function of the intraneural microvessels as related to trauma, edema formation and nerve function. J Bone Joint Surg. 1975;57A:938–948

Lundborg G, Rydevik B. Effects of stretching the tibial nerve of the rabbit: a preliminary study of the intraneural circulation and the barrier function of the perineurium. J Bone Joint Surg. 1973;55B:390–401

Luomajoki H, Kool J, De Bruin ED, Airaksinen O. Movement control tests of the low back: evaluation of the difference between patients with low back pain and healthy controls. BMC Musculoskelet Disord. 2008;9:170

Lutza U, Kohlmann T, Deck R, Raspe H. Influence of occupational factors on the relation between socioeconomic status and self-reported back pain in a population-based sample of German adults with back pain. Spine. 2000;25:1390–1397

Machado GC, Maher CG, Ferreira PH, Pinheiro MB, Lin CW, Day RO et al. Efficacy and safety of paracetamol for spinal pain and osteoarthritis: systematic review and meta-analysis of randomised placebo controlled trials. BMJ. 2015;31:350:h1225

Maier-Riehle B, Harter M. The effects of back schools: a meta-analysis. Int J Rehabil Res. 2001;24:199–206

Maigne JY, Deligne B. Computed tomographic follow-up study of 21 cases of nonoperatively treated cervical intervertebral disc herniation. Spine. 1994;19:189–191

Maigne JY, Rime B, Deligne B. Computed tomographic follow-up study of forty-eight cases of nonoperatively treated lumbar intervertebral soft disc herniation. Spine. 1992;17:1071–1074

Maitland G. Vertebral Manipulation. London: Butterworth; 1986

Maitland G. Manipulation der Wirbelsäule. Berlin: Springer; 1994

Maitland G. Manipulation der peripheren Gelenke. Berlin: Springer; 2000

Malmivaara A, Häkkinen U, Aro T. The treatment of acute low back pain—bed rest, exercises, or ordinary activity? N Engl J Med. 1995;332:351–355

Mannion AF, Müntener M, Taimela S, Dvorak J. A randomized clinical trial of three active therapies for chronic low back pain. Spine. 1999;24:2435–2448

Marshall J. Nerve stretching for the relief or cure of pain. BMJ. 1883;2:1173–1179

Matsui H, Kanamori M, Ishihara H, Yudoh K, Naruse Y, Tsuji H. Familial predisposition for lumbar degenerative disc disease. A case-control study. Spine. 1998;23:1029–1034

May S, Gardiner E, Young S, Klaber-Moffett J. Predictor Variables for a Positive Long-Term Functional Outcome in Patients with Acute and Chronic Neck and Back Pain Treated with a McKenzie Approach: A Secondary Analysis. The Journal of Manual § Manipulative Therapy 2008;16:155–160.

McCracken LM, Gross RT, Aikens J, Carnrike CLM. The assessment of anxiety and fear in persons with chronic pain: a comparison of instruments. Behav Res and Ther. 1996;34:927–933

McKenzie R. The Lumbar Spine: Mechanical Diagnosis and Therapy. Waikanae: Spinal Publications New Zealand; 1981, 2003

McKenzie R. Die lumbale Wirbelsäule. Mechanische Diagnose und Therapie. Zürich: Spinal Publications Switzerland; 1986

McKenzie R. The Cervical and Thoracic Spine. Mechanical Diagnosis and Therapy. Waikanae: Spinal Publications New Zealand; 1990, 2006

McKenzie R, May S. The Lumbar Spine: Mechanical Diagnosis and Therapy. Waikanae: Spinal Publications New Zealand; 2003

McMillan DW, Garbutt G, Adams MA. Effect of sustained loading on the water content of intervertebral discs: implications for disc metabolism. Ann Rheum Dis. 1996;55:880–887

Melzack R. The short form McGill Pain Questionnaire. Pain. 1987;30:191–197

Miyaguchi M, Nakamura H, Shakudo M, Inoue Y, Yamano Y. Idiopathic spinal cord herniation associated with intervertebral disc extrusion. A case report and review of the literature. Spine. 2001;26:1090–1094

Moneta GB, Videman T, Kaivanto K, Aprill C, Spivey M, Vanharanta H et al. Reported pain during lumbar discography as a function of anular ruptures and disc degeneration. A re-analysis of 833 discograms. Spine. 1994; 19:1968–1974

Montgomery GH, Kirsch I. Classical conditioning and the placebo effect. Pain. 1997;72:107–113

Morgan H, Abood C. Disc herniation at T1–2. Report of four cases and literature review. J Neurosurg. 1998;88:148–150

Moyad A. The placebo effect and randomized trials: analysis of conventional medicine. Uro Clin N Am. 2002;29:125–133

Mundt DJ, Kelsey JL, Golden AL, Panjabi MM, Pastides H, Berg AT et al. An epidemiologic study of sports and weight lifting as possible risk factors for herniated lumbar and cervical discs. Am J Sports Med. 1993;21:854–860

Nachemson A. Chronic pain: the end of the welfare state? Qual Life Res. 1994;(Suppl.)1:S11–S17

Nachemson A, Elfström G. Intravital dynamic pressure measurements in lumbar discs. Scand J Rehabil Med. 1970;1:1–40

Nadler SF, Malanga GA, Stitik TP, Keswani R, Foye PM. The crossed femoral nerve stretch test to improve diagnostic sensitivity for the high lumbar radiculopathy: 2 case reports. Arch Phys Med Rehabil. 2001;82:522–523

Nentwig CG, Krämer J, Ullrich CH. Die Rückenschule. Stuttgart: Enke; 1997

Nygaard OP, Kloster R, Solberg T. Duration of leg pain as a predictor of outcome after surgery for lumbar disc herniation: a prospective cohort study with 1-year follow up. J Neurosurg. 2000;92:131–134

Olmarker K, Nordborg C, Larsson K, Rydevic B. Ultrastructural changes in spinal nerve roots induced by autologous nucleus pulposus. Spine. 1996;21:411–414

Ordway NR, Seymour RJ, Donelson RG, Hojnowski LS, Edwards WT. Cervical flexion, extension, protrusion, and retraction. A radiographic segmental analysis. Spine. 1999;24:240–247

Ostelo RWJG, de Vet HCW, Waddell G, Kerckhoffs MR, Leffers P, Van Tulder M. Rehabilitation after lumbar disc surgery. Cochrane Database Syst Rev. 2007;2

Oswestry Low Back Pain Disability Questionnaire. Oswestry Disability Index. Available at: http://www.aadep.org/documents/resources/Appendix_D__The_Oswestry_Disability_477E-0AE6E8258.pdf; n.d. Accessed September 1, 2015

Pal B, Johnson A. Paraplegia due to thoracic disc herniation. Postgrad Med J. 1997;73:423–425

Palmgren T, Grönblad M, Virri J, Seitsalo S, Ruuskanen M, Karaharju E. Immunohistochemical demonstration of sensory and autonomic nerve terminals in herniated lumbar disc tissue. Spine. 1996;21:1301–1306

Pearce RH, Grimmer BJ, Adams M. Degeneration and the chemical composition of the human lumbar intervertebral disc. J Orthop Res. 1987;5:198–205

Petersen T, Kryger P, Ekdal C, Olsen S, Jacobsen S. The effect of McKenzie therapy as compared with that of intensive strengthening training for the treatment of patients with subacute or chronic low back pain. Spine. 2002; 27:1702–1709

Peul WC, van Houwelingen HC, van den Hout WB, Brand R, Eekhof JAH, Tans JTJ, Thomeer RTWM, Koes BW. Surgery versus prolonged conservative treatment for sciatica. New England Journal of Medicine 2007: 22:2245–2256

Pfingsten M, Hildebrandt J, Leibing E, Franz C, Saur P. Effectiveness of a multimodal treatment program for chronic low back pain. Pain. 1997;73:77–85

Pfingsten M, Kröner-Herwig B, Leibing E, Kronshage U, Hildebrandt J. Validation of the

German version of the Fear-avoidance Beliefs Questionnaire (FABQ). Eur J Pain. 2000;4: 259–266

Plass D, Vos T, Hornberg C, Scheidt-Nave C, Zeeb H, Krämer A. Trends in disease burden in Germany. Dtsch Ärztebl Int. 2014;111:629–638

Pope MH, Magnusson M, Wilder DG. Low back pain and whole body vibration. Clin Ortho Relat Res. 1998;354:241–248

Porter RW, Adams MA, Hutton WC. Physical activity and the strength of the lumbar spine. Spine. 1989;14:201–203

Postacchini F, Giannicola G, Cinotti G. Recovery of motor deficits after microdiscectomy for lumbar disc herniation. J Bone Joint Surg. 2002;84:1040–1045

Race A, Broom ND, Robertson P. Effect of loading rate and hydration on the mechanical properties of the disc. Spine. 2000;25:662–669

Rao R. Neck pain, cervical radiculopathy, and cervical myelopathy. Pathophysiology, natural history, and clinical evaluation. J Bone Joint Surg. 2002;84A:1872–1881

Rasmussen C, Rechter L, Schmidt I, Hansen VK, Therkelsen K. The association of involvement of financial compensation with the outcome of cervicobrachial pain that is treated conservatively. Rheumatol (Oxford). 2001;40:552–554

Razmjou H, Kramer JF, Yamada R. Intertester reliability of the McKenzie evaluation in assessing patients with mechanical low-back pain. J Orthop Sports Phys Ther. 2000;30:368–383

Reinhardt B. Die große Rückenschule. Nürnberg: Perimed; 1992

Reyentovich A, Abdu WA. Multiple independent, sequential, and spontaneously resolving lumbar intervertebral disc herniations. Spine. 2002;27:549–553

Richardson C, Hodges P, Hides J. Therapeutic Exercise for Lumbopelvic Stabilization. London: Churchill Livingstone; 2004

Rittner HL, Brack A, Stein C. Schmerz und Immunsystem: Freund oder Feind? Anästhesist. 2002;51:351–358

Roland M, Morris R. A study of the natural history of back pain. Spine. 1983;8:141–144

Ross JS. MR imaging of the postoperative lumbar spine. Magn Reson Imaging Clin N Am. 1999;7:513–524

Saal JA, Saal JS. Nonoperative treatment of herniated lumbar intervertebral disc with radiculopathy. An outcome study. Spine. 1989;14:431–437

Saal JA, Saal JS, Herzog RJ. The natural history of lumbar intervertebral disc extrusions treated nonoperatively. Spine. 1990;15:683–686

Sachse J. Manuelle Medizin: Eine Einführung in Theorie, Diagnostik und Therapie. Heidelberg: Springer; 1995

Sambrook PN, MacGregor AJ, Spector TD. Genetic influences on cervical and lumbar disc degeneration: a magnetic resonance imaging study in twins. Arthritis Rheum. 1999;42:366–372

Sato T, Kokubun S, Tanaka Y, Ishii Y. Thoracic myelopathy in the Japanese: epidemiological and clinical observations on the cases in Miyagi Prefecture. Tohoku J Exp Med. 1998;184:1–11

Satoh K, Konno S, Nishiyama K, Olmarker K, Kikuchi S. Presence and distribution of antigen-antibody complexes in the herniated nucleus pulposus. Spine. 1999;24:1980–1984

Sauer SK, Bove GM, Averbeck B, Reeh PW. Rat peripheral nerve components release calcitonin gene-related peptide and prostaglandin E2 in response to noxious stimuli: evidence that nervi nervorum are nociceptors. Neurosci. 1999;92:319–325

Schneider M, Erhard R, Brach J, Tellin W, Imbarlina F, Delitto A. Spinal palpation for lumbar segmental mobility and pain provocation: an interexaminer reliability study. J Manipulative Physiol Ther. 2008;31:465–473

Schünke M. Funktionelle Anatomie. Topographie und Funktion des Bewegungsapparats. Stuttgart: Thieme; 2000

Schwarzer AC, Aprill CN, Derby R, Fortin J, Kine G, Bogduk N. The prevalence and clinical features of internal disc disruption in patients with chronic low back pain. Spine. 1995;20:1878–1883

Scott SC, Goldberg MS, Mayo NE, Stock SR, Poitras B. The association between cigarette smoking and back pain in adults. Spine. 1999;24:1090–1098

Seferlis T, Nemeth G, Carlsson AM, Gillström P. Conservative treatment in patients sick-listed for acute low-back pain: a prospective randomised study with 12 months follow-up. Eur Spine J. 1998;7:461–470

Selim AJ, Ren XS, Fincke G, Deyo RA, Rogers W, Miller D et al. The importance of radiating leg pain in assessing health outcomes among patients with low back pain. Results from the Veterans Health Study. Spine. 1998;23:470–474

Siivola SM, Levoska S, Tervonen O, Ilkko E, Vanharanta H, Keinanen-Kiukaanniemi S. MRI changes of cervical spine in asymptomatic and symptomatic young adults. Eur Spine J. 2002;11:358–363

Slavin KV, Raja A, Thornton J, Wagner FC. Spontaneous regression of a large lumbar disc herniation: report of an illustrative case. Surg Neurol. 2001;56:333–336

Snook SH, Webster BS, McGorry RW, Fogleman MT, McCann KB. The reduction of chronic nonspecific low back pain through the control of early morning lumbar flexion. Spine. 1998;23:2601–2607

Sondell M, Lundborg G, Kanje M. Vascular endothelial growth factor has neurotrophic activity and stimulates axonal outgrowth, enhancing cell survival and Schwann cell proliferation in the peripheral nervous system. J Neurosci. 1999;19:5731–5740

Specchina N, Pagnotta A, Towsca A, Greco F. Cytokines and growth factors in the protruded intervertebral disc of the lumbar spine. Eur Spine J. 2002;11:145–151

Spencer D. The anatomical basis of sciatica secondary to herniated lumbar disc: a review. Neurol Res. 1999;(Suppl.)1:33–36

Stankovic R, Johnell O. Conservative treatment of acute low back pain. A 5-year follow-up study of two methods of treatment. Spine. 1995;20:469–472

Strauss-Blasche G, Ekmekcioglu C, Klammer N, Marktl W. The change of well-being associated with spa therapy. Forsch Komplementärmed Klass Naturheilkd. 2000;7:269–274

Sufka A, Hauger H, Trenary M, Bishop B, Hagen A, Lozon R et al. Centralization of low back pain and perceived functional outcome. J Orthop Sports Phys The. 1998;27:205–212

Sugar O. Victor Horsley, John Marshall, nerve stretching, and the nervi nervorum. Surg Neurol. 1990;34:184–187

Sunderland S. The nerve lesion in carpal tunnel syndrome. J Neurol, Neurosurg Psychiatry. 1976;39:615–626

Sunderland S. Advances in Neurology. New York: Raven Press; 1979

Sunderland S. The anatomy and physiology of nerve injury. Muscle Nerve. 1990;13: 771–784

Symington J. The physics of nerve stretching. BMJ. 1882;1:770

Takasaki H, May S, Fazey PJ, Hall T. Nucleus pulposus deformation following application of mechanical diagnosis and therapy: a single case report with magnetic resonance imaging. Journal of Manual and Manipulative Therapy 2010; 18: 153–158.

Tanou M, Yamaga M, Die J, Takagi K. Acute stretching of peripheral nerves inhibits retrograde axonal transport. J Hand Surg. 1996;21:358–363

Ten Brinke A, Van der Aa HE, Van der Palen J, Oosterveld F. Is leg length discrepancy associated with the side of radiating pain in patients with a lumbar herniated disc? Spine. 1999;24: 684–686

Thomas E, Silman AJ, Croft PR, Papageorgiou AC, Jayson MI, Macfarlane GJ. Predicting who develops chronic low back pain in primary care: a prospective study. BMJ (Clinical Research ed.). 1999;318:1662–1667

Toepfer M, Rieger J, Pfluger T, Hautmann H, Sitter T, Pfeifer KJ et al. Primäre hypertrophische Osteoarthropathie (Touraine-Solente-Gole-Syndrom). Dtsch Med Wochensch. 2002;127:1013–1016

Tokuhashi Y, Matsuzaki H, Uematsu Y, Oda H. Symptoms of thoracolumbar junction disc herniation. Spine. 2001;26:E512–E518

Tölle TR, Berthele A. Das Schmerzgedächtnis. In: Zenz M, Jurna I. Lehrbuch der Schmerztherapie. Stuttgart: Wissenschaftliche Verlagsgesellschaft; 2001

Trepel M. Neuroanatomie, Struktur und Funktion. München: Urban & Schwarzenberg; 1995

Troup JDG. Straight-leg-raising (SLR) and the qualifying tests for increased root tension. Spine. 1981;6:526–527

Turgut M. Spinal cord compression due to multiple thoracic disc herniation: surgical decompression using a "combined" approach. A case report and review of the literature. J Neurosurg Sci. 2000;44:53–59

Urban JPG, McMullin JF. Swelling pressure of the lumbar intervertebral discs. Influence of age, spinal level, compression, and degeneration. Spine. 1988;13:179–187

Van den Berg F. Angewandte Physiologie. Stuttgart: Thieme; 1999

Van der Heide B. Physiologische Reaktion auf einen Provokationstest der Neuralstrukturen in der oberen Extremität. Krankengymnastik. 2000;52:816–828

Van Tulder M, Becker A, Bekkering T, Breen A, del Real MTG, Hutchinson A et al. European guidelines for the management of acute nonspecific low back pain in primary care. Spine. 2006;15:169–191

Van Tulder MW, Esmail R, Bombardier C, Koes BW. Back schools for non-specific low back pain. Cochrane Database Syst Rev. 2000;2:CD000261

Van Tulder MW, Koes BW, Bouter LM. Conservative treatment of acute and chronic nonspecific low back pain. A systematic review of randomized controlled trials of the most common interventions. Spine. 1997;22:2128–2156

Vogelsang JP, Finkenstaedt M, Vogelsang M, Markakis E. Recurrent pain after lumbar discectomy: the diagnosis value of peridural scar on MRI. Eur Spine J. 1999;8:475–479

Volinn E. The epidemiology of low back pain in the rest of the world. A review of surveys in low- and middle-income countries. Spine. 1997;22:1747–1754

Von Strempel A. Die Wirbelsäule. Stuttgart: Thieme; 2001

Vos T, Flaxman AD, Naghavi M, Lozano R, Michaud C, Ezzati M et al. Years lived with disability (YLDs) for 1160 sequelae of 289 diseases and injuries 1990–2010: a systematic analysis for the Global Burden of Disease Study 2010. Lancet. 2012; 15;380:2163–2196

Vroomen P, De Krom M, Knottnerus JA. When does the patient with a disc herniation undergo lumbosacral discectomy? J Neurol, Neurosurg Psychiatry. 2000;68:75–79

Vucetic N, Mättänen H, Svensson O. Pain and pathology in lumbar disc herniation. Clin Orthop Rel Res. 1995;320:65–72

Waddell G. A new clinical model for the treatment of low back pain. Spine. 1987;12:632– 641

Waddell G. Low back pain: a twentieth century health care enigma. Spine. 1996;21:2820–2825

Waddell G. The Back Pain Revolution. London: Churchill Livingstone; 1998

Waddell G, Feder G, Lewis M. Systematic reviews of bed rest and advice to stay active for acute low back pain. Br J Gen Pract. 1997;47:647–652

Waddell G, McCulloch JA, Kummel E, Venner RM. Nonorganic physical signs in low-back pain. Spine. 1980;5:117–125

Waddell G, Newton M, Henderson I, Somerville D, Main CJ. A fear-avoidance beliefs questionnaire (FABQ) and the role of fear-avoidance beliefs in chronic low back pain and disability. Pain. 1993;52:157–168

Walach H, Sadaghiani C. Plazebo und Plazeboeffekte. Eine Bestandsaufnahme. Psychotherapie, Psychosomatik, Medizinische Psychologie. 2002;52:332–342

Weber H. Lumbar disc herniation. A controlled, prospective study with ten years of observation. Spine. 1983;8:131–140

Weber H. The natural history of disc herniation and the influence of intervention. Spine. 1994; 19:2234–2238

Weber H, Holme I, Amlie E. The natural course of acute sciatica, with nerve root symptoms in a double blind placebo-controlled trial evaluating the effect of piroxicam (NSAID). Spine. 1993;18:1433–1438

Weinstein JN, Tosteson TD, Lurie JD, Tosteson ANA, Hanscom B, Skinner JS et al. Surgical vs nonoperative treatment for lumbar disk herniation. The Spine Patient Outcomes Research Trial (SPORT): observational group. JAMA. 2006a;296:2451–2459

Weinstein JN, Tosteson TD, Lurie JD, Tosteson ANA, Hanscom B, Skinner JS et al. Surgical vs nonoperative treatment for lumbar disk herniation. The Spine Patient Outcomes Research Trial (SPORT): a randomized trial. JAMA. 2006b;296: 2441–2450

Weishaupt D, Zanetti M, Hodler J, Boos N. MR imaging of the lumbar spine: prevalence of intervertebral disk extrusion and sepuestration, nerve root compression, end plate abnormalities, and osteoarthritis of the facet joints in asymptomatic volunteers. Radiol. 1998;209:661–666

Werneke M, Hart DL, Cook D. A descriptive study of the centralization phenomenon. A prospective analysis. Spine. 1999;24:676–683

Whitcomb DC, Martin SP, Schoen RE, Jho HD. Chronic abdominal pain caused by thoracic disc herniation. Am J Gastroenterol. 1995;90:835–837

Wiesinger G, Nuhr M, Quittan M, Ebenbichler G, Wölfl G, Fialka-Moser V. Cross-cultural adaptation of the Roland-Morris questionnaire for German-speaking patients with low back pain. Spine. 1999;24:1099–1103

Wilke A, Wolf U, Lageard P, Griss P. Thoracic disc herniation: a diagnostic challenge. Man Ther. 2000;5:181–184

Wilke HJ, Neef P, Caimi M, Hoogland T, Claes LE. New in-vivo measurements of pressures in the intervertebral disc in daily life. Spine. 1999;24:755–762

Williams DA, Feuerstein M, Durbin D, Pezzullo J. Health care and indemnity costs across the natural history of disability in occupational low back pain. Spine. 1998;23:2329–2336

Winter SCA, Maartens NF, Anslow P, Teddy PJ. Spontaneous intracranial hypotension due to thoracic disc herniation. Case report. J Neurosurg. 2002;96:342–345

Witt TN, Stöhr M. Radikuläre Syndrome. In: Brandt T, Dichgans J, Diener HC. Therapie und Verlauf neurologischer Erkrankungen. Stuttgart: Kohlhammer; 2003

Woodhall B, Hayes GJ. The well-leg-raising test of Fajersztajn in the diagnosis of ruptured intervertebral disc. J Bone Joint Surg. 1950;32A:786–792

World Health Organization. International Classification of Impairments, Disabilities and Handicaps. Geneva: WHO; 1976:28

World Health Organization. WHO Expert Committee on Selection and Use of Essential Medicines—WHO Technical Report Series, No. 850, Annex 3 (Guidelines for Good Clinical Practice (GCP) for Trials on Pharmaceutical Products). Sixth Report, Annex 3. Geneva: WHO; 1995

Yorimitsu E, Chiba K, Toyama Y, Hirabayashi K. Long-term outcomes of standard discectomy for lumbar disc herniation: a follow-up study of more than 10 years. Spine. 2001;26:652–657

Yoshihara K, Shirai Y, Nakayama Y, Uesaka S. Histochemical changes in the multifidus muscle in patients with lumbar intervertebral disc herniation. Spine. 2001;26:622–625

Zentner J, Schneider B, Schramm J. Efficacy of conservative treatment of lumbar disc herniation. J Neurosurg Sci. 1997; 41:263–268

Zenz M, Jurna I. Lehrbuch der Schmerztherapie. Stuttgart: Wissenschaftliche Verlagsgesellschaft; 2001

Zieglgänsberger W. Schmerzwahrnehmung: ein dynamischer Prozess. Anästhesist. 2002;51:349–350

Zilles K, Rehkrämper G. Funktionelle Neuroanatomie: Lehrbuch und Atlas. Berlin: Springer; 1998

Zitting P, Rantakallio P, Vanharanta H. Cumulative incidence of lumbar disc diseases leading to hospitalization up to the age of 28 years. Spine. 1998;23:2337–2343

Zochodne DW. Epineural peptides: a role in neuropathic pain? Can J Neurol Sci. 1993;20: 69–72

Zung WWK. A self-rating pain and distress scale. Psychosom. 1983;24:887–894

Zung WWK, Wonnacott TH. Treatment prediction in depression using a self-rating scale. Biol Psychiatry. 1970;2:321–329

Zwart JA, Sand T, Unsgaard G. Warm and cold sensory thresholds in patients with unilateral sciatica: C fibres are more severely affected than A-delta fibres. Acta Neurol Scand. 1998; 97:41–45.

Index

Page numbers in *italics* refer to illustrations; those in **bold** refer to tables